Pediatric Endocrinology and Growth

2nd Edition

Commissioning Editor: *Judith Fletcher*
Project Development Manager: *Tim Kimber*
Project Manager: *Jess Thompson*
Illustration Manager: *Mick Ruddy*
Designer: *Andy Chapman*
Illustrator: *Tim Loughead*

Pediatric Endocrinology and Growth

2nd Edition

Dr Jeremy K. H. Wales
Senior Lecturer in Paediatric Endocrinology
The University Department of Paediatrics
Sheffield Children's Hospital
Sheffield, UK

Professor Jan-Maarten Wit
Professor of Pediatrics
Leiden University Medical Center
Leiden, The Netherlands

Professor Alan D. Rogol
Professor of Clinical Pediatrics
University of Virginia
Charlottesville, VA, USA

SAUNDERS

Edinburgh London New York Oxford Philadelphia St Louis Sydney Toronto 2003

SAUNDERS
An imprint of Elsevier Science Limited

First edition 1996
Second edition 2003

ISBN 0702026565

BRITISH LIBRARY CATALOGUING IN PUBLICATION DATA
A catalogue record for this book is available from the British Library

LIBRARY OF CONGRESS CATALOGING IN PUBLICATION DATA
A catalog record for this book is available from the Library of Congress

NOTE
Medical knowledge is constantly changing. Standard safety precautions must be followed, but as new research and clinical experience broaden our knowledge, changes in treatment and drug therapy may become necessary or appropriate. Readers are advised to check the most current product information provided by the manufacturer of each drug to be administered to verify the recommended dose, the method and duration of administration, and contraindications. It is the responsibility of the practitioner, relying on experience and knowledge of the patient, to determine dosages and the best treatment for each individual patient. Neither the Publisher nor the author assumes any liability for any injury and/or damage to persons or property arising from this publication.
The Publisher

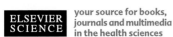

your source for books, journals and multimedia in the health sciences
www.elsevierhealth.com

The Publisher's policy is to use **paper manufactured from sustainable forests**

Printed in China

CONTENTS

PREFACE to the first edition

Pediatric endocrine and growth disorders lend themselves to a problem-oriented approach to diagnosis. They are also often associated with clinical signs that may be demonstrated photo- and radiographically. Children are growing beings and their growth charts also provide a wealth of information. We have collected together prime illustrations of examples of these disorders from two continents in a book that is designed as a manual for the primary care physician and the non-specialist. The text aims to give guidance for the diagnosis of endocrine and growth disorders and to allow referral to the appropriate local specialist for further diagnostic evaluation and management. We hope that specialist pediatric and adult endocrinologists and physicians in training will be able to use the book as a teaching resource.

Each chapter has a common lay-out, setting out brief details of physiology, a diagnostic classification, a work-up (including history, examination and investigations) together with a brief plan of management. Space does not allow for a detailed description of endocrine anatomy or biochemistry and the interested reader is referred to one of the excellent comprehensive texts on the subject.

Much endocrine therapy is highly specialized and the focus of active research and debate. We have restricted our descriptions to well-established treatments, but also indicated areas of controversy. There is a large overlap of pediatric endocrinology with clinical genetics. As it would be impossible to illustrate even a minority of clinical syndromes, particularly those associated with short stature, we have tried to outline a broad diagnostic approach rather than give specific details, except in the most common and most important examples.

We believe that the book is comprehensive and that it approaches some of the goals that we set out to achieve. We are grateful to colleagues in the United Kingdom, the Netherlands and the United States of America, some of who are detailed on the acknowledgement page, for their assistance and support and, of course, to the patients whose photographs and data form the bulk of the work.

PREFACE to the second edition

Why bother to produce a second edition to the Color Atlas in an interval as short as 6 years? There certainly is not time for a secular change, and the diseases described have not changed that much. We have produced a new edition because there has been a huge increase in the knowledge base regarding the genetic basis of many of the common (and not so common) endocrine disorders. Also, new hormones have been described, helping us to define some of the physiologic (and pathophysiologic) alterations in feedback axes and increasing our ability to describe the child as a whole – integrated – person. In addition we have striven to add illustrations for conditions for which we did not have appropriate photos in the first edition, and to replace others that were not of the highest photographic quality or that did not depict the issues desired as well as the replacement pictures.

Our intellectual discipline is visual in many aspects and often the gestalt of the whole child – the height, weight, body proportions and facial features – teach us more than the individual parts or even the sum of the individual features. We often have a partial differential diagnosis before we begin with the history and physical examination. This is quite unlike much of general pediatrics, and especially unlike general internal medicine.

Some of the knowledge gained since publication of the first edition has translated into diagnostic testing and is included in this new edition, as well as being summarized in the Appendix on endocrine system testing in children and adolescents. Among the new hormones described, such as leptin and resistin, are those related to adipose tissue as an endocrine organ concomitant with the greatly increased numbers of children with severe obesity presenting to the pediatric endocrinologist, either to exclude endocrinopathies or to treat the consequences of obesity such as type 2 diabetes mellitus. In fact, it is the group of very obese children that is increasing so rapidly: the 50th centile for weight has not changed nearly as much as the 85th centile and above. We have included an entirely new chapter on the Overweight Child. The opposite condition – failure to thrive – is a relatively common general pediatric problem that was not covered in the first edition. In the second edition we have corrected this oversight with a chapter on the Thin Child. Although often cared for in separate clinics, the commonest endocrine abnormality in childhood is type 1 diabetes mellitus. Often the separation is due to the specialized team approach required, especially with reference to diet, school and psychosocial functioning. Partly because of the great increase in obesity, most clinics that care for children with diabetes mellitus are evaluating an increasing proportion of children with type 2 diabetes mellitus. We have added a new chapter to focus on both types of diabetes, and have increased the profile of hyperinsulinism.

The chapters on the Short and Tall Child have been rewritten to account for the new ESPE (European Society for Paediatric Endocrinology) diagnostic classification produced by Michael Ranke, Chris Kelnar and one of our co-authors, Jan-Maarten Wit. As experience in pediatric imaging of the thyroid has become more common, we have added more information concerning this modality to some of the chapters.

We are extremely grateful to colleagues who have helped us in the preparation of the text and in permitting us to use some of their photographs of patients. We acknowledge them in the following list.

Dr Jeremy K. H. Wales
Professor Jan-Maarten Wit
Professor Alan D. Rogol
2002

ACKNOWLEDGEMENTS

Mr MJ Bell
Prof N Bishop
Dr J Bridson
Prof RM Blizzard
Dr CR Buchanan
Dr A Cant
Mrs S Carney
Dr J Challener
Dr T Clarke
Dr PE Clayton
Dr V Datta
Dr L Davis-Reynolds
Dr H Davies
Prof D Dunger

Dr S Farooqui
Mr RB Fraser
Dr EA Gouta
Dr AT Gibson
Dr A Hokken
Dr M Jansen
Dr MS Kibirige
Mr AE Mackinnon
Dr ML Maerin
Dr K Ong
Dr W Oostdijk
Mrs M Pickering
Dr KJ Price
Dr RA Primhak

Dr B Rikken
Prof M Saleh
Dr C Smith
Dr A Sprigg
Dr RG Stanhope
Prof MS Tanner
Prof JL Van der Brande
Dr S Variend
Dr JJJ Waelkens
Dr WG Wilson
Mr J Woodruff
Dr N Wright
Dr G Yeoman

Mr J Burke, Mr IM Strachan and the Orthoptic Department, Sheffield Children's Hospital.

The Medical Illustration Departments at Sheffield, Leiden, Utrecht and Charlottesville.

The Dutch Growth Foundation for the program 'Growth Analyser™' used in the production of the growth charts.

KEYS

Key to growth charts

All the charts in this book were created using the program 'Growth Analyser' version 1; ©The Dutch Growth Foundation 2001, PO Box 23608, 3001 KB, Rotterdam, The Netherlands, which kindly supplied the software.

The standards used are the 1997 Netherlands values from the Fourth Dutch Growth Study (Fredriks et al. Pediatric Research 2000; 47: 316–323) unless otherwise stated.

Target height (TH) is calculated in centimeters as follows:

Ht (boy) = [Ht (father) + Ht (mother) + 13]/2

Ht (girl) = [Ht (father) + Ht (mother) − 13]/2

In imperial units, measure height in inches and apply a correction of ± 5 inches.

A correction of 4.5 cm (1_ inches) has been added to target height to allow for secular trends.

Key to interpretation of clues

Throughout the book various combinations of symptoms, signs and investigations may indicate the strong likelihood of a particular diagnosis. This has been indicated by an equals sign ('='). Please bear in mind that there is always room for uncertainty in any diagnosis and it is rare for the most likely diagnosis to represent the only possible diagnosis.

The lines shown correspond to −2, −1, zero, +1 and +2 standard deviation score (SDS).

The Ullrich–Turner charts created by the software are derived from the German data of Ranke et al. Acta Paediatrica Scandinavica. Supplement 1988; 343: 22–30, and the achondroplasia charts are from Horton et al. Journal of Pediatrics 1978; 93: 435–438.

Mother's (pink) and father's (blue) heights are given as absolute values along with a target height (black).

Bone age is shown in yellow, and is connected to measuring points with a dotted line.

The red arrow plus the notation M2 in females and G2 in males indicates onset of puberty.

Therapies are described in the accompanying legend.

Chapter 1

History, Auxology and Examination

HISTORY

All diagnosis begins with a comprehensive history and examination. This chapter covers general points in the assessment of a child who may have an endocrine disorder; more specific points are included in subsequent sections.

First, explore in detail the presenting complaint as perceived by the parents. If old enough, ask patients whether *they* have any concerns, or whether there is a problem only for other family members or medical personnel.

Take details of the mother's pregnancy, including ill health or drug administration (prescribed or illicit), the gestational age, mode of delivery and any requirement for neonatal special care. All mothers can recall the birth weight of their offspring, but it may be possible to obtain birth length and head circumference from parental or hospital records. It is important to obtain information regarding growth rate in height and weight as recorded in past medical records or as perceived by the parents and child – has there been recent gain or loss of weight and is the child growing out of their clothes and shoes before they wear out, or going through a growth spurt?

Establish a family tree that records details of the heights (preferably measured directly), build and age

of sexual maturation of both parents, siblings and any more distant relations with aberrant stature. There is a tendency for both partners to overestimate their own size and for males to underestimate the height of their female partner, with females tending to overestimate their male partner's height. There is a particularly large bias to underestimating weight in familial obesity. Although estimates of predicted height based on reported size are usually a reasonable guide to genetic target height, there can occasionally be huge discrepancies and the measurement of even one parent (usually the mother) increases the accuracy of the prediction. Possible non-paternity (as much as 10% in some studies) should also be borne in mind.

Enquire whether there is parental consanguinity that may lead to an increased risk of autosomal recessive disorders. Ask whether there are any family members with ill health, especially autoimmune (rheumatoid, pernicious anemia, alopecia, vitiligo) or 'gland' problems, and then enquire specifically about thyroid disorders and diabetes mellitus. The pedigree can be used to record social details that may be vitally important when considering both etiology and subsequent treatment and prognosis (**Fig. 1.1**). Is the patient on any regular medication (including topical and inhaled preparations)? Ask about past medical events including

Fig. 1.1 Family pedigree.

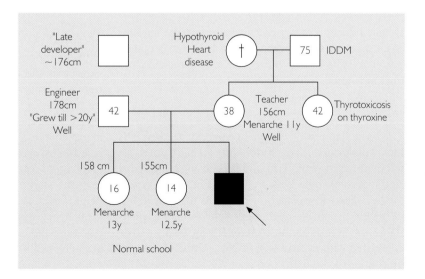

Details of presenting problem and level of concern

Details of mother's pregnancy and of delivery

Birth weight and length; other neonatal measurements if available

Family sizes, ages of sexual maturity

Family history of endocrine or autoimmune disease

Social details

Medication, by any route; past illnesses or operations

Diet in infancy and current food intake

Current growth – growing out of clothes or shoes? Make use of any past records of growth

Developmental or educational level

Bullying or peer pressure (especially related to size and appearance)

Any specific symptoms in chest, cardiovascular system, gastrointestinal, CNS, skin

Table 1.1 Essential points in the history

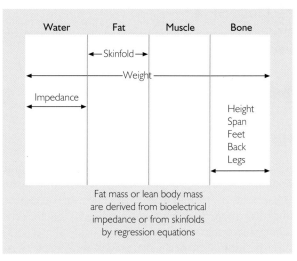

Fig. 1.2 Direct measurements of various body compartments are indicated by the arrows.

what might be perceived as minor surgical procedures such as hernia repair or orchidopexy. Enquire about the current and early diet, and any specific exclusions.

Depending on the age of the child, establish the developmental or educational level and ask about the ability to participate actively in sport. Is there any bullying from peers? Ask the adolescent about career plans. Finally, run through the other systems of the body not involved in the presenting complaint to exclude other pathology.

The main points that must be established from the history of a child presenting with an endocrine disorder are given in **Table 1.1**.

AUXOLOGY

Detailed measurements can give an immense amount of information when performed and charted properly. **Fig. 1.2** demonstrates the information obtained from each measurement described below.

WEIGHT

This is a deceptively simple measurement, which is often performed very badly. An infant should be weighed naked (**Fig. 1.3**) and a child in the minimal clothing compatible with modesty (**Fig. 1.4**). A wet modern disposable diaper can weigh as much as 450 g (1 lb) and the indoor clothing of a child wearing sports shoes and jeans weighs around 1.5 kg (3 lb 5 oz), contrasted with a mean weight gain in mid-childhood of 2–3 kg (4.5-6.5 lb) per year. All scales should be calibrated and serviced regularly. A struggling child's weight can be approximated by turning on electronic scales with the mother standing on them – this results in a 'zero' value that changes to the infant's weight when placed in the mother's arms.

LENGTH AND HEIGHT

Under the age of 2 years, and in children with a motor disability, it is usual to record supine length (**Fig. 1.5**). This requires two people, often the mother plus the auxologist. The head is held against the headboard with the face in a horizontal plane. The hips and knees are extended gently and the movable footboard is brought up to touch the soles of the feet held at 90°.

Standing height (**Fig. 1.6**) should be measured using a stadiometer or other rule, in bare feet with the heels in the same vertical plane as the measuring instrument. The arms should be held relaxed at the sides, and the face should be in the 'Frankfurt plane' with the outer canthus and upper ear horizontal. The subject should be asked to take a deep breath in, then out whilst the auxologist exerts *gentle* upward traction on the mastoid processes. It has been shown that the 'stretch' technique, where the traction is sufficient to lengthen the spine slightly, is unnecessary and may result in increased inter-observer error.

Height is read to the nearest complete millimeter at the end of the breath. If repeated measurements of height are taken to establish a growth velocity, then ideally they should be performed at the same time of day to avoid errors due to spinal compression; on average, height measured in the morning is 8 mm (about $\frac{1}{4}$ inch) more than the afternoon value. The

Fig. 1.3 (Right) Measurement of infant weight. The nappy is removed and calibration of the scales checked frequently.

Fig.1.4 (Far right) Measurement of weight; minimal clothing on calibrated electronic scales.

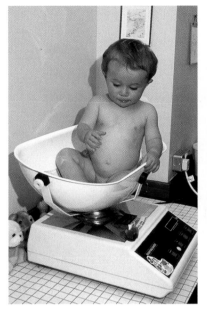
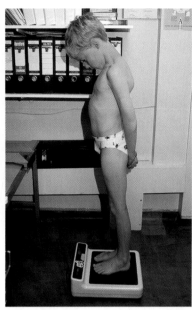

Fig. 1.6 Measurement of height, using a gentle stretch technique, with child in bare feet, and a wall-mounted stadiometer.

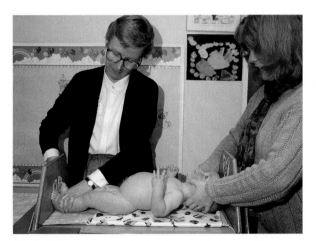

Fig.1.5 Measurement of infant length. Mother positions head horizontally; auxologist extends legs gently. First, the legs are lifted to reduce the lumbar lordosis and then the heels and feet are slid down the footplate.

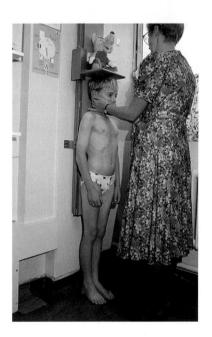

standard error of measurement of height on a single occasion in the hands of a trained auxologist is in the order of 0.2 cm.

CROWN–RUMP LENGTH OR SITTING HEIGHT

Estimation of the length of the back and head can be of great benefit in establishing the relative proportions of the body. In an infant the legs are drawn up to 90° and the footboard is brought into contact with the buttocks (**Fig. 1.7**). In an older child, using a specially designed instrument (**Fig. 1.8**) with the feet resting on a bar, the arms folded loosely in the lap and a similar gentle stretch technique to the one described above, it is possible to obtain precise estimates of sitting height. A simpler method uses a hard seat of known height and horizontal top placed under the height stadiometer. Crown–rump length or sitting height may then be subtracted from standing height to derive subischial leg length.

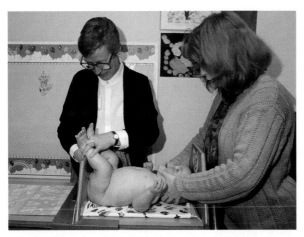

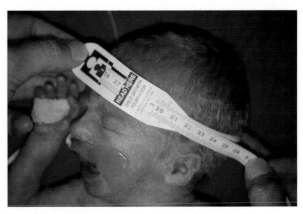

Fig. 1.9 Measurement of head circumference using non-stretchable lasso tape measure (Lasso-o™ Child Growth Foundation, UK).

Fig. 1.7 Measurement of infant crown–rump length. First lift the legs to reduce lumbar lordosis and then slide buttocks down the footplate.

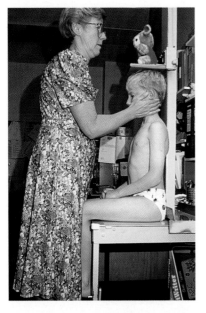

Fig. 1.8 Measurement of sitting height; gentle stretch technique, using purpose-built sitting-height table.

determined with the left arm loose at the side and a fold raised between the measurer's thumb and forefinger at the mid-point of the dorsum of the upper arm. The callipers are applied and, once the reading has stabilized (4–5 sec), the reading is made. The subscapular skinfold (Fig. 1.11) is raised at the tip of the shoulder blade, on the left, with the arms again relaxed at the sides. The biceps skinfold (Fig. 1.12) is determined as for the triceps skinfold but on the ventral aspect of the upper arm. The suprailiac fold (Fig. 1.13) is found at the maximum height of the iliac crest. The skinfold thicknesses give an estimation of the amount of subcutaneous fat, and its distribution, and may be used in various equations to estimate total body adiposity.

HEAD CIRCUMFERENCE

A non-stretchable paper or metal tape or lasso (e.g. the Lasso-o™ available from the UK Child Growth Foundation) should be used and three estimations made of the maximum occipitofrontal circumference (OFC) (Fig. 1.9). In children with abnormal head shape it may not be possible to obtain accurate readings.

SKINFOLD THICKNESS

A skinfold calliper is required that has a known strength of pinch and a known area of tip. Four sites are often chosen, of which the first two are in most common use. The triceps skinfold (Fig. 1.10) is

ARM AND WAIST/HIP CIRCUMFERENCES

Mid upper arm circumference (MUAC) may be measured using a flexible non-stretch tape measure as means of estimating undernutrition (see Ch. 4) and waist and hip circumferences (then expressed as a waist/hip ratio) as a measure of overnutrition (see Ch. 5).

MUAC is measured at a point half-way between elbow and shoulder (Fig. 1.14). Waist circumference is measured between the lower ribs and the ischial ridge, at the level of the umbilicus at the end of a normal expiration. Hip circumference is measured at the level of both greater trochanters.

BODY MASS INDEX

Another commonly used estimate of relative obesity is the body mass index (BMI), or Quetelet index, which can be estimated from the formula: Weight (kg)/Height (m)^2. BMI varies with age and must be

Figs 1.10–1.13 Measurement of triceps (top left), subscapular (top right), biceps (bottom left) and suprailiac (bottom right) skinfold thickness.

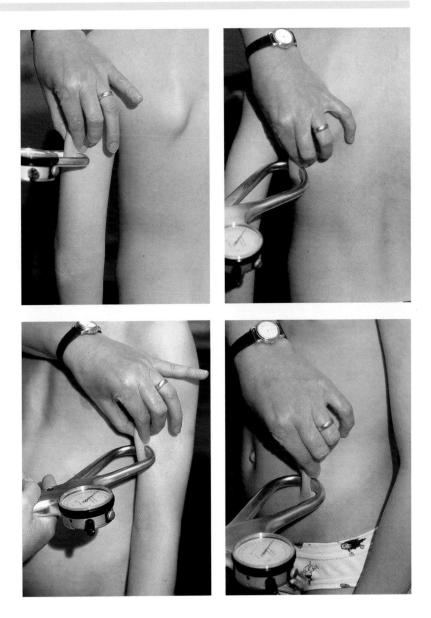

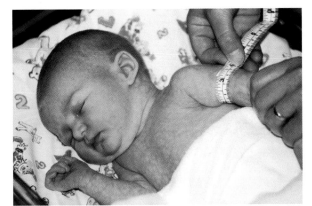

Fig. 1.14 Measurement of mid upper arm circumference, midpoint between elbow and shoulder.

compared with appropriate age- and sex-related standards (see Ch. 5).

OTHER MEASUREMENTS

It is sometimes helpful to assess other body sizes and their relationships directly; standard centile charts exist for almost every imaginable parameter.

Measurement of span is the value most likely to be of use in the endocrine clinic and may be estimated by measuring the fingertip to fingertip distance with the arms held horizontally (**Fig. 1.15**). The normal relationship of span to height is:

Span = Height ± 3.5 cm (1.5 inches)

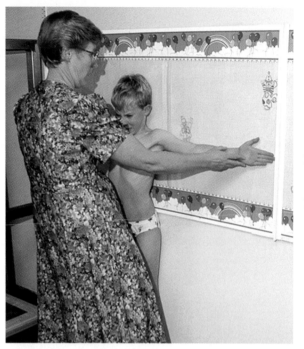

Fig. 1.15 Measurement of span. The arms are horizontal with the right fingertips held against a fixed vertical bar and the left against a movable vertical guide on calibrated graph paper.

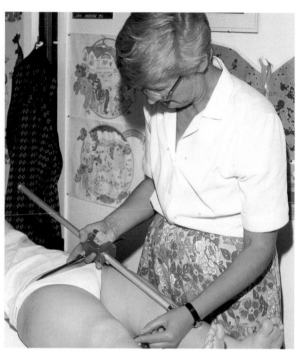

Fig. 1.16 Measurement of individual body segments in a child with short limbs, using an anthropometer.

In short-limbed conditions and if hemihypertrophy is suspected (see below), then direct measurement of limb segments using a specially designed anthropometer (**Fig. 1.16**) or a metal builder's tape measure may be of help.

GROWTH CHARTS

Up-to-date standards for height, weight, BMI and head circumference are available for many populations. Standards should be updated regularly to take secular changes in growth into account, and ideally patients from ethnic subgroups should be compared with appropriate charts, although this is not always possible. Standards for sitting height, leg length, skinfold thickness, span, etc. are less universally available, but published.

Most commonly used charts are sex specific and show the measured parameter on the vertical axis and age on the horizontal. Almost all scales are linear, except for skinfold thickness, where a vertical logarithmic axis is used, and in some charts extending into premature infancy where a non-linear age axis allows expansion of data in the early months.

Many charts use 'centile' lines spaced at varying intervals depending on the design of the chart. A common layout is to use the 0.4th, 2nd, 9th, 25th and 50th centiles with corresponding values above the mean to give nine centile lines, smoothed by a statistical method known as LMS. Thus only 1 in 250 children would fall below the 0.4th or above the 99.6th centile in a normal population, which may form the basis for a referral protocol.

Charts of height and weight have been published for many named syndromic conditions and should be used where necessary; there are also charts of limb length, height and OFC for many of the skeletal dysplasias.

The measured value should be plotted as a simple dot and other values, such as bone age (see below), plotted in a different color or a square symbol.

Whenever a standard centile chart is used, of whatever construction, it is possible rapidly to estimate the expected genetic potential of the subject by plotting the centile value of each parent on the right-hand y-axis. The mid-parental centile can then be drawn. Alternatively, for height only, the following simple calculations may be performed:

$$\text{Target height of boy in cm} = \frac{(\text{father's height} + \text{mother's height} + 13)}{2}$$

$$\text{Target height of girl in cm} = \frac{(\text{mother's height} + \text{father's height} - 13)}{2}$$

(For imperial units, give height in inches plus a correction of 5 inches.)

If a secular trend is expected, for example if the economic situation of the child is much better than that of the parents in their youth, 4.5 cm (approximately 1.75 inches) should be added to the target height. In 95% of cases the final height of the child is expected to be within the target height ±9 cm (4.5 inches), the so-called 'target range'. The centile position of the target height can then be compared with the centile position of the present height of the child. *This is the method used in illustrations throughout this book.*

As growth is a longitudinal process, change of height with time is even more important than absolute height at a particular timepoint. The final evaluation of growth in any parameter is made by connecting consecutive measurements on the growth chart and visually assessing any deviation upwards or downwards through the centile lines.

Growth rate can also be evaluated by calculating a velocity that can be compared with published height and weight velocity curves. Velocity is calculated by the formula:

$$\frac{Ht\ 2 - Ht\ 1}{Interval\ (decimal\ years)}$$

Because measurement error is magnified when two separately obtained values are used to calculate a velocity (95% confidence interval (CI) for velocity estimated from two measurements 1 year apart $= \pm$ [2SD of measurement (around 0.25 cm)] $\times \sqrt{2}$; for a 3-month interval the CI is four times this value), the use of this calculation is dependent on accurate measurements and improved by long intervals between estimates. The design of the reference charts means that optimal information will come from yearly estimations of height velocity (and in clinical practice a minimum period of 6 months).

To allow more precise quantification of any normally distributed parameter for which standards exist, it is common to use the Standard Deviation Score (SDS, or Z score), especially for values that lie outside the normal centile range. This technique allows comparison of the parameters for children of different age and sex.

$$SDS = \frac{x - \bar{x}}{SD}$$

where x is the measured value; $\bar{x}$ the mean, and SD the standard deviation for a given population. In a normally distributed population the SDS will have a mean of 0 and a SD of 1. A SDS of from −1 to +1 includes 68.26%, and from −2 to +2 includes 95.44% of the population. Only 0.13% of a population will have an SDS of more or less than 3. *The charts used throughout this book show the mean and ± 1 and 2 SD.*

EXAMINATION

The examination of the child can begin during the history-taking by observing their activity, demeanor and interaction with the parents or carers. It is then usual to begin with the hands, work up the arms to the head and neck, examine the chest and back, then the cardiovascular system followed by the abdomen and external inspection of the genitalia with an assessment of maturity. Finish with the central nervous system examination and inspection of the body and skin. These points are now described in more detail.

THE HANDS

The hands (and sometimes the feet) hold the clue to many endocrine disorders and syndromic malformations associated with abnormal stature. **Figs 1.17–1.45** show a number of abnormalities with their interpretation.

Abnormal dermatoglyphics (**Fig. 1.17**), such as a single palmar crease, are non-specific signs of possible syndromic malformations. The fingers and wrist may be conveniently used to demonstrate increased mobility and arachnodactyly (**Figs 1.18–1.21**), as may be seen in the Marfan syndrome and some of the collagen disorders, or stiffness in long-standing diabetes mellitus (**Fig. 1.22**) and some of the storage disorders (**Figs 1.23 & 1.24**). Fixed joint contractures, arthrogryposis (**Fig. 1.25**), may be restricted to one group of joints, or may be generalized: it is a non-specific sign of congenital neuromuscular disease and various syndromes. Generally short fingers (brachydactyly) are

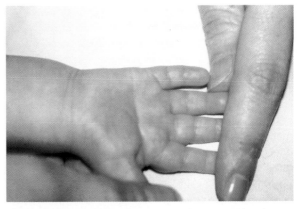

Fig. 1.17 Single palmar crease – may be a normal variant but can be a non-specific clue to look for other dysmorphic features.

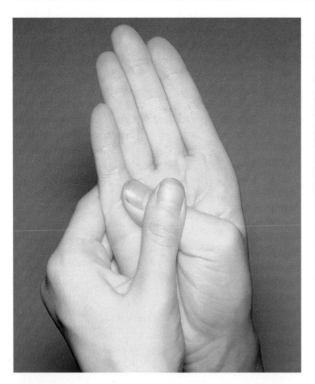

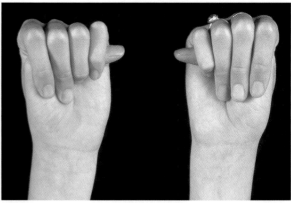

Figs 1.18, 1.19 Increased joint mobility in the Marfan syndrome shown by touching palm with length of thumb (left) and ability to enclose thumb, which protrudes from the other side, with the clenched hand (above).

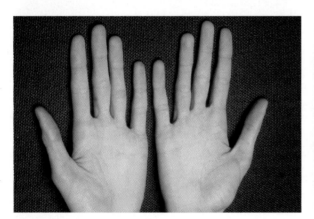

Fig. 1.20 Arachnodactyly in the Marfan syndrome.

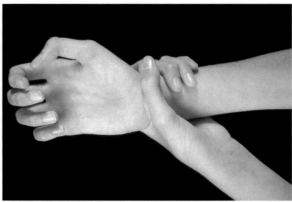

Fig. 1.21 The wrist sign, demonstrated by clasping one wrist with the opposite hand and noting overlap of the distal phalanges of thumb and middle finger.

seen in many syndromes associated with short stature (**Fig. 1.26**). Only the fifth finger may be shortened, as in Coffin–Siris syndrome (**Fig. 1.27**), or just one or two metacarpals as in pseudohypoparathyroidism (**Figs 1.28 & 1.29**). Fingers may show fusion (syndactyly), or duplication with or without fusion (polydactyly or polysyndactyly) (**Figs 1.30 & 1.31**), in some dysmorphic syndromes. Polydactyly or other finger abnormalities can be classed as pre-axial (radial/tibial side) or post-axial (ulnar/fibular) (**Fig 1.32**). All the fingers may be bent, as in various of the camptodactyly

syndromes associated with short stature (**Fig. 1.33**), or just the fifth finger (clinodactyly), which is a non-specific abnormality in many syndromic disorders (**Fig. 1.34**). A trident hand is seen in achondroplasia (**Fig. 1.35**). The thumb may be broad (**Fig. 1.36**), triphalangeal (**Fig. 1.37**) or low set (**Fig. 1.38**) in various syndromes. The fingertips and interphalangeal joints are broad in Aarskog syndrome (**Fig. 1.39**), an X-linked, dominantly inherited, condition associated with moderate short stature. The wrist is expanded in rickets for whatever causes (see Chs 4 & 11). Clubbing

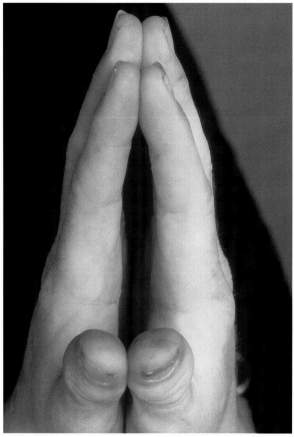

Fig. 1.22 Joint stiffness in a long-standing diabetic. The 'prayer sign' – an inability to oppose the palms of the hands – is caused by irreversible glycosylation of tissue proteins (see Ch. 10).

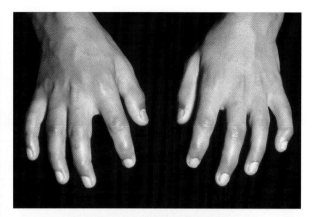

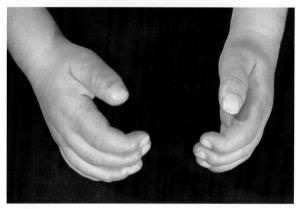

Figs 1.23, 1.24 'Claw hands' in two children with storage disorders: mucolipidosis 3 (top) and Hunter syndrome (bottom).

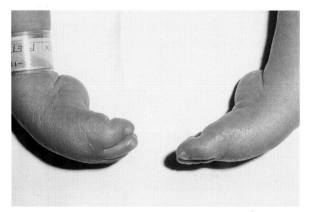

Fig. 1.25 Fixed joint contractures (or arthrogryposis), here presenting as bilateral talipes in a child with camptodactyly and short stature of prenatal onset.

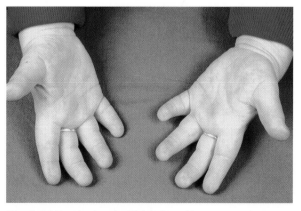

Fig. 1.26 Brachydactyly. This is found in many syndromes associated with short stature.

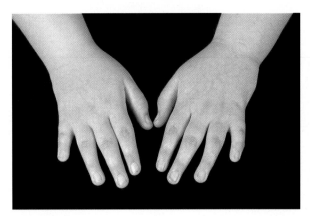

Fig. 1.27 Isolated short fifth digit in Coffin–Siris syndrome.

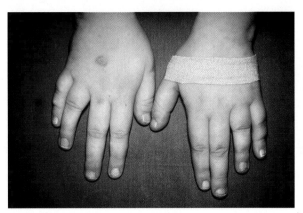

Fig. 1.28 Short fourth and fifth metacarpals in the hand of child with pseudohypoparathyroidism.

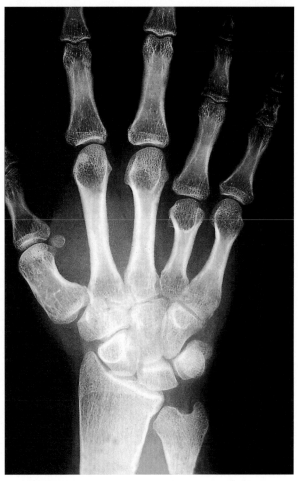

Fig. 1.29 Corresponding radiograph of the child in Fig. 1.28.

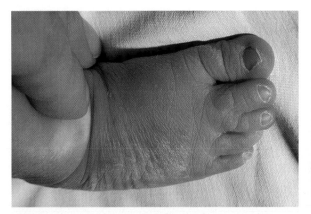

Fig. 1.30 Syndactyly. A common, often familial, variant and a non-specific clue to look for other dysmorphic features. In association with ambiguous genitalia in an XY individual, this may raise the possibility of Smith–Lemli–Opitz syndrome.

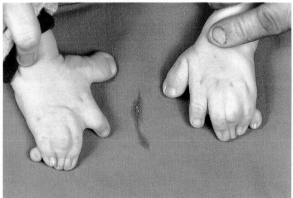

Fig. 1.31 Polysyndactyly, here in the Carpenter syndrome.

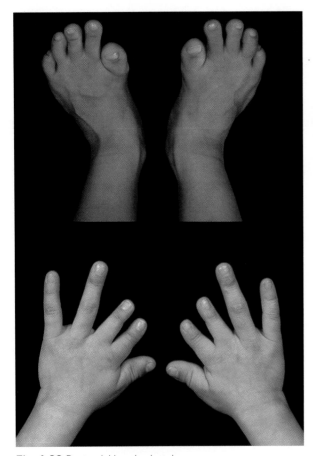

Fig. 1.32 Post-axial brachydactyly.

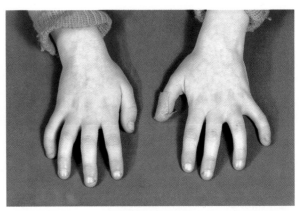

Fig. 1.34 Clinodactyly. This is found in many syndromes associated with short stature.

Fig. 1.35 Trident hand in achondroplasia.

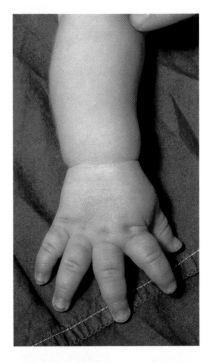

Fig. 1.33 Camptodactyly. There is a group of camptodactyly syndromes associated with short stature and scoliosis.

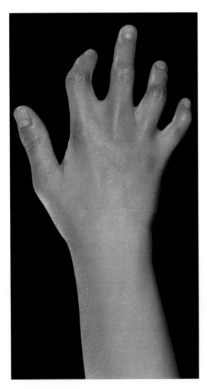

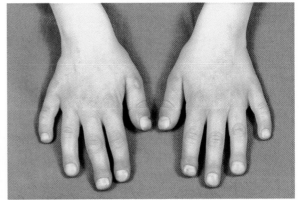

Fig. 1.36 Broad thumb as seen in Rubinstein–Taybi syndrome.

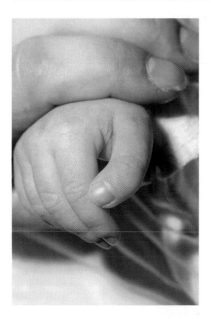

Fig. 1.37
Triphalangeal
thumb.

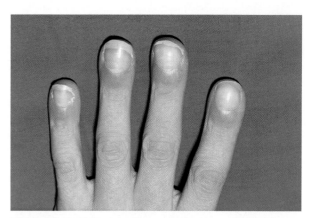

Fig. 1.40 Clubbing, here in a patient with cystic fibrosis.

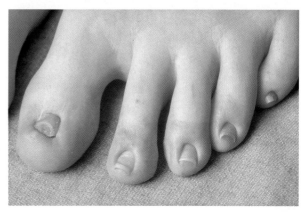

Fig. 1.41 Deep-set nails in Sotos syndrome.

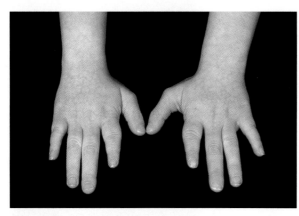

Fig. 1.38 Low-set thumb.

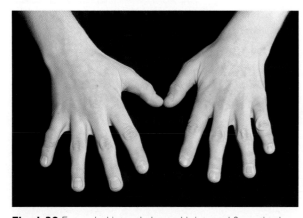

Fig. 1.39 Expanded interphalangeal joints and fingertips in the X-linked recessive Aarskog syndrome associated with short stature.

is seen in chronic cyanotic heart disease, chronic purulent respiratory disorders and inflammatory bowel disease, as well as occurring dominantly in families (**Fig. 1.40**). The nails may be deep set in the Sotos syndrome of cerebral gigantism (**Fig. 1.41**) and hypoplastic in ectodermal dysplasia and those syndromes characterized by early lymphedema such as the Ullrich–Turner syndrome (**Figs 1.42 & 1.43**). The palms show redness in chronic liver disorders and a yellowish discoloration in true pituitary gigantism (**Fig. 1.44**) and in hypothyroidism, where the knuckles are yellow in contrast to the generalized pallor (**Fig. 1.45**).

THE ARMS

The relative length of the arms can be assessed by measurement of span, as described above. Fixed flexion of the elbow and wrist may be seen with arthrogryposis, and limited rotation of the forearm in some of the skeletal dysplasias (**Fig. 1.46**). Radial aplasia or hypoplasia and distal digital ray abnormalities may be seen in some dysmorphic short-stature syndromes and

Fig. 1.42
Hypoplastic nails
as seen in around
40% of girls with
Ullrich–Turner
syndrome.

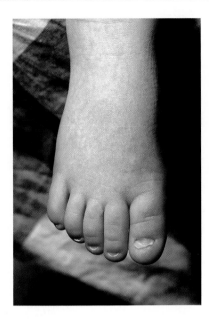

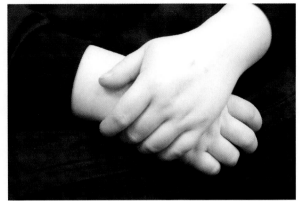

Fig. 1.45 Extremely pale skin and yellow knuckles in hypothyroidism.

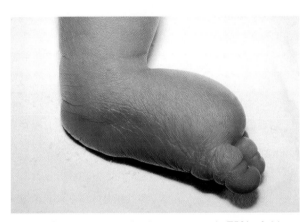

Fig. 1.43 Neonatal lymphedema, as seen in 75% of girls with Ullrich–Turner syndrome.

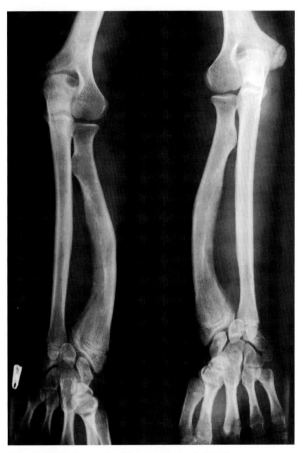

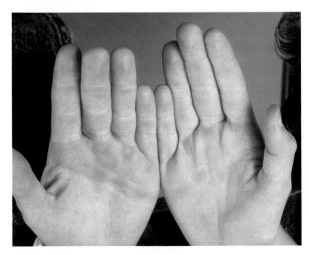

Fig. 1.44 Yellow palmar discoloration in pituitary gigantism.

Fig. 1.46 Radiograph of forearm in Leri–Weill dyschondrosteosis with bowed radius producing limited forearm rotation – the Madelung deformity.

associated with congenital heart defects, renal or hematologic abnormalities (**Fig. 1.47**). An increased carrying angle (**Fig. 1.48**) is classically seen in the Ullrich–Turner syndrome, although it is absent in 50% of cases and may be present in other syndromes.

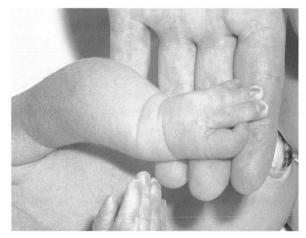

Fig. 1.47 Radial hypoplasia and digital ray abnormality in Holt–Oram syndrome, associated with atrial and ventricular septal defects.

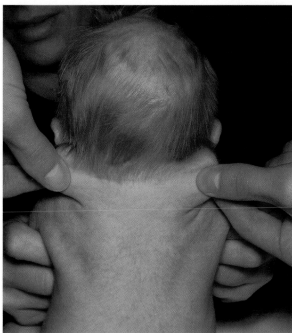

Fig. 1.49 Loose skin of neck in neonate with Down syndrome.

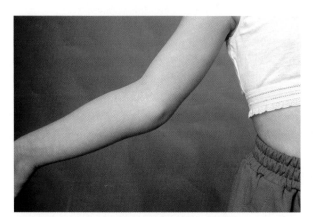

Fig. 1.48 Increased carrying angle as seen in 40–50% of girls with Ullrich–Turner syndrome.

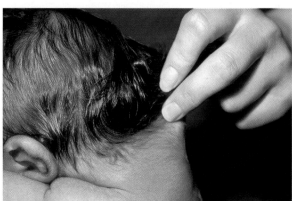

Fig. 1.50 Loose skin of neck in neonate with Ullrich–Turner syndrome.

THE HEAD AND NECK

There are many abnormalities of this region that may indicate pathology, and a selection of these is given in **Figs 1.49–1.86**.

Redundant skin at the site of previous fetal nuchal edema is a feature of the Down, Ullrich–Turner and other chromosomal syndromes in the neonatal period (**Figs 1.49 & 1.50**) and may be more obvious than webbing at this stage. Webbing of the neck (**Fig. 1.51**) is seen in 70% of cases of Ullrich–Turner syndrome, although it is not a specific finding, and a short neck with a low hairline (**Figs 1.52 & 1.53**) is also seen in many dysmorphic syndromes (**Fig. 1.54**).

The shape of the skull should be assessed. Mild brachycephaly or plagiocephaly is common, but if craniosynostosis (**Figs 1.55 & 1.56**) is suspected there should be palpable suture lines and a typical radiographic appearance (**Figs 1.57 & 1.58**).

Around the eyes hypertelorism (**Fig. 1.59**), heavy supraorbital ridges (**Fig. 1.60**) or the presence of epicanthic folds, ptosis (**Fig. 1.61**), blepharophimosis, microphthalmia and exophthalmos (**Fig 1.62**) due to thyrotoxicosis should be assessed. There may be prolapsing of the temporal horn into the orbit, producing exophthalmos in neurofibromatosis (**Figs 1.63 & 1.64**) and syndromes affecting the depth of the orbit such as Apert syndrome.

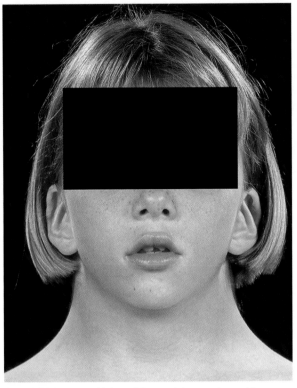

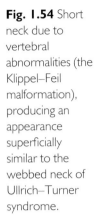

Fig. 1.54 Short neck due to vertebral abnormalities (the Klippel–Feil malformation), producing an appearance superficially similar to the webbed neck of Ullrich–Turner syndrome.

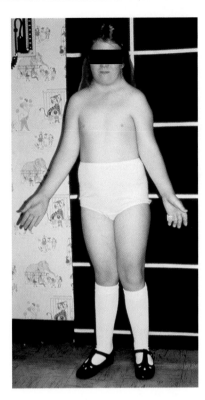

Fig. 1.51 Later webbing of the neck in a patient with Noonan syndrome (as seen to some degree in 70% of girls with Ullrich–Turner syndrome). Note abnormal ears, seldom seen in Ullrich–Turner syndrome.

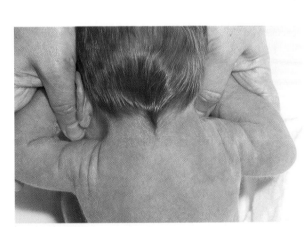

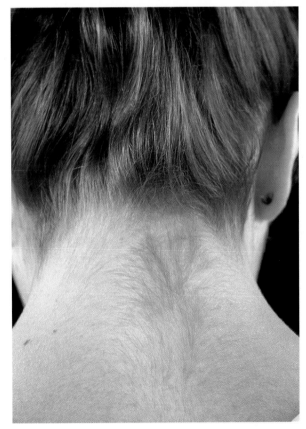

Figs 1.52, 1.53 Low hairline with midline extension seen in 75% of girls with Ullrich–Turner syndrome, shown in a neonate (above) and in late childhood (right).

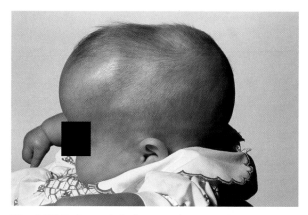

Fig. 1.55 Dolicocephaly from craniosynostosis.

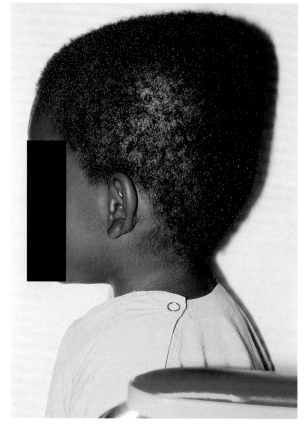

Fig. 1.56 Turricephaly from craniosynostosis.

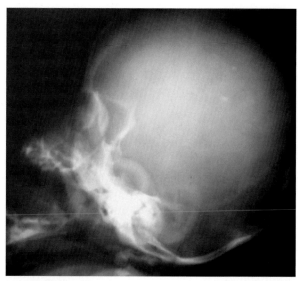

Fig. 1.57 Radiograph of coronal craniosynostosis showing absent suture lines with sclerosis and abnormal head shape.

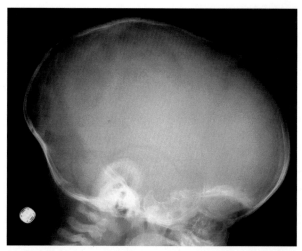

Fig. 1.58 Radiograph of sagittal craniosynostosis showing absent suture lines with sclerosis and abnormal head shape.

Look at the mouth and palate. Submucous cleft palate may be revealed only by palpation. Any abnormalities of the midline are especially significant as they may indicate an associated abnormality of the pituitary gland (**Fig. 1.65**). Holoprosencephaly with microcephaly, hypotelorism and palatonasal abnormalities is due to a mutation of a midline patterning gene and there will be failure of fusion of the midline cerebral structures, often with associated hypopituitarism

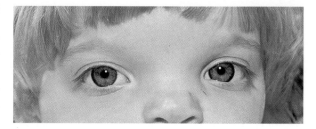

Fig. 1.59 Severe hypertelorism.

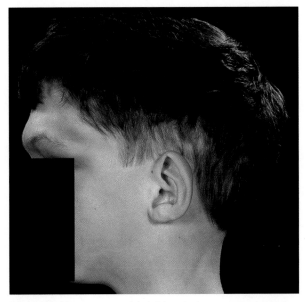

Fig. 1.60 Heavy supraorbital ridges in frontometaphyseal dysplasia.

Fig. 1.62
Exophthalmos in thyrotoxicosis.

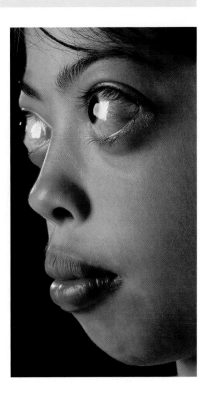

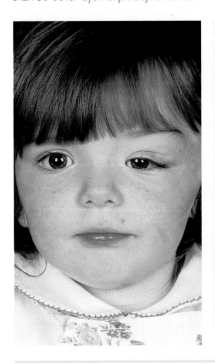

Fig. 1.61 Ptosis, seen in 25% of girls with Ullrich–Turner, the majority of children with Noonan syndrome, and more than 50 other dysmorphic syndromes.

(**Figs 1.66 & 1.67**). A less severe but related abnormality produces the single central incisor and growth hormone deficiency syndrome (**Fig 1.68**).

Cleft palate is part of the Smith–Lemli–Opitz syndrome, in which there may be associated genital ambiguity (**Fig. 1.69**). A high arched palate may be seen

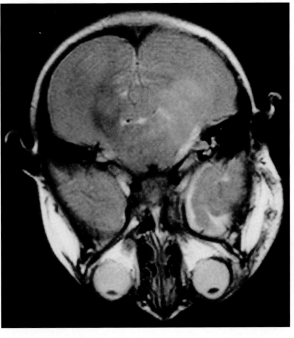

Figs 1.63, 1.64
Exophthalmos in neurofibromatosis (left) secondary to prolapsing temporal horn into orbit (right).

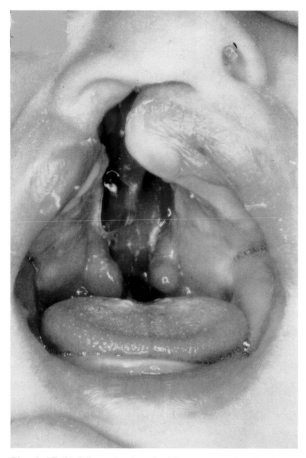

Fig. 1.65 Cleft lip and palate, in this case associated with panhypopituitarism.

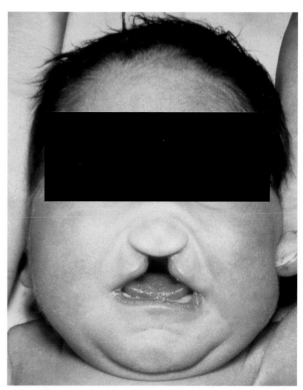

Fig. 1.66 Midline cleft and abnormal nose in holoprosencephaly. There may be associated panhypopituitarism.

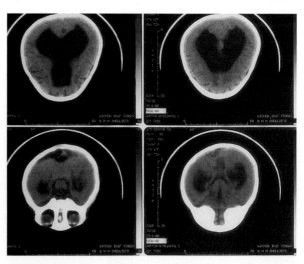

Fig. 1.67 Computed tomogram of the patient in Fig. 1.66, demonstrating abnormal midline structures and cloverleaf ventricles.

in the Marfan, the Ullrich–Turner and some other dysmorphic syndromes (**Fig. 1.70**).

The tongue is smooth (**Fig. 1.71**) in iron deficiency of any cause and, in older age groups, in pernicious anemia, where it may be associated with other autoimmune disease. Both the tongue and lips may show neuromata in neurofibromatosis and in the multiple endocrine neoplasia (MEN) type IIb syndrome (**Fig. 1.72**). The lips may be swollen and 'fish-like' in Crohn's disease (**Fig. 1.73**) and MEN-IIb. Oral candidiasis outside the neonatal period (**Fig. 1.74**) may signal type 1 diabetes mellitus, immunodeficiency associated with hypoparathyroidism in DiGeorge syndrome and the autoimmune polyglandular type I or 'HAM' syndrome of hypoparathyroidism, adrenal failure and moniliasis.

The teeth may be unusually soft and carious in disorders affecting collagen, fibrin and calcium metabolism, and peg-like in ectodermal dysplasia (**Fig. 1.75**). They are an abnormal shape in the Rubinstein–Taybi syndrome (**Fig. 1.76**). They may be stained or rotted by drugs and bilirubin (**Fig. 1.77**). After chemotherapy for malignancy there may be enamel hypoplasia (**Fig. 1.78**). An assessment of the presence and number of the primary dentition and appearance of

Fig. 1.68 Single central incisor, associated with congenital growth hormone deficiency.

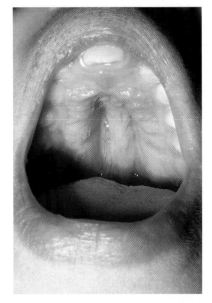

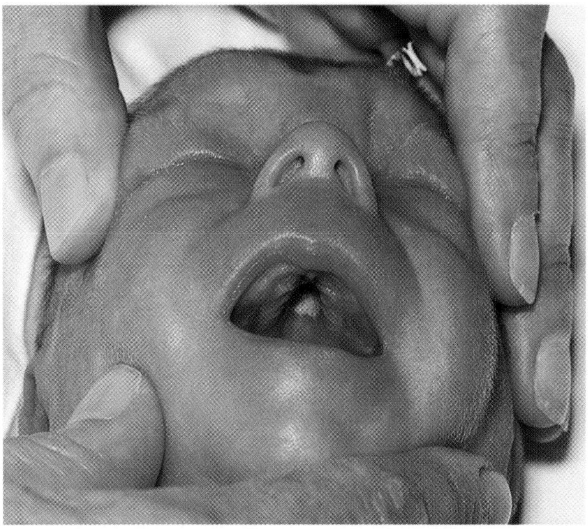

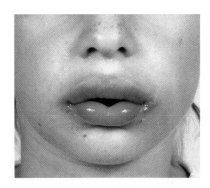

Fig. 1.69 Isolated cleft palate in Smith–Lemli–Opitz syndrome.

Fig. 1.70 High arched palate seen in 75% of girls with Ullrich–Turner syndrome and in most patients with Marfan syndrome.

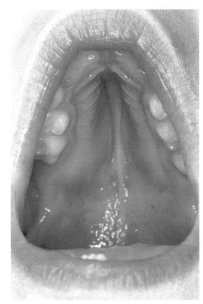

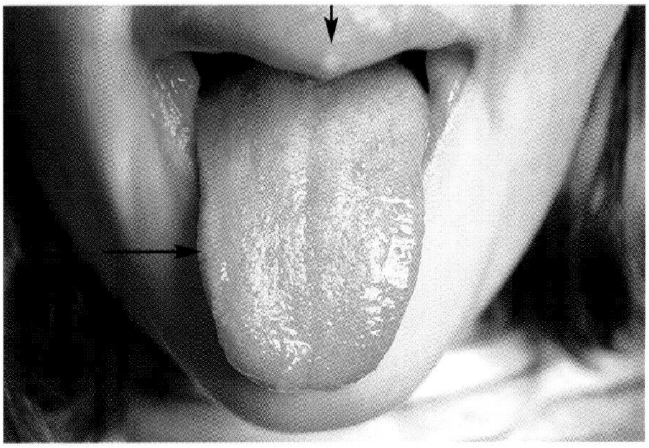

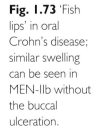

Fig. 1.72 Labial and glossal neuromas in MEN type IIb.

Fig. 1.73 'Fish lips' in oral Crohn's disease; similar swelling can be seen in MEN-IIb without the buccal ulceration.

Fig. 1.71 Smooth tongue in severe iron deficiency.

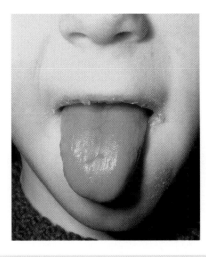

the secondary teeth may give clues to skeletal age and physiological maturity (see below). Delayed eruption of the teeth is seen in any disorder that delays physical maturation (especially chronic disease, hypothyroidism and hypopituitarism), in cleidocranial dysostosis

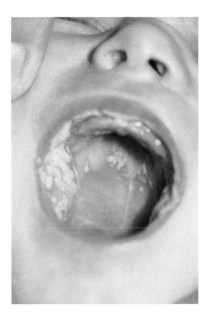

Fig. 1.74 Oral candidiasis. If seen outside infancy, diabetes mellitus, immunodeficiency and autoimmune disease need to be excluded.

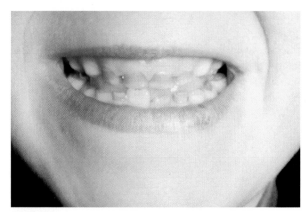

Fig. 1.77 Bilirubin staining after severe jaundice in an ex-premature neonate with sustained growth failure.

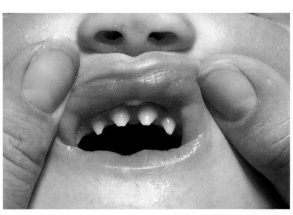

Fig. 1.75 Peg-like teeth in ectodermal dysplasia.

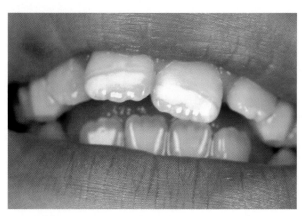

Fig. 1.78 Enamel hypoplasia secondary to chemotherapy.

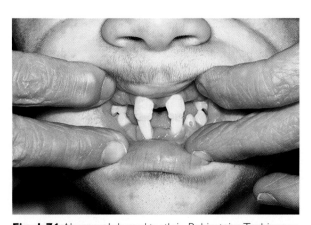

Fig. 1.76 Abnormal shaped teeth in Rubinstein–Taybi syndrome.

(**Fig. 1.79**) and in some other dysmorphic syndromes associated with short stature. Early loss of teeth is seen in Down and Ehlers–Danlos syndromes.

The ears are low set with or without rotation (**Fig. 1.80**), or folded in an abnormal manner (**Fig. 1.81**) in a host of dysmorphic syndromes associated with short stature.

Head hair may be abnormally sparse or curled in several syndromic and metabolic disorders, and in progeria (**Fig. 1.82**). It may show abnormal patterns of whorl formation with underlying CNS malformation. Alopecia may indicate autoimmune disease (**Fig. 1.83**) and temporal hair loss is a feature of hypo-thyroidism (**Fig. 1.84**).

Palpation of the neck, from behind the patient, will allow assessment of the size and shape of the thyroid gland, which should also be measured at its widest point across the isthmus and from top to base on both sides of the midline. Most goiters in childhood (see Ch. 9) are smooth, although nodular enlargement

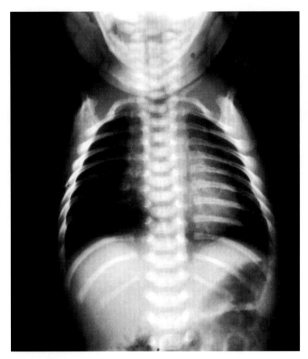

Fig. 1.79 Extreme delay of dental eruption is seen in cleidocranial dysostosis (severe hypothyroidism may produce similar delay).

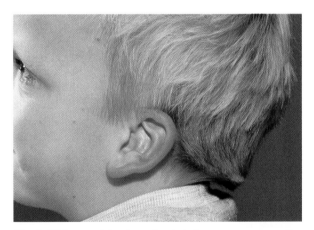

Fig. 1.80 Low-set, backward, rotated ears – a non-specific finding in many dysmorphic syndromes.

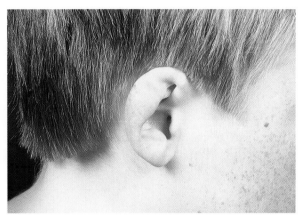

Fig. 1.81 Abnormal helical pattern of ear in pseudohypoparathyroidism.

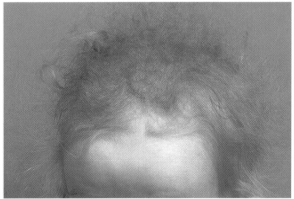

Fig. 1.82 Sparse head hair in the Russell–Silver syndrome

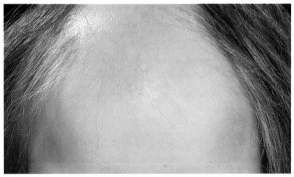

Fig. 1.83 Alopecia areata in autoimmune disease.

may rarely occur. They move upwards on swallowing and it is useful to have a glass of water in the examination room for this purpose. Aberrant lingual thyroid tissue may be visible in the mouth at the root of the tongue on swallowing (**Fig. 1.85**). Retrosternal thyroid tissue can be identified by ultrasonography or lateral radiography of the thoracic inlet. Thyroglossal cysts are usually near the midline, solitary and transilluminate (**Fig. 1.86**).

THE CHEST, ABDOMEN AND CARDIOVASCULAR SYSTEM

These systems should be examined to exclude any organic disorders that could produce poor growth or mimic an endocrinopathy. It is especially important to measure the blood pressure, as hypertension may be a feature of pheochromocytoma, CNS tumors, neuro-

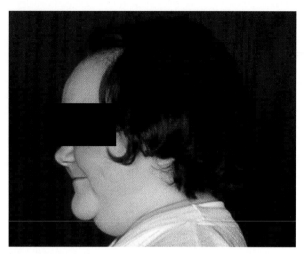

Fig. 1.84 Temporal thinning of the hair in severe hypothyroidism.

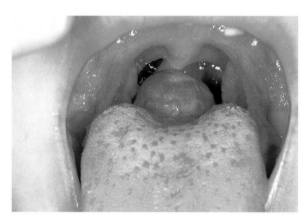

Fig. 1.85 Goitrous lingual thyroid.

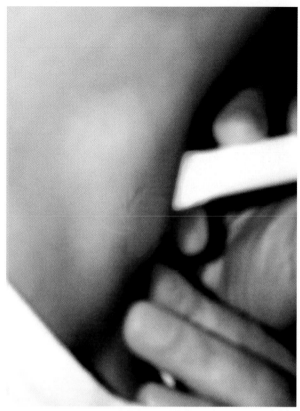

Fig. 1.86 Thyroglossal cyst.

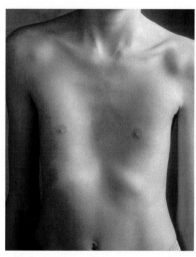

Fig. 1.87 Pectus excavatum in the Marfan syndrome.

fibromatosis, the Cushing and Conn syndromes, ovarian tumors and some disorders of adrenal steroid biosynthesis. Hypertension in the right arm is also a feature of coarctation of the aorta, which may be present in 40% of girls with Ullrich–Turner syndrome, and so the femoral pulses must also be assessed. A wide pulse pressure (with tachycardia) is a feature of thyrotoxicosis. Low blood pressure with postural hypotension can be seen in adrenal insufficiency.

Major heart malformations and abnormal chest shape, such as pectus excavatum or pectus carinatum (**Figs 1.87 & 1.88**), may be seen in many syndromes associated with both short and tall stature. A rachitic rosary may be seen in vitamin D deficiency (see **Fig. 11.24**). Many of the storage disorders, syndromic malformations, and disorders of bone and collagen metabolism may show a scoliosis or kyphoscoliosis (**Fig. 1.89**). There is an accentuated lumbar lordosis or gibbus in achondroplasia (**Fig.**

1.90). The degree of angulation of the spine can be assessed radiographically (**Fig. 1.91**) or by surface mapping techniques (**Fig. 1.92**), and the loss of height quantified by measurement of sitting height.

There may be abdominal organomegaly in some of the storage disorders, thalassemia and Beckwith–Wiedemann syndrome, where an umbilical hernia or

Fig. 1.88 Pectus carinatum in the Noonan syndrome.

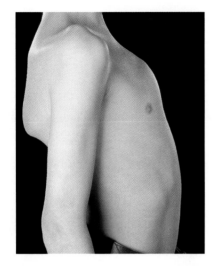

Fig. 1.89 Scoliosis with plexiform neuroma in neurofibromatosis.

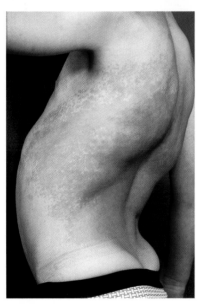

Fig. 1.90 Lumbar gibbus in achondroplasia.

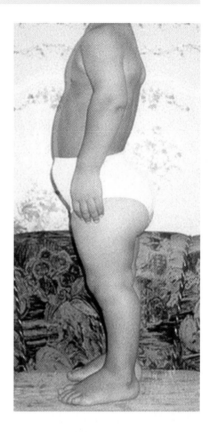

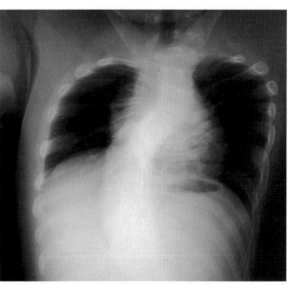

Fig. 1.91 Radiograph of scoliosis in camptodactyly syndrome of the Tel–Hashomer variety.

omphalocele can also be seen (**Fig. 1.93**) (see Ch. 3). Adrenal carcinomas producing virilization are often large and palpable (**Fig. 1.94**). Inspection of the anal margin may reveal signs of sexual abuse or chronic inflammatory bowel disease (**Fig. 1.95**).

THE BREASTS

Breast tissue and the pectoralis major muscle may be absent congenitally in the Poland sequence (**Fig. 1.96**) (there may also be associated heart, renal and vertebral defects). It may be damaged or destroyed after bilateral neonatal breast abscess (**Fig. 1.97**), or after surgery for abscess or physiologic neonatal gynecomastia (**Fig. 1.98**). Physiologic gynecomastia in the adolescent male is common and may be seen especially in the obese individual (**Fig. 1.99**). It is also

often unilateral (**Fig. 1.100**) and in any case may possibly require surgical resection and/or liposuction. Pathologic causes of early breast development are discussed in Chapter 6. Virginal breast hypertrophy (juvenile fibroadenoma) is uncommon but dramatic (**Fig. 1.101**). Accessory nipples are common (**Fig.**

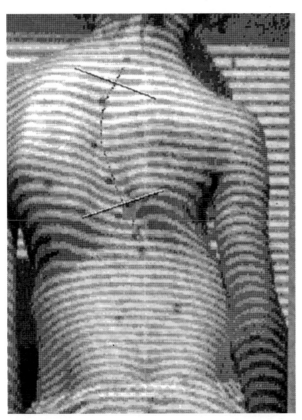

Fig. 1.92 Assessing scoliosis using optical surface mapping.

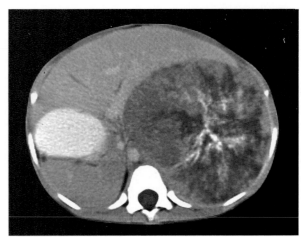

Fig. 1.94 Massive adrenal carcinoma presenting as abdominal mass with virilization.

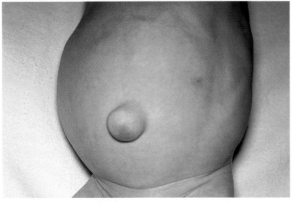

Fig. 1.93 Umbilical hernia and visible organomegaly in Beckwith–Wiedemann syndrome.

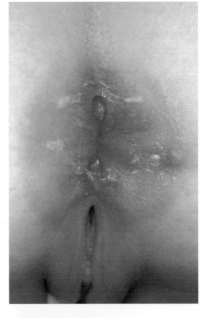

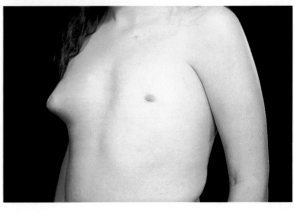

Fig. 1.95 (Left) Anal signs of Crohn's disease. Fig. 1.96 (Bottom) Poland sequence. There is absence of the left pectoralis major and breast tissue. This child was referred with unilateral breast enlargement – a good example of normal stage 4 breast development.

1.102); it is rare, but possible, for them to overlie significant breast tissue.

THE GENITALIA

Many endocrine disorders have associated abnormalities of the genitalia; these are dealt with in detail in Chapters 6, 7 & 8.

In both sexes look especially for signs of hernia (or the scars of their repair early in life). In all patients

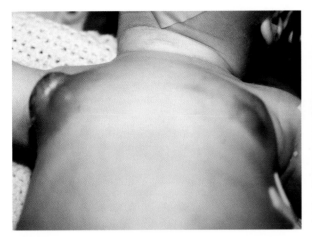

Fig. 1.97 Neonatal breast abscess. Delayed antibiotic therapy or mistaken surgical intervention can lead to later amastia.

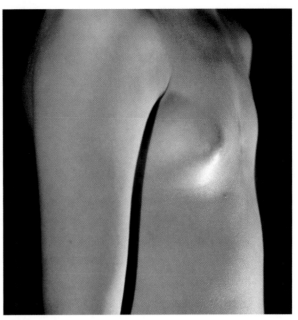

Fig. 1.100 Unilateral male gynecomastia, not uncommon but difficult to explain in the absence of a history of trauma.

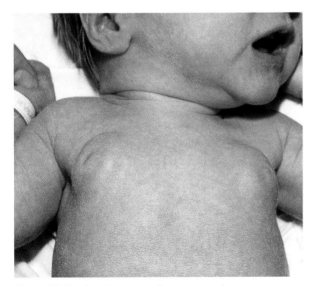

Fig. 1.98 Physiologic neonatal gynecomastia.

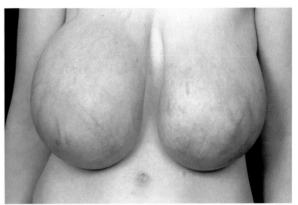

Fig. 1.101 Virginal breast hypertrophy (juvenile fibroadenoma).

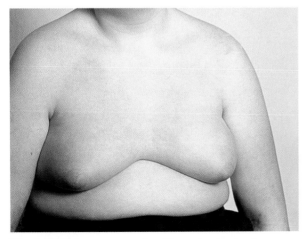

Fig. 1.99 Male gynecomastia with moderate obesity.

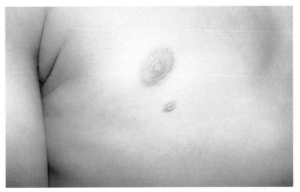

Fig. 1.102 Accessory nipple.

	Male	Female
Pubic hair		
I	None	None
2	Barely visible at base of penis or on scrotum	Barely visible on mons or labia
3	More visible, darker, same sites as (2)	More visible, darker, same sites as (2)
4	More extensive and dark, extending to suprapubic region	More extensive and dark, extending to suprapubic region
5	Adult triangle with extension on to medial aspect of thighs	Adult triangle
5+	Extension upwards in midline	Extension upwards in midline and on to medial aspect of thighs
Male genital stages		
I	Prepubertal penis	
2	Beginning of enlargement, more in length than breadth. Scrotal skin thickens	
3	Further enlargement and early separation of contour of glans from shaft	
4	Near adult shape, not fully grown. Scrotal skin dark and thick	
5	Adult penis	
Testicular volume	Recorded directly by comparison to an orchidometer (Fig. 1.105). Onset of puberty (≥3.5 mL testis) is followed by the onset of the pubertal growth spurt after approx. 6 months. Peak height velocity is attained with 12–14 mL testicular volume	
Female breast stages[a]		
I		Prepubertal
2		Breast bud palpable
3		Obvious elevation of breast tissue
4[b]		Areola and nipple separate on enlarging breast
5		Adult size and shape; areola and nipple merge
Menarche		Recorded as an all-or-nothing event (although regular periods may take time to establish)
Growth potential (cm)[c]		
Stage 2 – PHV	12.5 (2.9–28.7)	6.8 (0.0–16.3)
Stage 2 – final	27.9 (17.9–41.2)	21.0 (11.6–29.4)
Stage 3 – final	20.3 (3.9–30.1)	13.7 (6.1–21.6)
PHV – final	15.7 (9.6–22.6)	14.4 (8.6–23.0)
Stage 4 – final	14.6 (1.1–25.2)	7.5 (2.7–13.7)
Stage 5 – final	8.4 (0.0–20.5)	3.8 (0.0–10.0)
Menarche – final	–	5.8 (1.0–12.7)

[a]The onset of the pubertal height spurt is concurrent with the appearance of stage 2 breast development, and peak height velocity (PHV) is usually associated with stage 3 breast development.

[b]Some normal girls will not pass this stage of development.

[c]Values are mean (range) for stage of puberty. To convert centimeters to inches, multiply by 0.394. Data from J.M.H. Buckler, with permission.

Table 1.2 Stages of sexual maturation

presenting with a possible endocrine disorder, a full assessment of physical maturity is mandatory. It is usual to stage the appearance of the pubic hair, penis and testicular volume in the male, and the appearance of the breast, pubic hair and the onset of menstruation in a girl. Details of this staging are given in **Table 1.2** and **Figs 1.103–106**.

Other secondary sexual characteristics should be noted, such as acne (**Fig. 1.107**), axillary hair, vaginal discharge and an adult body odor. Any discrepancy between the stages of sexual development in an individual is of particular importance (**Figs 1.108 & 1.109**) (see Ch. 6).

Shawl scrotum, where the root of the penis lies within the upper scrotum, which is often bifid (see Ch. 8), is seen in several dysmorphic syndromes, including the Aarskog syndrome. Other apparently minor abnormalities of genital architecture may have significance in the context of other physical findings.

CENTRAL NERVOUS SYSTEM AND EYES

Examination here should concentrate on an assessment of developmental or educational level and an exclusion of major neurologic abnormality. It is particularly important to examine the optic discs, which might demonstrate

Fig. 1.103 Female pubic hair, stages 1–5+.

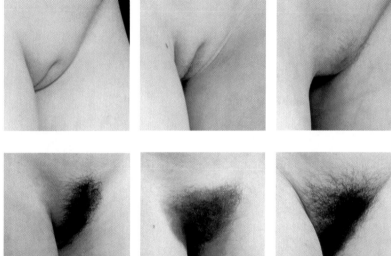

Fig. 1.104 Male penis and pubic hair development, stages 1–5+.

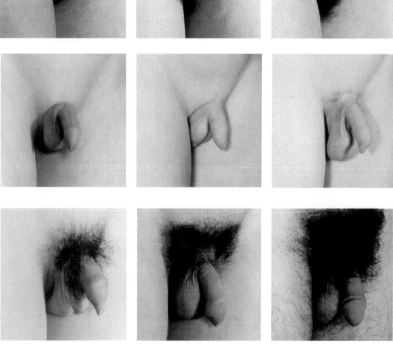

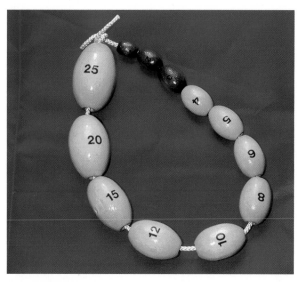

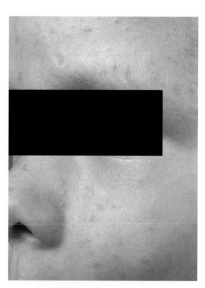

Fig. 1.107 Early acne in a 2-year-old child with precocious puberty.

Fig. 1.105 Prader orchidometer graded from 1 to 25 mL. The achievement of pubertal 4-mL testes is shown by a change from blue to yellow beads.

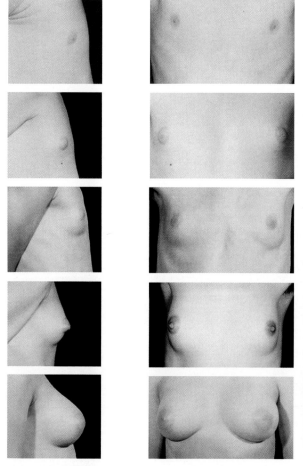

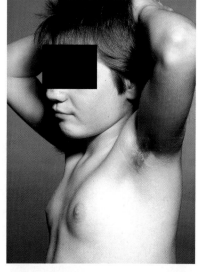

Fig. 1.108 Excess adrenal steroids – acne and axillary hair are excessive for the stage of breast development.

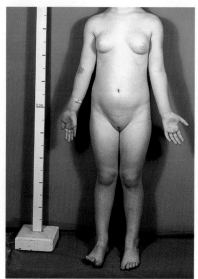

Fig. 1.109 Ovarian tumor with breast development in the absence of any pubic hair.

Fig. 1.106 Female breast development, stages 1–5.

papilledema (**Fig. 1.110**) secondary to raised intracranial pressure. Growth hormone therapy may occasionally result in benign raised intracranial hypertension that results in dramatic papilledema. The pallor of optic atrophy (**Fig. 1.111**) may be secondary to compression by a local tumor or raised intracranial pressure, or found in the DIDMOAD syndrome of Diabetes Insipidus, Diabetes Mellitus, Optic Atrophy and Deafness (see Ch. 10). The visual fields (**Figs 1.112 & 1.113**) may show bitemporal restriction in the presence of compression of the optic chiasm by a craniopharyngioma. The retina may be dysplastic with small optic nerve heads in septo-optic dysplasia (**Figs 1.114–1.116**) associated with panhypopituitarism or isolated pituitary hormone deficiencies and/or midline brain abnormalities.

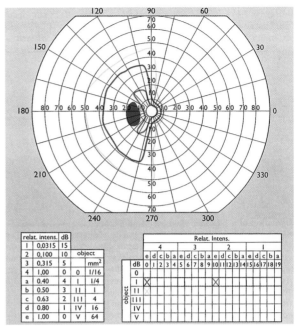

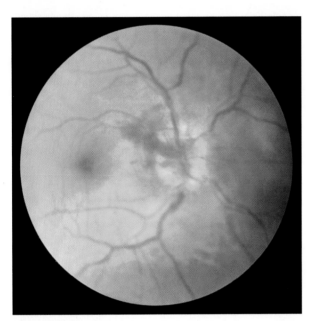

Fig. 1.110 Papilledema in craniopharyngioma.

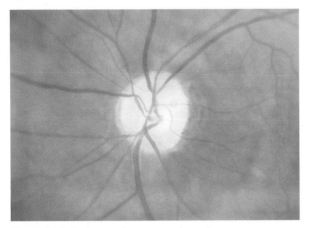

Fig. 1.111 Optic atrophy, as seen in optic nerve compression or DIDMOAD syndrome.

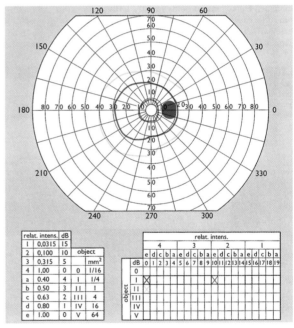

Figs 1.112, 1.113 Visual fields in a child with craniopharyngioma – temporal hemianopia in the left eye (top) and generalized restriction of vision in the right eye (bottom) secondary to compression of the optic chiasm. This formal plotting is possible in older, cooperative children. In the young child the presence of temporal field loss can be demonstrated by confrontation or by bringing a small, interesting, object inwards from the periphery, close to the child's face and noting when there is a reaction.

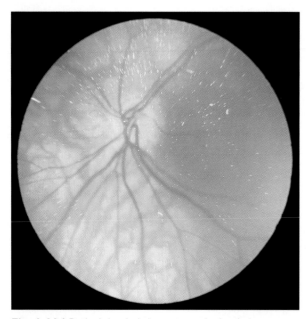

Fig. 1.114 Retinal dysplasia in septo-optic dysplasia (de Morsier syndrome).

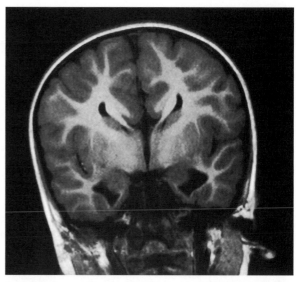

Fig. 1.116 Absent corpus callosum in septo-optic dysplasia – MRI view.

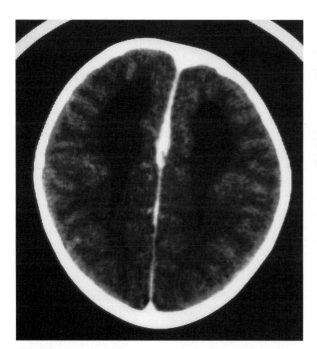

Fig. 1.115 Absent midline structures in the patient in Fig. 1.114; CT scan showing parallel ventricles.

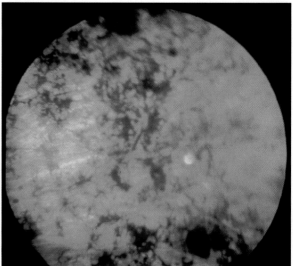

Fig. 1.117 Retinitis pigmentosa, in the Laurence–Moon syndrome.

Retinitis pigmentosa (**Fig. 1.117**) is seen in several syndromes associated with short stature, for instance the Laurence–Moon (with obesity, spasticity, learning difficulties and hypogonadism) or similar Bardet–Biedl (with obesity, polydactyly, learning difficulties and hypogonadism) syndromes. Storage deposits may be visible in either the retina (**Fig. 1.118**) or lens. The lens shows dislocation or loose fixation in the Marfan syndrome (said to be more commonly upwards) and in homocystinuria (said to be more commonly downwards) (**Fig. 1.119**).

The eyes might show abnormal blue coloration of the cornea in disorders of collagen formation, such as osteogenesis imperfecta (**Fig. 1.120**). A nevus of Ota can be associated with intracranial hamartomas and

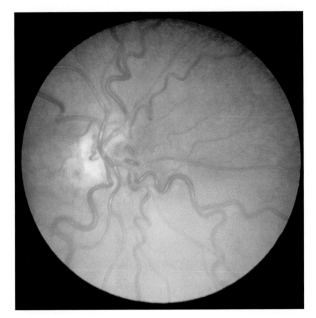

Fig. 1.118 Pseudopapilledema caused by abnormal storage deposits in geleophysic dwarfism.

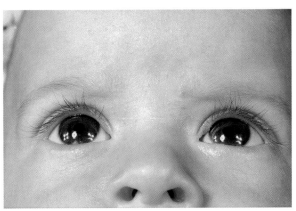

Fig. 1.120 Blue sclerae in the commonest (type I) osteogenesis imperfecta.

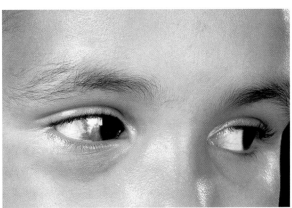

Fig. 1.121 Nevus of Ota, in this case associated with gigantism and sexual precocity due to hypothalamic dysfunction.

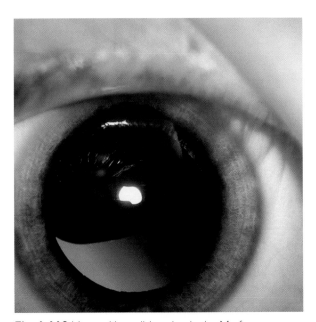

Fig. 1.119 Upward lens dislocation in the Marfan syndrome.

sexual precocity (**Fig. 1.121**). Heterochromia is seen in several syndromes associated with short stature and hypogonadism (**Fig. 1.122**). There may be abnormal sparsity, duplication or luxuriance of the eyelashes in several short stature syndromes and in severe chronic ill health (**Fig. 1.123**).

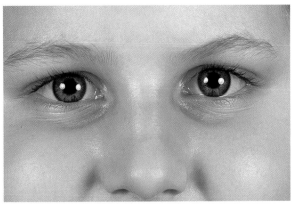

Fig. 1.122 Heterochromia.

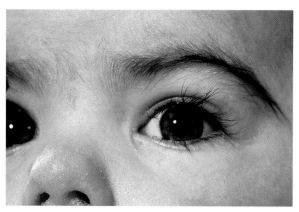

Fig. 1.123 Long eye lashes in De Lange syndrome.

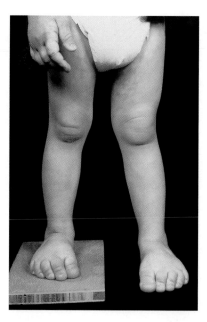

Fig. 1.125
Generalized left-sided hemihypertrophy.

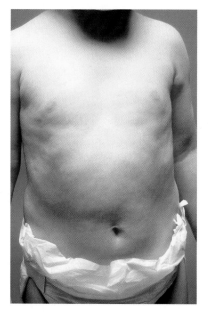

Fig. 1.124
Abnormal dimpled abdominal fat in hypopituitarism.

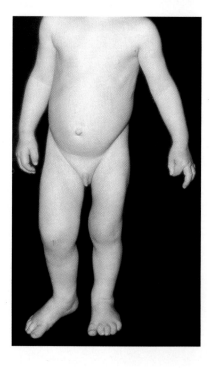

Fig. 1.126
Isolated hemihypertrophy of right leg.

BODY SHAPE AND THE SKIN

Look at the general shape of the body and at the distribution of muscle and fat. Abnormal muscularity may be seen in non-salt-losing males with the adrenogenital syndrome and in anabolic steroid abuse in young adolescents. Generalized lipodystrophy is seen in progeria and in the 'leprechaun' and related syndromes, where there may be associated insulin resistance (see Ch. 4); there are also some localized lipoatrophy syndromes, which can be both congenital and acquired (and may be related in the latter case to glomerulonephritis and protease inhibitors for treating human immunodeficiency virus).

Localized lipoatrophy is seen in relation to injection sites of (usually) animal insulin and lipohypertrophy in relation to human insulin and growth hormone (see Ch. 10). Excess adiposity is a feature of many endocrine disorders and may show a peculiar dimpled appearance in hypopituitarism (**Fig. 1.124**).

Hemihypertrophy may affect the whole body (**Figs 1.125 & 1.127**) or isolated areas such as one side of the face or one limb (**Fig. 1.126**). Asymmetry is associated with Russell–Silver syndrome and Beckwith–Wiedemann syndrome, and in the isolated form may also increase the risk of Wilms tumor. Hemiatrophy may be seen in VATER syndrome (**Fig. 1.127**). Local hypertrophy of a limb in association with hemangiomata

Fig. 1.127
Hemiatrophy in
Vertebral Anal
Tracheoesophageal
fistula Renal
abnormalities
(VATER) syndrome.

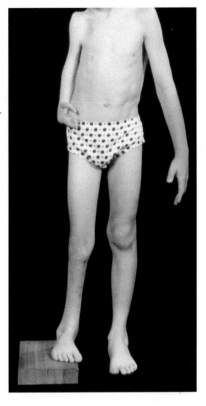

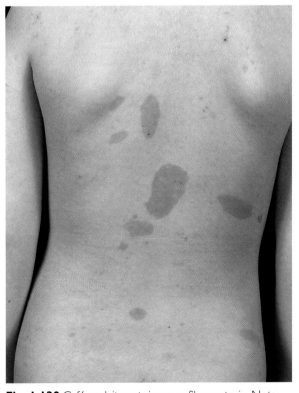

Fig. 1.129 Linear pigmentation in the Proteus syndrome, overgrowth of left foot.

Fig. 1.128 Limb
overgrowth in
Klippel–Trenaunay
–Weber
syndrome.

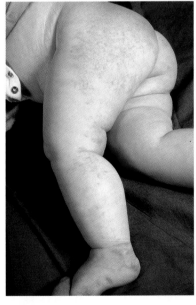

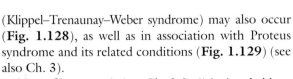

(Klippel–Trenaunay–Weber syndrome) may also occur (**Fig. 1.128**), as well as in association with Proteus syndrome and its related conditions (**Fig. 1.129**) (see also Ch. 3).

Neurofibromatosis (see Chs 2 & 6) is signaled by a large number of café-au-lait spots, axillary freckling (**Fig. 1.130**) and neuromas (**Fig. 1.131**) – usually

Fig. 1.130 Café-au-lait spots in neurofibromatosis. Note the relatively smooth outline.

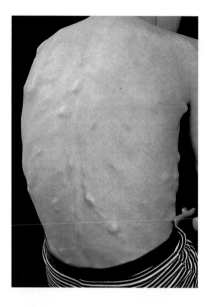

Fig. 1.131 Multiple neuromas in neurofibromatosis.

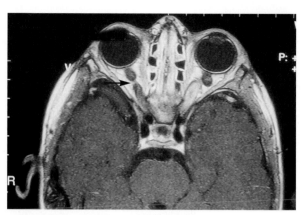

Fig. 1.134 Optic gliomas in neurofibromatosis involving both optic nerves.

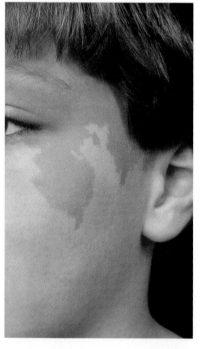

Fig. 1.135 Café-au-lait spot in McCune–Albright syndrome. Note irregular border.

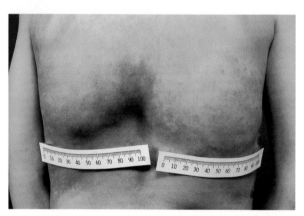

Fig. 1.132 Plexiform neuroma in neurofibromatosis.

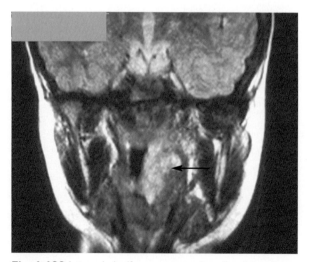

Fig. 1.133 Internal plexiform neuroma invading thoracic inlet.

more often in young adult life, although small or solitary neuromas may be palpated in young children. The café-au-lait patches may be discrete or large and plexiform (**Fig. 1.132**), and may then be external or involve deeper structures (**Figs 1.63, 1.64, 1.89 & 1.133**). There may be unilateral or bilateral optic gliomas (**Fig. 1.134**) with reduced visual fields, disk pallor or sexual precocity (see Ch. 6). The edge of these spots is said to be relatively smooth, like the coastline of California. The café-au-lait spot in McCune–Albright syndrome (**Fig. 1.135**) associated with sexual precocity (see Ch. 6) has a rough outline like the coast of Maine. Multiple pigmented nevi (**Fig. 1.136**) are associated

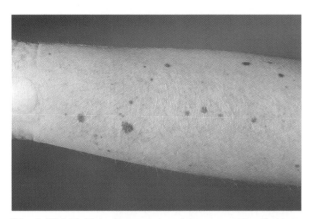

Fig. 1.136 Multiple pigmented nevi, here associated with Ullrich–Turner syndrome.

Fig. 1.137
Segmental nevi in
Turner syndrome
indicating tissue
mosaicism.
A similar
appearance with
café-au-lait spots
can be seen in
segmental
neurofibromatosis.

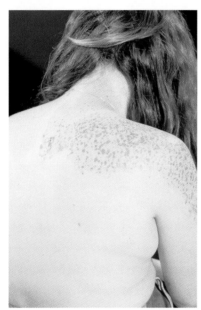

Fig. 1.138
Generalized (and
in abdominal scars)
hyperpigmentation
in Nelson
syndrome.

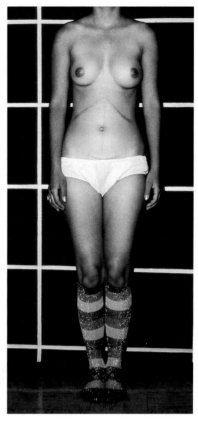

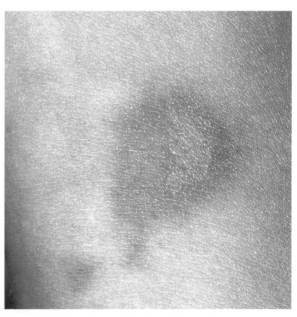

Fig. 1.139 Scar pigmentation in Addison's disease.

with the Ullrich–Turner syndrome and a number of syndromic malformations and neuroectodermal tumors. Nevi and café-au-lait spots may show a segmental distribution, indicating tissue mosaicism (**Fig. 1.137**).

Skin pigmentation may be abnormally increased with oversecretion of adrenocorticotropic hormone (ACTH) as in Addisonism and Nelson syndrome (see Chs 2 & 11), and this may be generalized (**Fig. 1.138**) or localized to scar tissue (**Fig. 1.139**). Coal-black discoloration of the axillae or neck (**Fig. 1.140**) (acanthosis nigricans) is associated with insulin resistance and obesity (see Chs 5 & 10). Vitiligo (**Fig. 1.141**) is commonly an isolated disorder but may be associated with several of the polyglandular syndromes (see Ch. 11).

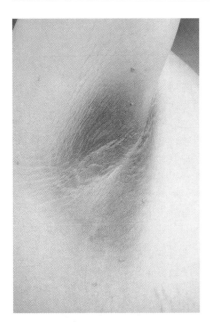

Fig. 1.140 Axillary acanthosis nigricans associated with insulin resistance.

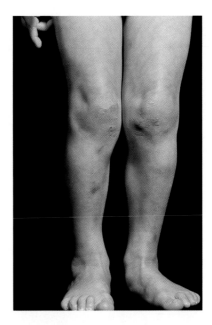

Fig. 1.142 Tissue paper scars from excess skin fragility in Ehlers–Danlos syndrome.

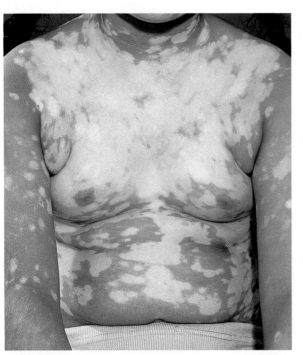

Fig. 1.141 Severe vitiligo in polyglandular syndrome type I.

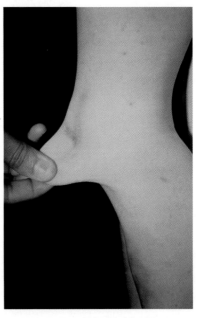

Fig. 1.143 Extensible skin in Ehlers–Danlos syndrome.

Easy bruising and skin fragility are seen in the tissue paper scarring of Ehlers–Danlos syndrome (**Fig. 1.142**), where there is also increased skin and joint laxity (**Figs 1.143 & 1.144**). Non-accidental bruising and burns indicate physical abuse (**Fig. 1.145**).

The Cushing syndrome in childhood is often associated with easy bruising. A particular feature of childhood-onset Cushing syndrome is marked hirsutism (which is also a feature of other disorders of the adrenal gland and ovary characterized by overproduction of testosterone; see Chs 3, 6, 8 & 11). Hirsutism is also seen as part of the fetal alcohol syndrome (see below). Treatment with some drugs, such as metyrapone, can also cause hirsutism. The use of diazoxide in hyperinsulinism (**Fig. 1.146**) (see Ch. 11) causes hypertrichosis (generalized and non-pigmented). Retention of excess lanugo hair may be seen in Aarskog syndrome (**Fig. 1.147**) and in anorexia nervosa. Striae are a feature of especially iatrogenic Cushing syndrome

Fig. 1.144
Hypermobile
joints in
Ehlers–Danlos
syndrome.

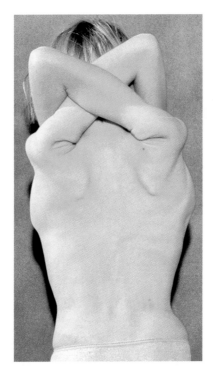

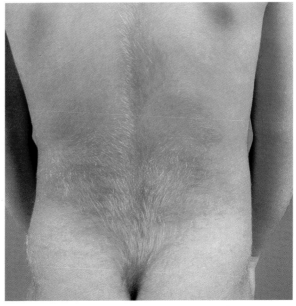

Fig. 1.146 Hypertrichosis secondary to diazoxide
treatment. Also seen with ciclosporin.

Fig. 1.145 Child
abuse. Multiple
bruises. (Note
characteristic
shortened lower
body segment
which may mimic
hypochondroplasia.)

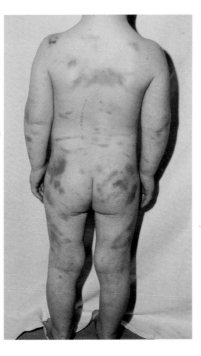

Fig. 1.147
Downy body hair
in the X-linked
recessive Aarskog
syndrome
associated with
short stature.

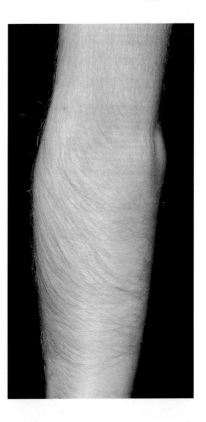

(**Fig. 1.148**) and may be also seen in nutritional
obesity and in tall stature (see Chs 3 & 5).

Dry skin is seen in atopic disorders, ectodermal
dysplasia and some other dysmorphic syndromes.
Excessive lichenification is seen in the X-linked metabolic
disorder placental sulfatase deficiency (**Fig. 1.149**) when
the affected fetus will be post-mature and maternal
estriol levels will have been undetectable during
pregnancy. Dry fissured reddening of the palms and
soles is seen in the 3A syndrome of **adrenal** failure,
alacrima and **achalasia**, where there may also be

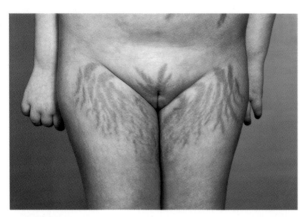

Fig. 1.148 Striae in iatrogenic Cushing syndrome.

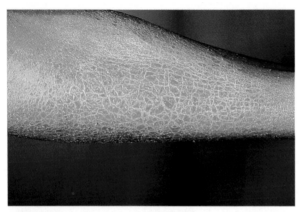

Fig. 1.149 Ichthyotic skin in placental sulfatase deficiency.

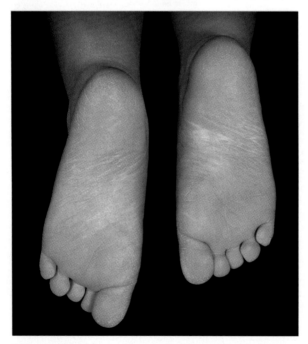

Fig. 1.150 Red fissured feet in the 3A syndrome.

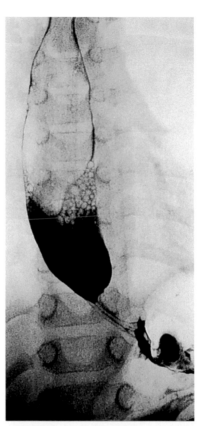

Fig. 1.151 Achalasia in the 3A syndrome.

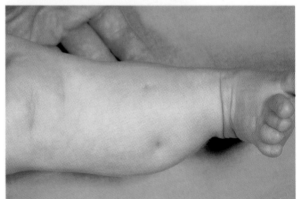

Fig. 1.152 Dimpling over tibia in hypophosphatasia.

progressive nerve degeneration (**Figs 1.150 & 1.151**). Necrobiosis lipoidica and granuloma annulare have associations with insulin-dependent diabetes mellitus (see Ch. 10). Dimpling of the skin is seen in hypophosphatasia, where there is undermineralization of the skeleton and teeth and, in the childhood form, short stature (**Fig. 1.152**).

THE PARENTS

It is important to examine the parents briefly, if at all possible; they may provide valuable clues as to

Fig. 1.153
Familial Noonan
syndrome in
parent and child.

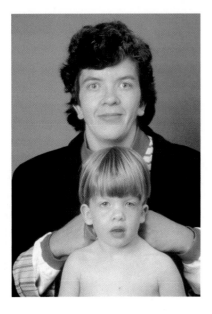

Auxology (including parents) and bone age
Any abnormalities of the hands, feet, nails or arms
Any abnormalities of the head and neck (with special
reference to the midline, mouth, tongue and thyroid)
Any chest wall (including breast) or spine abnormalities
Any cardiovascular or respiratory abnormalities
Any abdominal abnormalities? (must include external
genital inspection)
Stage of sexual maturation
Any abnormal skin or fat signs
Any abnormal body shape or asymmetry
Any eye abnormalities including lens, visual field and retina
Any abnormal appearance of either of the parents

Table 1.3 Summary of essential points on physical
examination

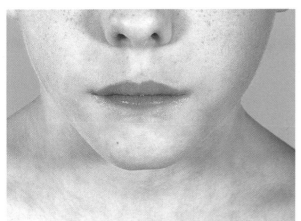

Fig. 1.154 Fetal alcohol syndrome in later childhood
showing typical appearance of lower face.

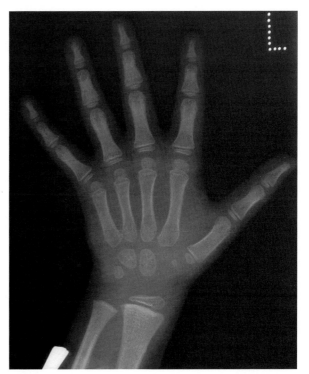

Fig. 1.155 Left hand and wrist radiograph for bone age
estimation.

the diagnosis. Many skeletal dysplasias and some
dysmorphic syndromes associated with both tall and
short stature are dominantly inherited, and may be
more obvious in later life (**Fig. 1.153**). A parent, more
often the mother, may show signs of undiagnosed
hypothyroidism or hyperthyroidism, and the mother
may be mildly affected by a metabolic disorder, such
as phenylketonuria or myotonic dystrophy, which has
affected the infant severely. A wide philtrum and a
thin upper lip may be seen in the offspring of heavy
drinkers during pregnancy, along with short stature,
learning difficulties, hirsutism and limb abnormalities
(**Fig. 1.154**).

The cardinal features to include in the examination
of a child with a possible growth or endocrine disorder
are summarized in **Table 1.3**.

SKELETAL MATURITY

Although not strictly part of the examination of a child,
it is pertinent to discuss a complementary, radiographic,
means of establishing physiologic maturity. The most
commonly used methods involve assessing the number
and degree of development of the bones of the left
hand and wrist (**Fig. 1.155**) (although other growth

centers can be used, including the jaw and teeth). Several methods exist for scoring or 'aging' the individual ossification centers in comparison to a standard atlas or by means of a computer recognition system. It is then possible by using published equations incorporating current height, or in some cases height and recent height velocity, to calculate a predicted adult height (with a range of error of ± 2 SD). *In this book the Tanner–Whitehouse 2 (TW2) method has been used in the creation of the charts*, although an updated version (TW3) has recently become available.

Chapter 2

The Short Child

PHYSIOLOGY

Human growth hormone (hGH) or somatotropin is a single-chain 191-amino-acid polypeptide that circulates complexed to a binding protein (see below), or is unbound ('free'). Multiple molecular forms of GH with various biological activities arise from post-translational processing. At all ages – from fetal through adult – GH is secreted in an intermittent, pulsatile pattern largely as a result of the reciprocal interactions of two hypothalamic peptides: growth hormone releasing hormone (GHRH) and somatostatin or somatropin release inhibiting factor (SRIF). As well as growth hormone itself there are a number of peptides, such as insulin-like growth factor (IGF-1), and neurotransmitters that control somatotropin release. Additionally novel compounds such as Ghrelin, released from the gut, and other GH-related peptides (GHRPs) may help to regulate GH release. During childhood there are apparently no differences between the sexes, although several investigators have noted significant correlations between height or height velocity and the amount of GH secreted throughout the day.

Growth hormone interacts with its receptor to generate IGF-I, the main mediator of GH action, in the liver and in most other tissues, including the epiphyses. This receptor, the extracellular domain of which is identical with the circulating GH binding protein, must link up with a second receptor molecule through a two-site GH bridge. This two receptors–one hGH molecular complex permits IGF-1 generation. In addition the circulating half-life of GH is virtually doubled by the presence of the binding protein.

Many of the effects of GH are mediated by IGF-1, which circulates in the plasma bound to one of a series of binding proteins called IGFBPs. These proteins circulate and modify IGF-1 action, either as stimulators or as inhibitors. Although there are at least six of these compounds, IGFBP-3 is the major circulating form.

This complex system subserves the process of growth. At puberty the pulsatile release of GH is increased 2–3-fold, predominantly by increased amounts of GH released at each secretory episode. Along with increasing amounts of sex steroid hormones, this accounts for the majority of the pubertal growth spurt following which the secretion of GH returns toward prepubertal values. As the levels of the GH binding protein do not increase as much as GH secretion, there is an apparent imbalance between the amounts of GH and its binding protein, permitting more GH to circulate in the active ('free') form. Theoretically, this increase also drives the local (e.g. epiphyseal) production of IGF-1 and its binding proteins and directly augments long bone growth.

Secretion of GH may be mediated by input from higher centers, allowing for modification of growth rate by environmental and emotional factors. The process of growth is also dependent on adequate nutrition, normal bone structure and biochemistry, normal thyroxine and other endocrine secretion as well as general health. Disruption of normal growth may therefore be an indication of many pathologies.

A number of genes, acting sequentially from the time of formation of the anterior neural ridge at 3–5 weeks of gestation, determine the development of the anterior pituitary gland. Some, such as Sonic (*Shh*), *LHX3* and *HESX1* which act early, help to determine the midline structure of the forebrain and often have a variable phenotype. Others, acting later, determine the development of specific cell lineages as straightforward single-gene defects, for instance *Prop1* and *Pit1* (presently called *POU1F1*) for lactotrophs, somatotrophs and thyrotrophs, *Kal1* for gonadotrophs. Other gene defects may result in the absence of a specific hormone or its receptor (e.g. recessive or dominantly inherited growth hormone deficiency (GHD), Laron syndrome and GHRH receptor mutations).

Estrogen from the ovary, or from aromatase production in the male, acts at the pituitary to augment GH pulsatility and produce the pubertal growth spurt, as well as acting on the epiphyseal growth plate to cause eventual bony fusion.

Environmental influences account for about 25% of birth weight variance modulated through maternal nutrition, social factors and other mechanisms. Both placental and fetal genes can influence birth size, although subsequently genetic size is determined largely by inheritance from the parents. The mechanisms underlying this programming of stature are obscure.

ETIOLOGY

There are many classifications of short stature, all with their advantages and disadvantages. None is perfect, as any group of disorders can be viewed as a spectrum in which dividing lines are often difficult to establish. In this chapter the diagnostic classification is based on that of the European Society for Paediatric Endocrinology.

GROWTH HORMONE DEFICIENCY

GHD may be idiopathic and of hypothalamic or pituitary origin. Neurosecretory dysfunction is defined by the lack of bursts of GH secretion on an overnight profile. There are genetic defects of the GHRH gene and receptor, the GH gene and other, very rare, abnormalities of GH structure and function. The gene sequence required for the formation of the anterior pituitary gland may be disturbed (*Ptx1*; *Hesx1*; *P-Lim*; *Prop1*; *POU1F1/Pit1*) and some of the central malformations producing GHD may be related to these abnormalities, such as septo-optic dysplasia (some *Hesx1*) (**Fig. 2.1**) and single central incisor (Sonic) (see **Fig. 1.68**). Any midline defect of the face, brain and head is of significance, for instance Rieger syndrome (hypodontia, mid-face hypoplasia and eye abnormalities), as it may imply malformation of the pituitary. Congenital infections may sometimes lead to GHD.

The growth-promoting actions of GH are mediated largely by the generation of local cartilage and possibly hepatic IGF-1. The various genetic mutations in the

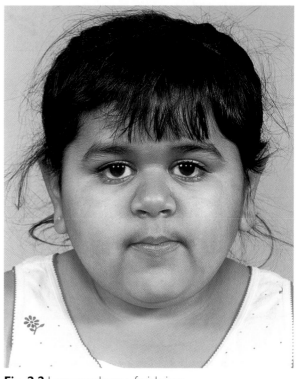

Fig. 2.2 Laron syndrome, facial view.

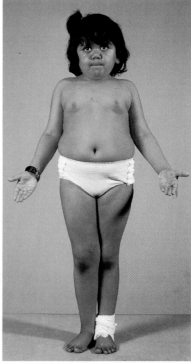

Fig. 2.3 Laron syndrome, whole body – note obesity and mid-face hypoplasia.

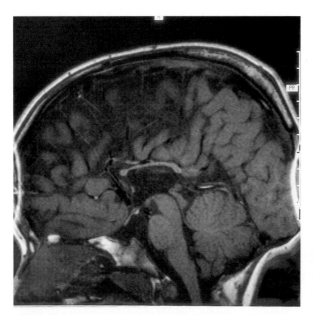

Fig. 2.1 Hypoplastic corpus callosum in septo-optic dysplasia associated with *HESX1* mutation.

Fig. 2.4 Severe growth retardation (adult height −5.1 SDS) secondary to chemotherapy and irradiation for a bone marrow transplant in T-cell acute lymphoblastic leukemia (ALL). There was growth hormone deficiency and diabetes mellitus (both treated from 9.25 years) as well as hypothyroidism (from 12 years). Gonadotropin secretion was not affected. The height of the donor identical twin is shown to illustrate the development and magnitude of the height loss.

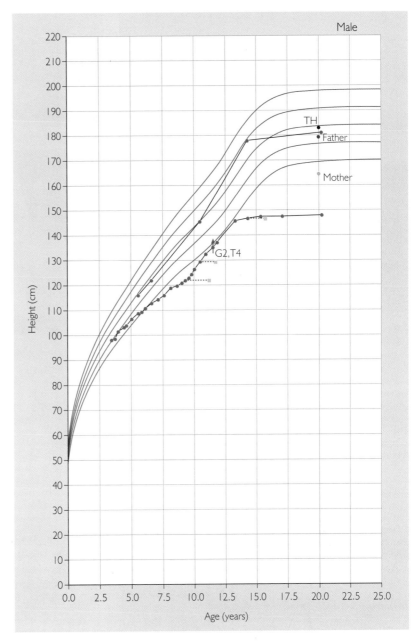

GH receptor that prevent generation of IGF-1 produce the rare Laron syndrome of GH resistance, in which there is clinical GHD in the presence of normal or high GH levels and low IGF-1 concentration (**Figs 2.2 & 2.3**). IGF-1 deficiency has been described.

GHD may be acquired as a result of tumors in the hypophyseal area (e.g. craniopharyngioma, germinoma, hamartoma) or may be secondary to effects from more distant CNS tumors or treatment of malignancy. The increasing number of survivors of childhood malignancy who have received cranial irradiation and have subsequently developed GHD means that this is a common cause of GHD (**Fig. 2.4**), although use of cranial irradiation in leukemia protocols is currently diminishing. Head trauma, meningitis, histiocytosis and hydrocephalus can damage the vulnerable pituitary stalk (**Fig. 2.5**).

GH deficiency may indeed be complete, for instance in familial gene deletion cases or after surgical removal of the pituitary gland with craniopharyngioma. It is more often a relative lack that may be defined in terms of response to various provocation tests or from the frequency and amplitude of overnight secretory episodes. The more minor degrees of deficiency merge

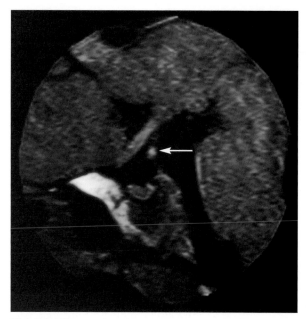

Fig. 2.5 MRI scan showing magnified view of ectopic pituitary tissue (arrow) and stalk disruption.

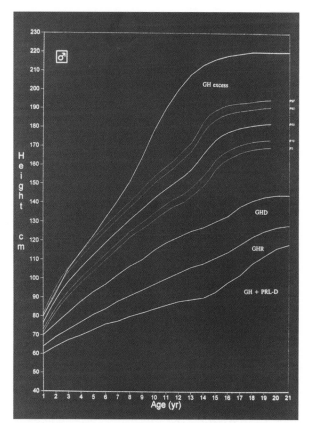

Fig. 2.6 Stylized growth curves for multiple hormone deficiency, growth hormone insensitivity, isolated GHD and GH excess compared to normal.

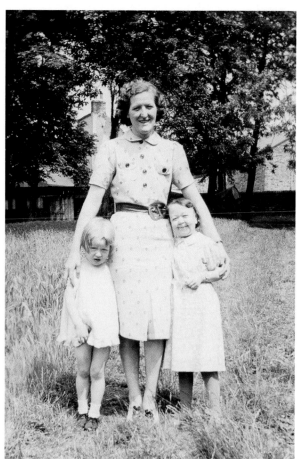

Fig. 2.7 Classic growth hormone deficiency. Normal 2-year-old in comparison to mother and 50-year-old affected aunt.

with the lower end of the normal range and idiopathic short stature (**Fig. 2.6**).

Unequivocal GHD from an early age historically produced an adult height of between 130 and 140 cm (around 4 feet 5 inches, or approximately 5 standard deviations (SD) below the population mean) (**Fig. 2.7**) and was not uncommon (estimates vary between 1 in 4000 and 1 in 20 000 of the population depending on the definition of severity). It may still present late with markedly short stature (**Fig. 2.8**), but more commonly presents with relatively mild short stature and a slow rate of growth. There is relative obesity (**Fig. 2.9**).

IDIOPATHIC SHORT STATURE

Idiopathic short stature is defined by the absence of abnormalities in the history and physical examination. More specifically, birth weight and length are normal, as well as body proportions; there is no chronic ill health, no severe psychosocial disturbance, and a normal food intake.

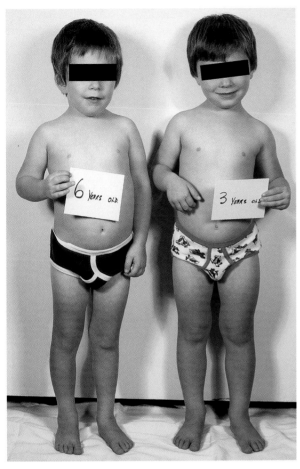

Fig. 2.8 Growth hormone deficiency age 6 years, with sibling age 3.

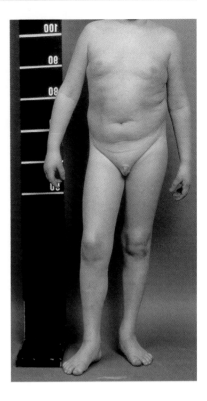

Fig. 2.9 Relative obesity in isolated GHD (note dimpled abdominal fat).

If growth velocity is normal, there is no need to exclude GHD or other pathologies by formal testing. If the growth curve deviates clearly, for example more than 0.3 SD over 1 year, or more than 0.5 SD over 2 years, or if the calculated height velocity is below the 25th centile twice in a row (with an adequate measurement interval), then a GH provocation test or measurement of serum levels of IGF-1 and its binding protein (IGFBP-3) is undertaken, along with the screening tests described below. Idiopathic short stature can be subclassified into two groups, familial and non-familial short stature, each of which may be divided into a further two subgroups.

Familial short stature

This is characterized by:

- short stature (less than −2 SDS, where SDS is the standard deviation score; see Ch. 1) during the growth period and a reduced adult height compared with the normal mean.

- a height within the target range defined by parental size. (As a cut-off limit, the parent-specific lower limit of height SDS is given by: [0.5 × (mother's height SDS + father's height SDS)/ 1.61] − 1.73. A similar equation is also available as a simple chart for screening purposes.)

In many cases the following characteristics are also present (not obligatory):

- a normal height velocity (varying around the 25th centile). As the height centile lines diverge with increasing age, a short child on the 3rd height centile will show a velocity that varies around the 25th velocity centile. Similarly a tall child on the 97th centile will show variation around the 75th centile. The majority of children with 'normal' stature and an adequate gap between measurements will have a velocity that fluctuates within these limits.)
- bone age consistent with (within ±2 SD) chronological age.

Familial short stature can further be subdivided into a group with a normal age at onset of puberty and a group with delayed puberty. (The cut-off limit for delayed puberty should ideally be based on recent population references. For the 1997 Dutch nation-wide growth study, the 97th centile in girls for B2 is 12.7 years and for G2 in boys 13.4 years.)

Non-familial short stature

This is characterized by:

- short stature (height less than –2 SDS) during childhood.
- stature below the range defined by parental size (for cut-off limit, see equation above).

In many cases the following characteristics are also present (not obligatory):

- a retarded bone age (>2 SD below chronological age).

- a reduced height velocity (<25%) in the later childhood years (see familial short stature, above).

Again, this group can be further subdivided into a subgroup with normal onset of puberty and a subgroup with delayed puberty. The latter subgroup has usually been called constitutional delay of growth and adolescence. Adult height is generally in the normal range. Often there is a positive family history of delayed puberty in the same sex parent. Strictly speaking, this diagnosis can be made only after the normal, but late, onset of puberty. However, the combination of above four criteria strongly suggests this diagnosis (see Ch. 7).

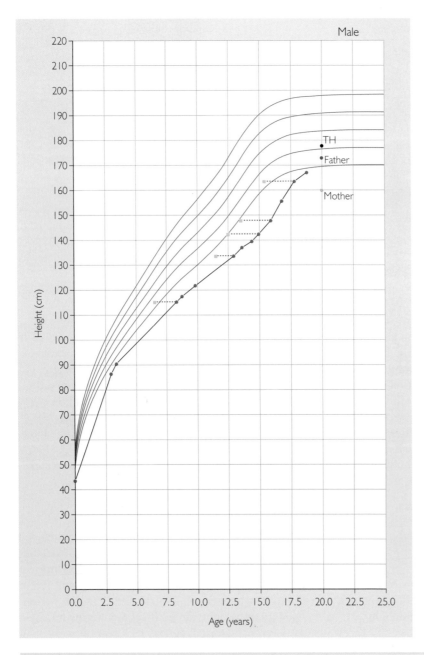

Fig. 2.10 Combined familial short stature and delay of growth and puberty. Both parents are short but the 3-year delay in onset of puberty produces a fall from a height of –3.4 SDS at 12 years to –4 SDS at 15 years, with eventual recovery to within the genetic range for adult height (–2.2 SDS).

The condition presents much more commonly in boys.

In many cases a short child is short because of the genetic influence of its parents, in combination with delayed puberty (**Fig. 2.10**). Children with this combined form frequently present for medical assessment at a relatively young age and, because height can be markedly reduced in adolescence, give rise to much concern. Mistaken or concealed paternity may be present in some cases.

PRIMARY GROWTH FAILURE

Five groups of disorders are found in this broad category.

1. Clinically defined syndromes with chromosomal abnormalities

This groups includes the Ullrich–Turner syndrome (see also Chs 5 & 7) and Down syndrome. As the Ullrich–Turner syndrome is relatively common (1 in 2500 female births) and is one of the few chromosomal or syndromic (see below) conditions in which the height deficit is potentially remediable, it will be described in detail.

The majority of fetuses with Ullrich–Turner syndrome do not survive to term, but chromosomal analysis is not performed routinely on all miscarriages. The exact chromosomal make-up is very variable with just over half being due to the classic 45X karyotype and the remainder to a variety of mosaics, chromosomal deletions and rings. Whatever the karyotype, the phenotypic features are similar, including a reduced adult height potential (see below), although the chances of spontaneous puberty may be greater in the mosaic forms.

Nuchal edema (also present in Down syndrome) may be seen on second-trimester ultrasonography and lead to diagnosis on amniocentesis.

Neonatal lymphedema (**Fig. 2.11**) and the related nail dysplasia (see **Fig. 1.42**) may allow an early diagnosis, which should be suspected in all females with coarctation of the aorta (**Fig. 2.1**). The major features of the condition are given in **Table 2.1**, but it is important to note that up to 40% of girls will show no external features apart from reduced height (**Figs 2.13 & 2.14**). Thus the diagnosis must be suspected in any girl presenting with short stature.

Adult height in the condition is reduced to a mean of around 145–147 cm (depending on the population), but is related to parental height in the same way as that of a normal child. Abnormalities of the *SHOX* gene (short stature on X chromosome) may be involved

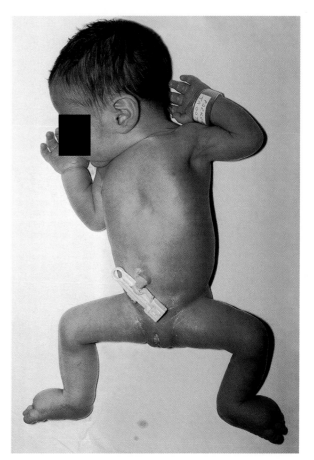

Fig. 2.11 Neonatal lymphedema in Ullrich–Turner syndrome.

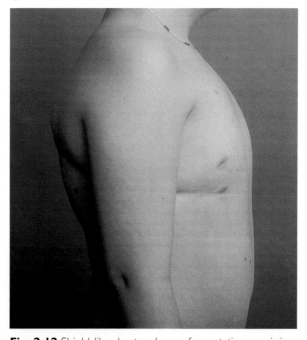

Fig. 2.12 Shield-like chest and scar of coarctation repair in Ullrich–Turner syndrome.

	Noonan	Ullrich–Turner
Sex	Either	Female
Chromosomes	Normal. Dominant inheritance	45X, mosaic or abnormal X chromosome
Performance	Mild reduction in approx. 20%	Normal, some isolated performance defecits
Mean final height	Male 162 cm	146 cm
	Female 152 cm	
Heart	Right-sided abnormalities (80%) and cardiomyopathy (10–20%)	Left-sided abnormalities, including coarctation Later aortic disection
Gonads	Males sometimes cryptorchid, females normal	Streak ovaries
Eyes	Ptosis majority	Ptosis-minority
Other	Café-au-lait spots, abnormal bleeding (70%)	Renal abnormalities

Table 2.1 Features of, and dissimilarities between, the Noonan and Ullrich–Turner syndromes

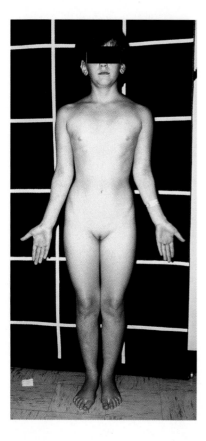

Fig. 2.13 Broad chest, wide carrying angle and sexual infantilism in Ullrich–Turner syndrome, age 15.5 years.

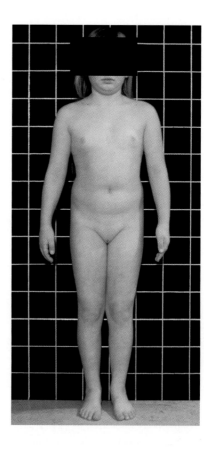

Fig. 2.14 Normal face and body phenotype (slightly broad chest) in Ullrich–Turner syndrome.

in the near universal growth failure seen in this condition. (SHOX is a transcription factor on the pseudoautosomal region of the X chromosome expressed in osteogenic cells of the mid-portion of the limbs and in the first and second pharyngeal arches. Leri–Weill dyschondrosteosis (see **Fig. 1.146**) results from complete deletion. In Ullrich–Turner syndrome there is haplo-insufficiency. A Y chromosome homolog is present to produce two functioning copies of the gene in the male. There are published centile charts for the condition, and so a predicted adult height may be obtained as described in Chapter 1, using the centile of both parents plotted on the adult centile position of the Ullrich–Turner centiles.

The main features of Prader–Labhart–Willi syndrome are given in **Table 2.2** and **Figs 2.15 & 2.16**. It is due to deletion of the paternal component of chromosome 15q11 (or maternal uniparental isodisomy).

2. Clinically defined syndromes without known chromosomal abnormalities

There are literally thousands of clinically defined syndromes without currently known chromosomal abnormalities that are associated with short stature. Some of the features that may point to one of this multitude are given in Chapter 1.

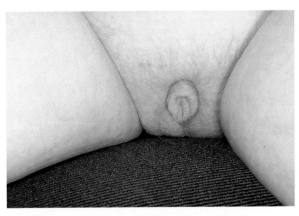

Fig. 2.16 Prader–Labhart–Willi syndrome showing hypogonadism, age 14.5 years.

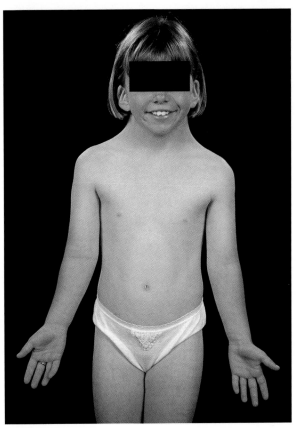

Fig. 2.17 Noonan syndrome.

An exact description of the majority of these disorders is beyond the scope of this text, but the reader may be aided by some of the commercially available computerized diagnostic databases or texts cited in the Foreword.

Amongst the commonest and most important of these syndromes presenting primarily with short stature are the Noonan (**Fig. 2.17**) and Russell–Silver (**Fig. 2.18, Table 2.2**) syndromes.

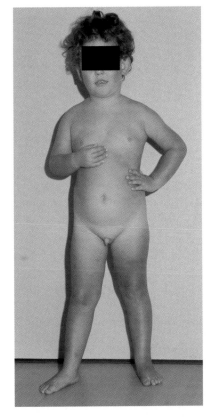

Fig. 2.15 Prader–Labhart–Willi syndrome showing early moderate obesity.

Prader–Labhart–Willi

Short stature, usually from birth, certainly from mid-childhood, with small feet and hands

Early poor feeding and weight gain followed by overeating and obesity from early childhood

Almond-shaped eyes and high forehead, squint

Hypotonia

Poor performance with behavior problems, especially related to food

Hypogonadism, osteoporosis, premature adrenarche

Diabetes mellitus (usually type 2, non-insulin-dependent)

Partial deletion of the long arm of paternal chromosome 15 or evidence of maternal disomy

Russell–Silver

Small from birth with delayed bone maturation

Hemihypertrophy/atrophy

Clinodactyly

Small triangular lower face, the corners of the mouth may turn down

Mild blue sclerae

Thin or sparse head hair

Café-au-lait spots

Some cases associated with maternal uniparental isodisomy of chromosome 7

Table 2.2 Features of the Prader–Labhart–Willi and Russell–Silver syndromes, two of the more common short stature syndromes

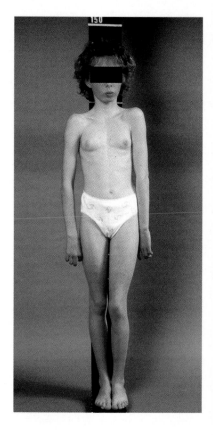

Fig. 2.18 Russell–Silver syndrome – note left-sided hypertrophy. There was a previous history of low birth weight.

Noonan syndrome is common, with an incidence of around 1 in 2000 individuals. It is dominantly inherited (see **Fig. 1.153**) with variable expression, and recently the responsible gene mutation was identified. As the Noonan syndrome shares many phenotypic features of Ullrich–Turner syndrome, these are contrasted in **Table 2.1**. There is an overlap of some cases of the Noonan syndrome and neurofibromatosis, with some children showing multiple café-au-lait spots.

Some syndromes have no known cause, are associated with normal intelligence and only relatively mild dysmorphic features and yet can produce the most striking degrees of short stature (an example of which, geleophysic dwarfism, is given in **Fig. 2.19**).

3. Intrauterine growth retardation with failure to demonstrate catch-up growth in height or weight

About 80% of children with intrauterine growth retardation (IUGR) or smallness for dates (birth weight less than the third percentile for gestational age) attain a height and weight in the normal centiles within the first 1 or 2 years of postnatal life. Asymmetric IUGR with low birth weight but normal length is often caused by events late in pregnancy and usually has a good outcome. Symmetric smallness (low weight and length) is less likely to recover (**Fig. 2.20**) and often hints at more severe, earlier or inherent problems, such as:

- genetic or metabolic disorders, e.g. chromosomal abnormalities and syndromes as described above, including Silver–Russell and Seckel syndrome (**Fig. 2.21**).
- damage *in utero* by environmental agents (infections, drugs, alcohol) (see **Fig. 1.154**).
- growth potential permanently restricted by severe placental dysfunction (**Fig. 2.22**).

The majority of premature infants born at less than 32 weeks will show growth failure with a severity related to the degree of prematurity and the presence of chronic lung disease. There is catch-up of length and weight in the majority by 5 years of age.

4. Skeletal dysplasias

In general, body dimensions are abnormal in these disorders, which mostly show relatively short limbs. There is a spectrum of severity of relatively common

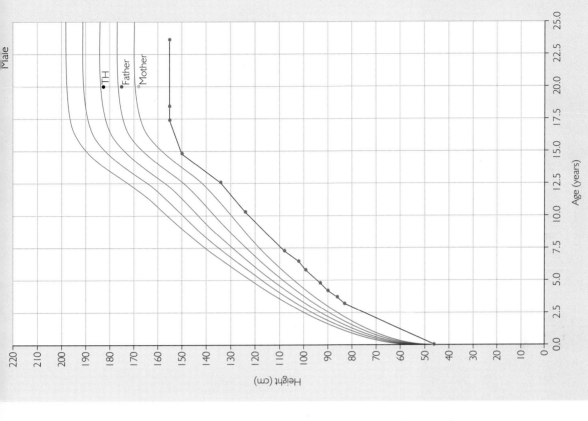

Fig. 2.19 Severe short stature as a result of a rare disorder, 'geleophysic nanism'. Growth hormone was given between 6 and 7 years with no benefit. Death occurred at 13 years as a result of mitral valve involvement, height −10.2 SDS.

Fig. 2.20 IUGR untreated. Low birth length and weight with no evidence of catch-up and reduced adult height (−4.1 SDS); compare with Fig. 2.85.

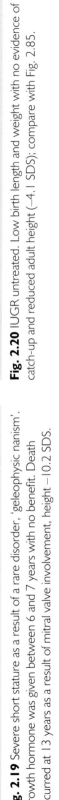

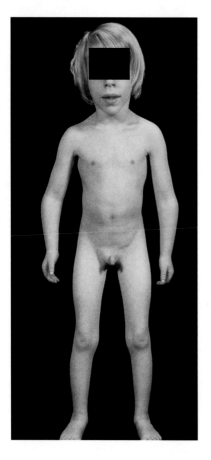

Fig. 2.21 Seckel syndrome – severe IUGR with later markedly reduced stature and 'bird-like' facies (form of 'primordial short stature').

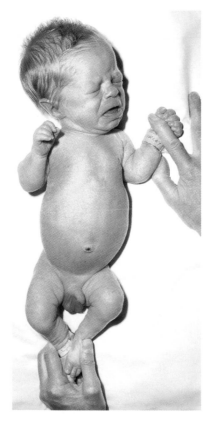

Fig. 2.23 Achondroplasia at birth.

short-limbed dwarfing disorders from the severe achondroplasia to the milder hypochondroplasia (**Figs 2.23–2.27**). The incidence of this group of disorders is around 1 in 15 000 live births. Achondroplasia is due to a single point mutation on chromosome 4p, which affects the fibroblast growth factor receptor 3, causing poor division of bone-forming fibroblasts. It is likely that many of the other conditions in this spectrum share quantitatively and qualitatively similar defects.

In the various types of spondyloepiphyseal dysplasia and spondylometaphyseal dysplasia (and the combined forms), the spine is affected along with specific areas of the long bones, producing variable shortening of the body segments and spinal deformity.

There are also many specific syndromes with bony dysplasia – some with dysmorphic features that overlap those described above. The growth retardation seen in the Ullrich–Turner syndrome is considered by some to be due to an underlying skeletal dysplasia, providing further overlap.

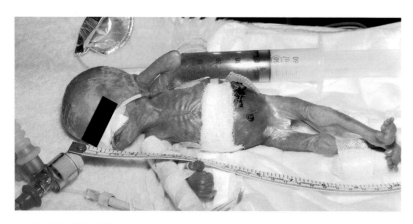

Fig. 2.22 Severe smallness for dates (540 g) and prematurity (29 weeks); 60-mL syringe and tape measure for comparison. This combination of events has a poor eventual size prognosis.

Fig. 2.24 Achondroplasia, age 2 years – note trident hand.

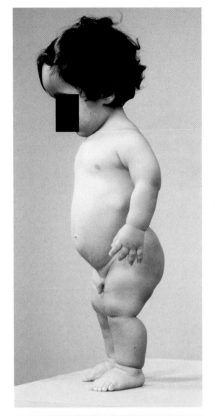

Fig. 2.26 Mild hypochondroplasia presenting with disproportionate short stature (–3 SDS).

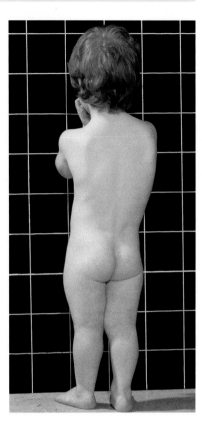

Fig. 2.25 Moderately severe hypochondroplasia as young adult, final height 125 cm (4 ft 1 in).

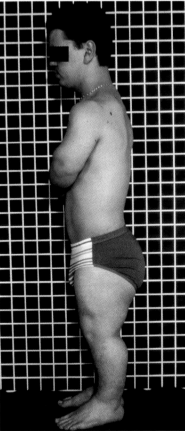

The diagnosis of these disorders is often difficult and may require expert radiographic review (see below). In general, there is no medical therapy even with a more specific diagnosis, but a diagnosis can be important for prognosis and genetic counseling.

5. Disorders of bone metabolism

Disorders of bone metabolism are rare and include mucopolysaccharidoses, mucolipidoses and others that may have profound effects on the bony skeleton and other tissues. Of those that present primarily with short stature as opposed to their CNS or metabolic consequences, the most important are the Morquio syndrome (mucopolysaccharidosis type 4); muco-lipidosis type 3, which often presents first to rheumatologists because of the claw hands (see **Figs 1.23 & 1.24**); and the juvenile form of Hunter syndrome (mucopolysaccharidosis type 2) (**Fig. 2.28**), in which short stature and a large jaw may be the only presenting feature before adult life, when more severe complications ensue.

These disorders characteristically all have a major impact on the individual and there are also genetic implications. They are almost all characterized by a back that is relatively short when compared with the legs (**Figs 2.29 & 2.30**).

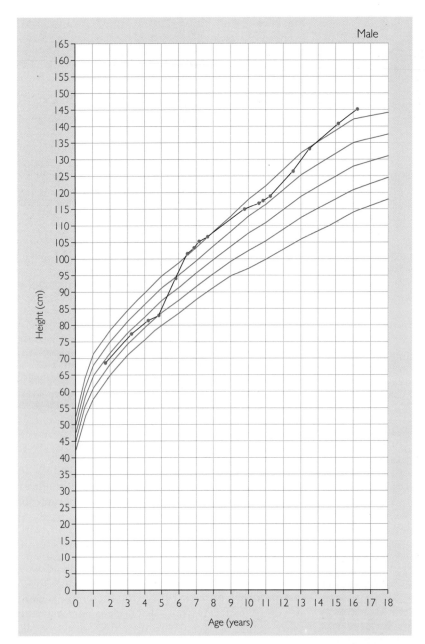

Fig. 2.27 Achondroplasia growth chart – two episodes of femoral and tibial leg lengthening at 5 and 10.5 years. Height gain from −1 to +2.4 SDS on achondroplasia chart.

Fig. 2.28
Juvenile Hunter syndrome (mucopolysaccharidosis type 2). White cell enzyme assay showed zero activity of iduronosulfate sulfatase. Presented in mid-teens with short stature and noted to have prognathism and a short back (−3.7 SDS) compared with legs (−2.5 SDS), which led to the diagnosis.

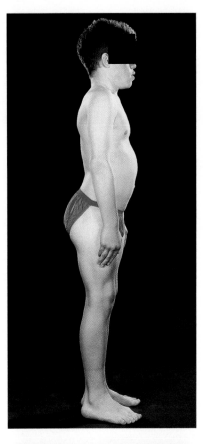

Fig. 2.30
Morquio syndrome (mucopolysaccharidosis type 4).

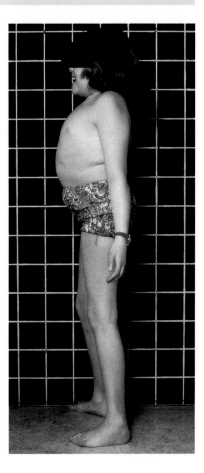

Fig. 2.29
Mucopolysaccharidosis 2 emphasizing the relatively long legs compared with the back.

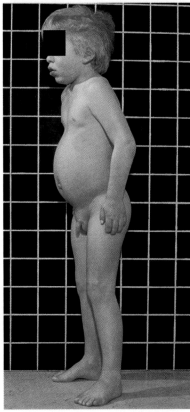

SECONDARY GROWTH FAILURE

In this category there are six subgroups.

1. Disorders in specific systems

The specific systems include cardiac, lung, liver, intestinal, renal, hematologic, CNS and generalized inflammatory disease. Often the diagnosis is made before the short stature is noted but, even in the asymptomatic child, it is important to rule out hidden organic pathology. The disorders that are most important to exclude are renal failure (**Fig. 2.31**); chronic anemia; chronic infections (HIV, tuberculosis) and chronic inflammatory bowel diseases (e.g. Crohn's disease) (see **Figs 1.85, 2.32 & 2.33**). Chronic asthma produces short stature (**Fig. 2.34**) and delayed puberty, usually with later catch-up, but the treatment of asthma with inhaled steroids can also produce growth suppression in some individuals (see **Fig. 2.53**).

Gluten enteropathy (**Figs 2.35–2.38**), in susceptible populations, may present very late in childhood – although it is more usual to present in infancy with

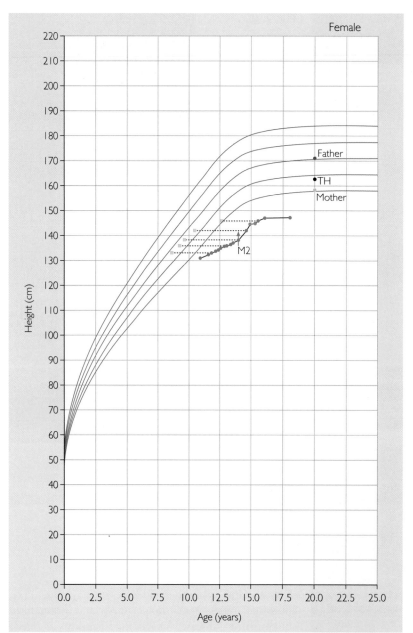

Fig. 2.31 Short stature (−2.6 SDS) and poor growth rate as presenting feature of juvenile nephronophthisis causing renal failure, age 10.9 years. Treatment with estrogens was given to induce puberty at 14 years but the adult height is much reduced (−3.5 SDS).

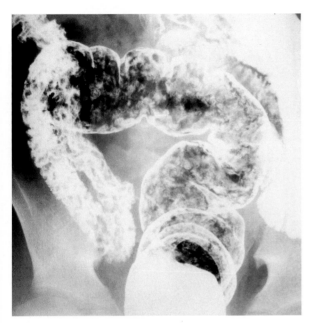

Fig. 2.32 Ulcerative colitis – double-contrast barium enema showing extensive colonic ulceration.

Table 2.3 Causes of Cushing syndrome in childhood and adolescence, in order of frequency

anemia and failure to thrive – and have poor growth as its only feature. There may be abdominal distension and wasting of the buttocks, and hypocalcemia may be present; however, a high index of suspicion is required for the diagnosis.

All of the above will tend to produce thinness (see Ch. 4), which may be even more pronounced than the short stature or poor growth rate, documented as a weight 'centile below the height 'centile, no matter what the absolute height (or a reduced weight for height on a weight-for-height chart).

2. Endocrine disorders

The main endocrine disorders causing short stature in children are hypothyroidism, GH deficiency and Cushing syndrome. Patients with hypogonadism (see Ch. 7) can be short in the pubertal age range. Relative obesity is often a feature of all of these conditions.

Hypothyroidism

Untreated congenital hypothyroidism (**Fig. 2.39**) (see Ch. 11), which is seen less commonly since the advent of neonatal screening, produces an adult height similar to that in severe GHD (see **Fig. 11.7**).

In the much more common acquired hypothyroidism (**Fig. 2.40**) there is growth retardation with obesity and delayed skeletal maturation and dentition. Usually puberty is delayed (see Ch. 7), but can be precocious with lactorrhea (see Ch. 6). The cause in iodine-sufficient areas is usually autoimmune thyroiditis, but the condition may occur in response to therapeutic irradiation. Isolated central hypothyroidism is rare (see Ch. 11).

Cushing syndrome

Other than being caused by the administration of topical, oral, inhaled or injectable steroids, Cushing syndrome is rare in childhood. The causes are summarized in **Table 2.3**. Very little excess cortisol or other steroid is required to inhibit growth; hence growth failure is almost universal (except in rare cases of adrenal tumor where testosterone production predominates, causing a 'pubertal' growth pattern). The most striking feature of hyperadrenocorticism is a rapid increase in body fat (**Figs 2.41–2.43**), particularly the abdomen, cervical fat pad ('buffalo hump') (**Fig. 2.44**) and the face ('moon face') (**Fig. 2.45**).

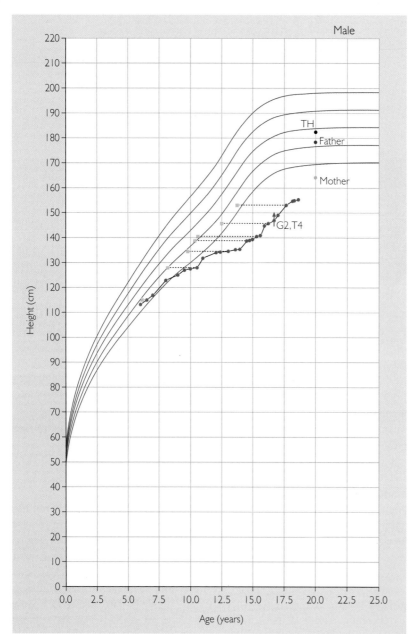

Fig. 2.33 Crohn's disease diagnosed at 6 years of age (−1 SDS). No growth response to hemicolectomy, parenteral nutrition or elemental diet. Pubertal spurt, 16.5–18.5 years, induced by depot testosterone, but adult height −3.9 SDS.

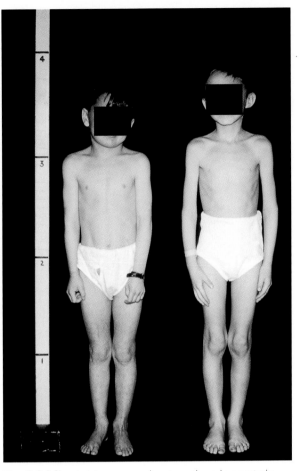

Fig. 2.34 Short stature secondary to asthma in one twin.

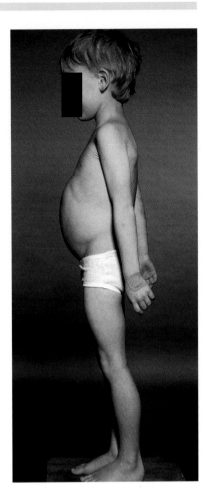

Fig. 2.35 Late-onset celiac disease with abdominal distension.

A thinning of the skin causes striae, which are especially prominent in the iatrogenic syndrome (**Fig. 2.46**), and capillary friability leads to ecchymoses. There is weakness and a decreased muscle mass, but this appears less striking in children than in adults. Hypertension is usually, but not always, present. Demineralization of bones occurs, and may be demonstrated by dual-energy X-ray absorptiometry (DEXA) (**Fig. 2.47**). In non-iatrogenic forms of the syndrome, the secretion not only of glucocorticoids, but also of androgens, is increased, and signs of hyper-androgenization (excessive hair, acne and cliteromegaly) may be present.

In adulthood the differentiation of nutritional obesity from Cushing syndrome may be difficult, but in childhood, although some of the features may be similar (**Fig. 2.48**), the relatively tall stature that is almost always associated with overeating means that there is seldom diagnostic confusion.

Other endocrine disorders, such as poorly controlled diabetes, gonadal disorders, precocity with early

Fig. 2.36 Wasting of the buttocks in celiac disease.

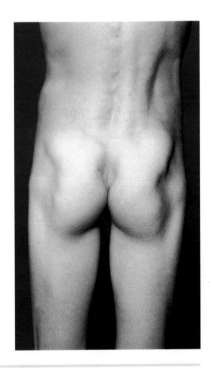

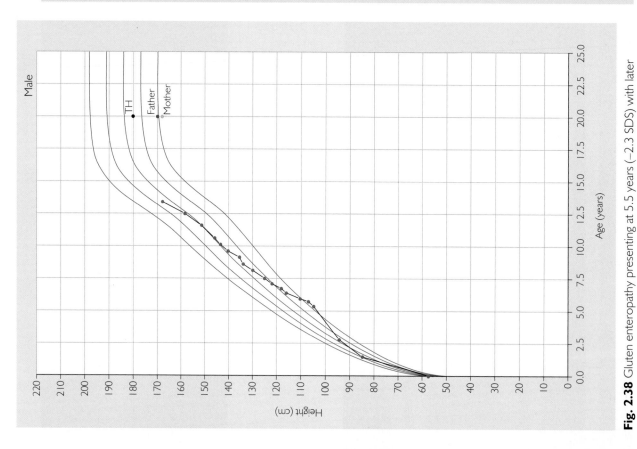

Fig. 2.38 Gluten enteropathy presenting at 5.5 years (−2.3 SDS) with later

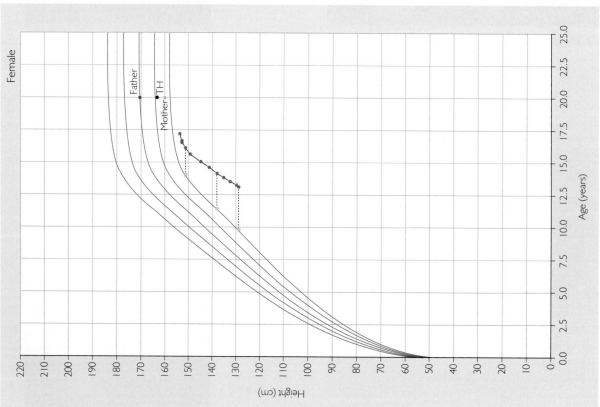

Fig. 2.37 Gluten enteropathy presenting as short stature (−4.8 SDS) at 13.2

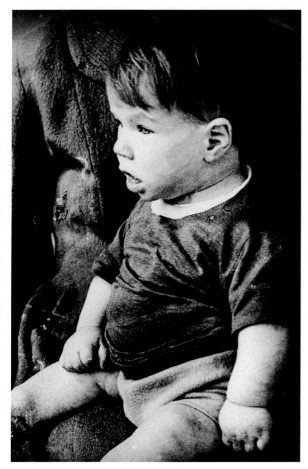

Fig. 2.39 Untreated congenital hypothyroidism – 'cretinism'.

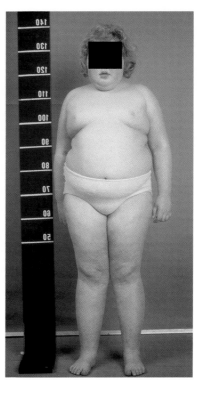

Fig. 2.41
Cushing disease due to pituitary adenoma – gross obesity.

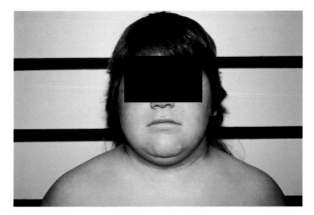

Fig. 2.40 Gross acquired hypothyroidism.

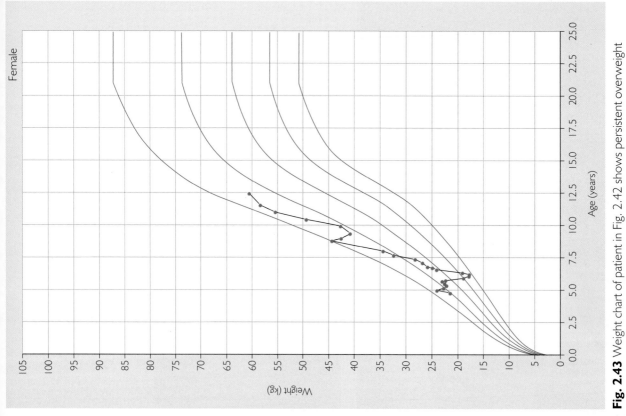

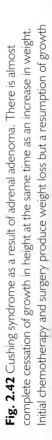

Fig. 2.43 Weight chart of patient in Fig. 2.42 shows persistent overweight (+1.5 SDS).

Fig. 2.42 Cushing syndrome as a result of adrenal adenoma. There is almost complete cessation of growth in height at the same time as an increase in weight. Initial chemotherapy and surgery produce weight loss but a resumption of growth

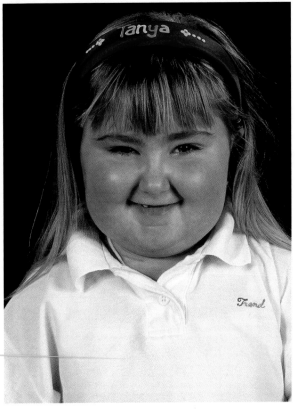

Fig. 2.45 Severe cushingoid facies in patient whose charts are shown in Figs 2.42 & 2.43.

Fig. 2.46 Iatrogenic Cushing syndrome secondary to treatment for dermatomyositis.

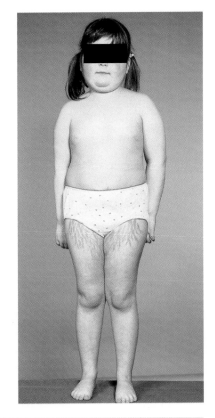

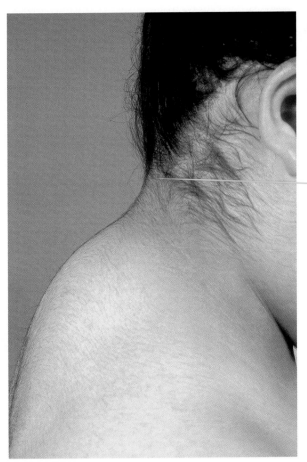

Fig. 2.44 Cushing syndrome with buffalo hump and hirsutism.

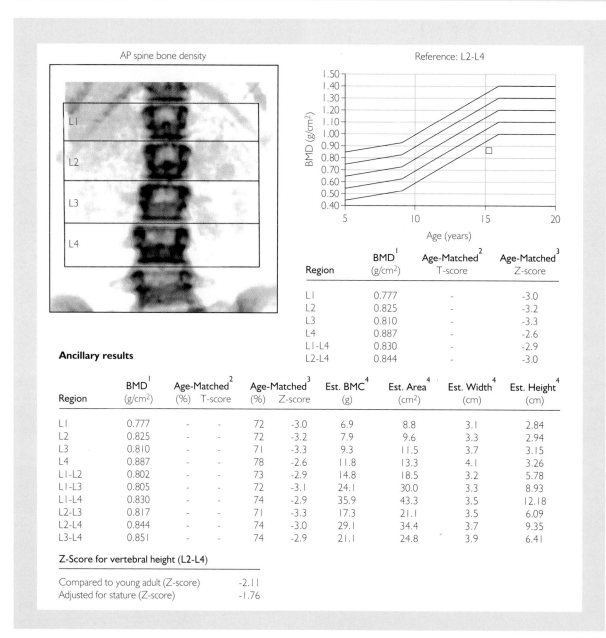

AP spine bone density

Reference: L2-L4

Region	BMD[1] (g/cm²)	Age-Matched[2] T-score	Age-Matched[3] Z-score
L1	0.777	-	-3.0
L2	0.825	-	-3.2
L3	0.810	-	-3.3
L4	0.887	-	-2.6
L1-L4	0.830	-	-2.9
L2-L4	0.844	-	-3.0

Ancillary results

Region	BMD[1] (g/cm²)	Age-Matched[2] (%)	T-score	Age-Matched[3] (%)	Z-score	Est. BMC[4] (g)	Est. Area[4] (cm²)	Est. Width[4] (cm)	Est. Height[4] (cm)
L1	0.777	-	-	72	-3.0	6.9	8.8	3.1	2.84
L2	0.825	-	-	72	-3.2	7.9	9.6	3.3	2.94
L3	0.810	-	-	71	-3.3	9.3	11.5	3.7	3.15
L4	0.887	-	-	78	-2.6	11.8	13.3	4.1	3.26
L1-L2	0.802	-	-	73	-2.9	14.8	18.5	3.2	5.78
L1-L3	0.805	-	-	72	-3.1	24.1	30.0	3.3	8.93
L1-L4	0.830	-	-	74	-2.9	35.9	43.3	3.5	12.18
L2-L3	0.817	-	-	71	-3.3	17.3	21.1	3.5	6.09
L2-L4	0.844	-	-	74	-3.0	29.1	34.4	3.7	9.35
L3-L4	0.851	-	-	74	-2.9	21.1	24.8	3.9	6.41

Z-Score for vertebral height (L2-L4)

Compared to young adult (Z-score)	-2.11
Adjusted for stature (Z-score)	-1.76

Fig. 2.47 DEXA scan showing bone mineral density of −3.1 SDS in male child with an adrenocorticotropic hormone (ACTH)-secreting adenoma. This areal density needs to be compared to height SDS which, in this case, was −1.2 SDS, indicating moderately severe osteoporosis.

epiphyseal fusion, etc., can produce short stature and are described elsewhere in the text.

3. Metabolic disorders

Many inborn errors of metabolism are associated with short stature but present primarily with neurologic signs, or signs in other systems. Glycogen storage disease type Ia produces short stature with truncal obesity and thin limbs, a 'doll-like' face and hepatomegaly, and there may be macroscopic hyperlipidemia (**Figs 2.49 & 2.50**).

4. Disorders of calcium and phosphate metabolism, and disorders of bone

Pseudohypoparathyroidism

This is a rare heterogeneous disorder of post-receptor activation where variable hypocalcemia is associated with moderate short stature, obesity, 'moon face' and shortening of the metacarpals (most often the IVth (**Fig. 2.51**) with cone-shaped epiphyses). The hypocalcemia is resistant to treatment with parathyroid hormone (PTH)

Fig. 2.48 Pseudo-Cushing syndrome secondary to nutritional obesity. Note the high cheek color and central obesity. There was also hypertension and easy bruising. Height was, however, at top-end of familial range and there was supranormal growth rate with slightly early puberty.

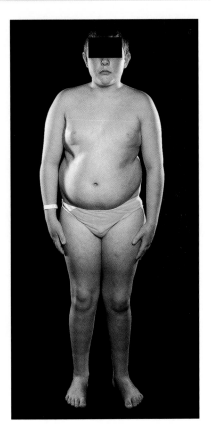

Fig. 2.50 Type I glycogen storage disease with hyperlipidemia.

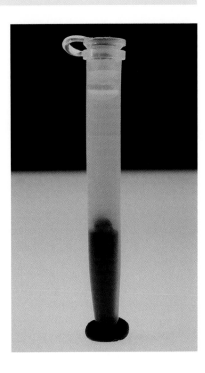

Fig. 2.49 Type I glycogen storage disease.

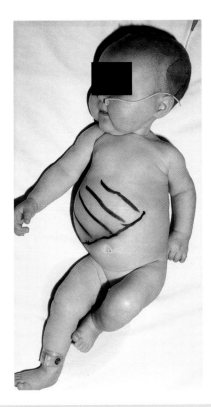

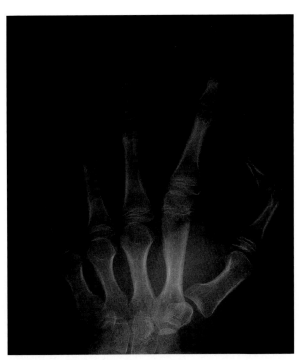

Fig. 2.51 Pseudohypoparathyroidism with short third to fifth metacarpals and cone epiphyses.

and may result in learning difficulties, cataracts and ectopic calcification. Primary hypoparathyroidism and central hypogonadism may coexist. (Differentiation between pseudohypoparathyroidism (with hypocalcemia) and pseudo-pseudohypoparathyroidism (without hypocalcemia) has been abandoned because the hypocalcemia is variable and both types have been described in the same family.)

Hypophosphatemic rickets

This condition (**Fig. 2.52**) is described in Chapter 11.

Osteogenesis imperfecta

Osteogenesis imperfecta (**Fig. 2.53**) and other disorders affecting collagen and fibrin production, such as the various Ehlers–Danlos syndromes, may also be included in this category.

5. Iatrogenic short stature

This may be either a result of treatment of childhood malignancy or caused by glucocorticoid treatment. The dose of steroids that may produce growth failure is far less than that needed to produce the other features of Cushing syndrome, and all children taking steroids – topical, inhaled or oral – should have their growth monitored regularly (**Fig. 2.54**).

6. Psychosocial short stature

An extremely poor emotional environment causes psychosocial short stature – also called emotional or psychosocial dwarfism. Although there is usually relative thinness, this is not always the case and there can be considerable diagnostic confusion between deprivation dwarfism and GHD. Hyperphagia may occur as a component of the syndrome. The GH response to stimulation testing can be severely, but reversibly, blunted and there is diminished spontaneous overnight GH secretion. There is a lack of response to GH therapy and a rapid catch-up is seen with a change of caregiver (**Figs 2.55 & 2.56**). There is commonly a preservation of more infantile body proportions than may be expected from the age of the child (see **Fig. 1.145**).

More minor degrees of short stature are a consequence of more minor deprivation, which may contribute to the well-known social class gradient in height.

DIAGNOSTIC WORK-UP OF SHORT STATURE

MEDICAL HISTORY AND PHYSICAL EXAMINATION

The following are the most relevant points to include when taking the history of a child presenting with short stature (see also Ch. 1):

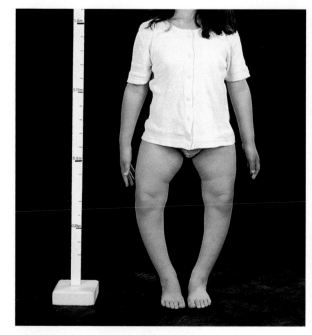

Fig. 2.52 Hypophosphatemic rickets.

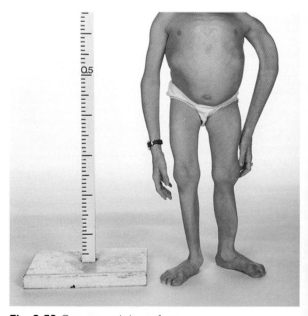

Fig. 2.53 Osteogenesis imperfecta.

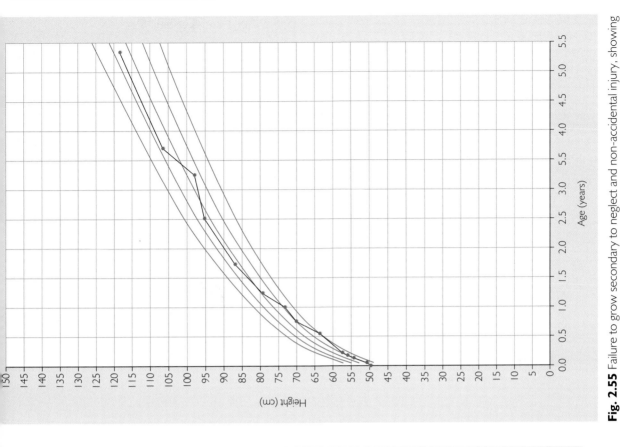

Fig. 2.54 Growth failure secondary to treatment with inhaled beclometasone dipropionate, 200 μg twice daily from 6 to 12 years of age, nadir −3.5 SDS. There is also constitutional short stature that led to the clinical presentation of this case. Adult height is within the target range (−2.5 SDS).

Fig. 2.55 Failure to grow secondary to neglect and non-accidental injury, showing complete catch-up in height.

Fig. 2.56 Patient in Fig. 2.55, showing weight after child was fostered (then subsequently adopted) at 0.7 years of age. Change in height −2 to +0.6 SDS; change in weight −3.0 to − 0.5 SDS.

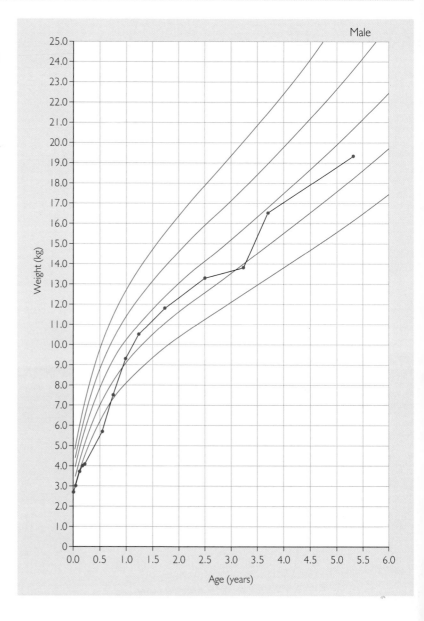

- Pattern of growth in height and weight. Include birth weight and length (in relation to duration of pregnancy).
- Presentation at birth (breech delivery is associated with GHD and many syndromic disorders).
- Parental heights: calculate the target height and compare its centile position with the patient's height centile. (Beware the dominantly inherited, relatively mild disorders of growth that may be undiagnosed in one parent, such as hypochondroplasia.)
- Family history: ask about the onset of puberty of the mother (age at menarche) and father (late onset? – the father may remember that he continued to grow in late teenage life or shaved later than his friends did).
- Milestones of puberty in the patient (onset of breast development, menarche; onset of penile enlargement, pubic hair).
- Nutritional assessment.
- Previous diseases and operations.
- Drug administration including inhaled and topical preparations, over-the-counter medication and herbal remedies.
- Neurologic symptoms; especially headache and disturbance of vision).
- Gastrointestinal, pulmonary, cardiac, urogenital symptoms.
- Psychosocial situation.

A full physical examination has to be performed, with special emphasis on the following:

- Accurate measurements of height, weight, sitting height, head circumference. Other special measurements may be required.
- Calculate the ratio between sitting height and leg length, and compare this with reference values.
- Nutritional state, fat distribution – skinfold thickness if possible.
- Pubertal stage.
- Dysmorphic stigmata in the hands, feet, head and neck, etc.
- Heart, lungs and abdomen to exclude other organic diagnoses.
- Neurologic examination (including fundoscopy and visual fields; see **Figs 1.112 & 1.113**). Relaxation of the Achilles tendon reflex is slow in hypothyroidism. Hypotonia and developmental delay are a feature of some dysmorphic syndromes.
- Skin signs.
- Palpation of the thyroid gland (see Ch. 9).

INTERPRETATION OF THE CLUES

If height is below the third centile and no physical abnormalities are found, there are several possibilities:

- Height is concordant with the target height centile = familial short stature unless a parent has a demonstrable pathology.
- Height is discordant with parental height = non-familial idiopathic short stature, including constitutional delay of growth and adolescence or mistaken paternity.
- Isolated growth hormone deficiency and late-presenting celiac disease may be very silent in their manifestations.

Clues that point to one of the primary growth disorders include:

- Specific dysmorphic features and/or intellectual impairment = one of the syndromic causes of short stature.
- Low birth weight and length for gestational age = intrauterine growth retardation with failure to catch up.
- Body disproportion: (1) legs < back = skeletal dysplasias; (2) back < legs = disorders of bone metabolism, spondyloepiphyseal dysplasia and storage disorders (but also to a more minor degree can be seen in delayed puberty of whatever cause).
- Hypogonadism = Ullrich–Turner syndrome, Prader–Labhart–Willi syndrome.

Pointers to chronic disease are:

- Specific signs in any system.
- Low growth rate or short stature accompanied by thinness.
- Anemia.

Pointers to an endocrinopathy include:

- A history of breech position and prolonged jaundice. The finding of a low height velocity, frontal bossing, increased abdominal fat, delayed puberty and a high-pitched voice = GHD (± signs of an additional pituitary deficiency).
- Low height velocity, obesity, sparse hair, discordant pubertal development, delayed bone age, irregular or heavy periods, constipation, goiter, pretibial myxedema, slow relaxation of the Achilles tendon reflex = hypothyroidism.
- Low height velocity, sudden rapid weight gain with a centripetal distribution, hirsutism, hypertension, weakness, glycosuria, striae, bruising and 'moon face' = Cushing syndrome.

Lateral skull
Chest
Lateral lumbar spine
Hips and pelvis including lower lumbar spine
Left hand and wrist (also for bone age)
One long bone – tibia and fibula are the best
Forearm bones if any limitation of movement or external abnormality

Table 2.4 Radiographs to be taken as part of a limited skeletal survey

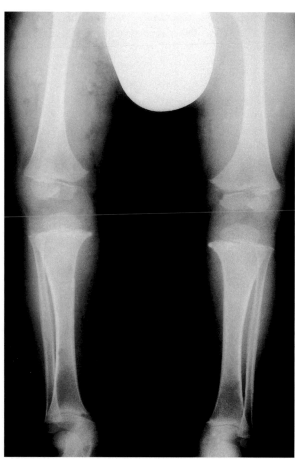

Fig. 2.58 Hypochondroplasia – less marked shortening of bones than in achondroplasia, fibula relatively long.

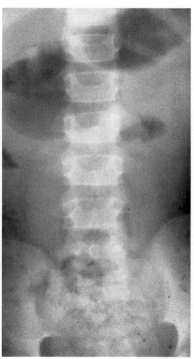

Fig. 2.59 Hypochondroplasia – lack of widening of the lumbar interpeduncular distance.

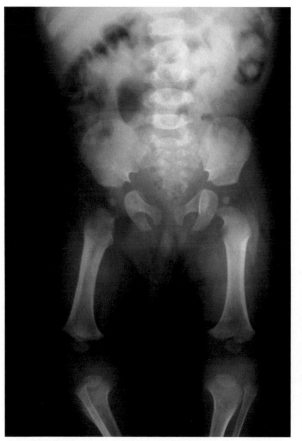

Fig. 2.57 Achondroplasia, short tubular bones, metaphyseal flare, square 'beaked' pelvis.

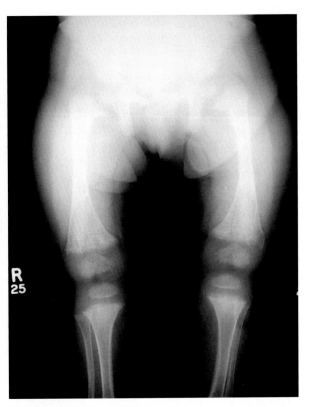

Fig. 2.60 Hypophosphatemic rickets.

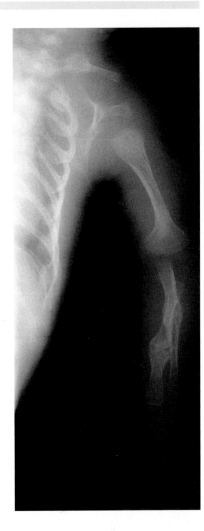

Fig. 2.62 The common (80% of all cases) type I, dominantly inherited, osteogenesis imperfecta.

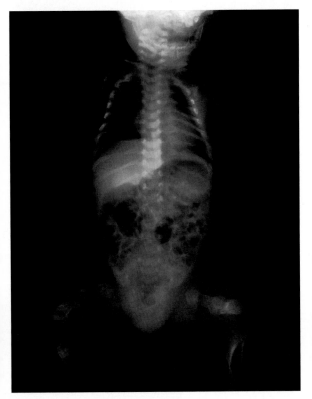

Fig. 2.61 Severe type 3, autosomal recessive, osteogenesis imperfecta.

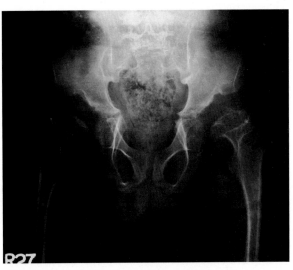

Fig. 2.63 Dysostosis multiplex in mucolipidosis 3.

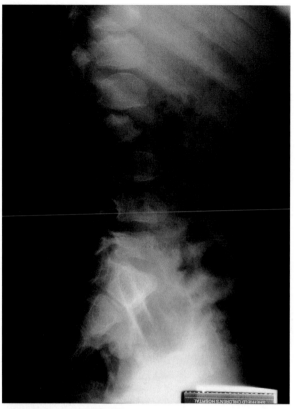

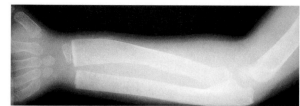

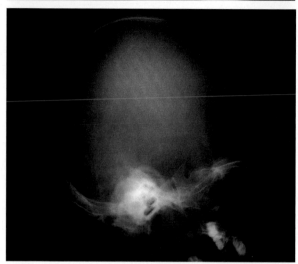

Figs 2.66, 2.67 Limb bone and skull radiograph in craniometaphyseal dysplasia. Note thickened base of skull.

Fig. 2.64 Dysostosis multiplex with abnormal beaked vertebra in mucolipidosis 3.

Fig. 2.68 Wrist bones in spondylometaphyseal dysplasia.

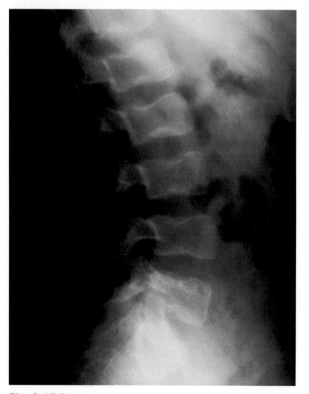

Fig. 2.65 Platyspondyly in spondylometaphyseal dysplasia.

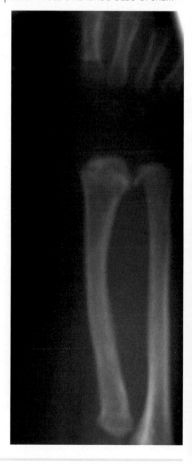

Fig. 2.69 Long bones and pelvis in spondylometaphyseal dysplasia.

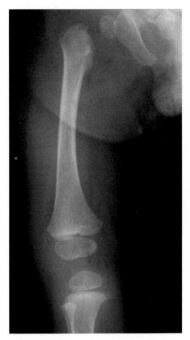

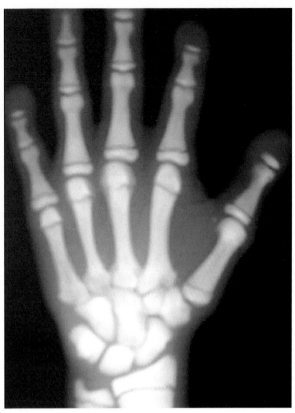

Fig. 2.71 Pyknodysostosis – an autosomal recessive disorder characterized by short stature and fractures. Note osteosclerosis and osteolysis of distal phalanges.

RADIOLOGICAL AND LABORATORY INVESTIGATIONS

(See Appendix for normal values and diagnostic test procedures)

If the clinical assessment and analysis of the growth curve indicate a pathological growth pattern, further investigations are warranted. In such cases a radiograph of the left hand and wrist for bone age should always be performed. Other investigations should be aimed at confirming or ruling out the most likely diagnoses.

Disproportion present

▪ In cases with body disproportion or obvious skeletal abnormalities, a limited skeletal survey should be performed (**Table 2.4, Figs 2.57–2.71**).

▪ If a storage disorder is likely, several urine specimens should be collected for analysis of mucopolysaccharides, and consideration should be given to an assay of white cell enzyme levels; a simpler screening test may be to ask for

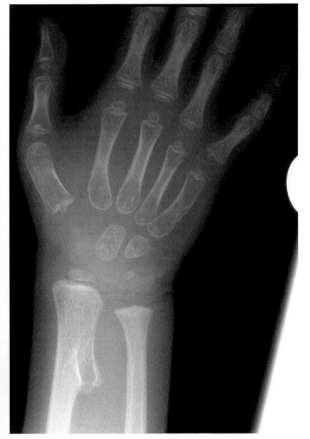

Fig. 2.70 Exostosis in Langer–Geidon (tricho-rhino-phalangeal) syndrome associated with short stature and small deletion of long arm of chromosome 8.

Full blood count and film

Renal and liver function tests, calcium/phosphate, alkaline phosphatase and acid–base status

Urinalysis

Stool analysis for fat globules, *Giardia* cysts, red blood cells, etc.

Thyroid stimulating hormone $\pm$ FT_4

IGF-1 and IGFBP-3

Antigliadin antibodies (or antiendomysial antibodies and IgA levels)

Chromosome analysis

Table 2.5 Suggested brief screening program for investigation of proportionate short stature

examination of a blood film, looking for vacuolation of lymphocytes.

- Serum calcium, phosphate and alkaline phosphatase levels are measured to evaluate bone diseases. Assays of collagen metabolites or genetic studies may be available in specialist centers.

Proportionate short stature

If no body disproportion is present, a short screening program can be carried out (**Table 2.5**), consisting of:

- Full blood count, mean corpuscular volume (MCV) and erythrocyte sedimentation rate (ESR). Anemia may be present, especially in inflammatory bowel disease, celiac disease and renal failure, although it may be associated with almost any prolonged illness. Microcytosis is an indication of nutritional deficiency and blood loss, and macrocytosis may indicate malabsorption.
- Acid–base status, urea and electrolytes, creatinine, liver function, calcium, phosphate and alkaline phosphatase levels. These will exclude occult renal failure and hepatic disease, the Bartter syndrome and metabolic bone disease.
- Urine analysis (simple biochemistry and microscopy).
- Stool analysis (giardiasis can produce profound growth retardation and may be picked up only if the stool is inspected microscopically for cysts). Test for reducing substances to exclude lactose intolerance. The presence of red blood cells and fat globules may point towards celiac disease and the need for a jejunal biopsy.
- Thyroid stimulating hormone (TSH) $\pm$ free thyroxine (FT4). FT4 levels are preferable to total

T4 levels as they are not prone to interference with drugs, renal or hepatic disease; see Chs 9 & 11).

- IGF-1 and IGFBP-3 (see below).
- Antigliadin antibody screen.
- Chromosome analysis.

Proportionate short stature with relative overweight

The consensus opinion of the Growth Hormone Research Society is that the GH axis should be tested if height is more than 3 SD below the mean or more than 1.5 SD below target height centile. Additionally investigations should be performed if height is more than 2 SD below the mean and height velocity over 1 year is more than 1 SD below the mean for 2 years (or more than 2 SD over 1 year), or if there are signs of other pituitary hormone deficiency or intracranial pathology.

If GHD is suspected, further testing of the GH–IGF-1/IGFBP-3 axis should be performed. Normal levels of IGF-1 or IGFBP-3 largely (but not completely) exclude GHD. Normal levels of IGFBP-3 are often seen in post-irradiation GHD. Low levels of IGF-1 may be due to several causes, including nutritional inadequacy, and do not prove GHD; hence one or two GH provocation tests should be performed at an experienced center (see Appendix).

Plain skull radiographs may show abnormalities suggestive of raised intracranial pressure or craniopharyngioma (**Fig. 2.72**), *but may also be normal and*

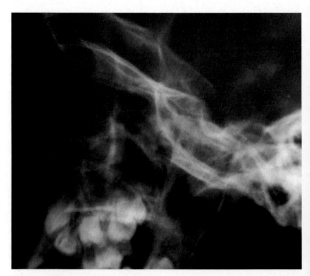

Fig. 2.72 Plain skull radiograph of craniopharyngioma. There is erosion of the posterior clinoid process and suprasellar calcification. The plain radiograph may be normal, however, and should not be relied upon in the investigation of short stature or hypopituitarism.

are thus unreliable as a primary investigation. Magnetic resonance imaging (MRI) or computed tomography (CT) is thus advisable in all cases of proven deficiency to exclude craniopharyngioma (**Figs 2.73–2.75**) or other tumors (**Fig. 2.76**) and to document anatomic abnormalities such as empty sella, ectopic pituitary tissue or stalk disruption (**Figs 2.77–2.79**). Cysts of Rathke's cleft (**Fig. 2.80**) can occasionally expand and produce hypopituitarism, and midline defects of the brain are associated with the septo-optic dysplasia sequence (**Fig. 2.81**). Hydrocephalus or hydranencephaly (**Fig. 2.82**) can also be associated with hypopituitarism (sometimes with sexual precocity).

In the Laron syndrome there is a failure to generate IGF-1 in response to normal or high levels of GH, which may be confirmed by an IGF-1 generation test (see Appendix).

The commonest forms of hypothyroidism may be detected by raised TSH levels in the preliminary screen. If found, this should prompt assay of antithyroid antibody levels. Isolated central hypothyroidism is rare but will be detected by the low–normal TSH level at the same time as a low free T_4 level. Further details of thyroid function testing are given in Chapters 9 & 11, and in the Appendix.

If Cushing syndrome is suspected, an estimation of 24-h urinary free cortisol (UFC) should be obtained

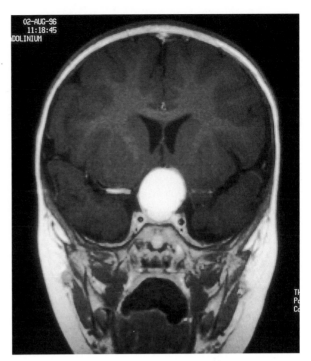

Fig. 2.74 Matching MRI scan of the patient in Fig. 2.73, showing a lipid-filled cyst.

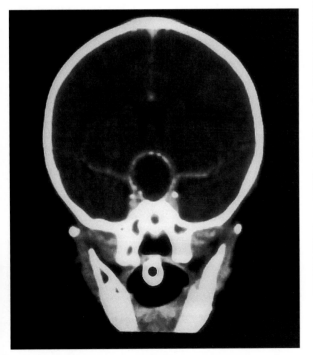

Fig. 2.73 Vertical CT scan of patient with a cystic craniopharyngioma, showing rim calcification.

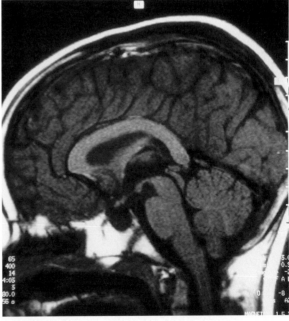

Fig. 2.75 Small craniopharyngioma (may well be missed if only CT is used).

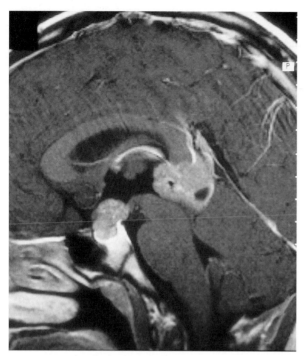

Fig. 2.76 MRI scan of bifocal germinoma presenting with panhypopituitarism.

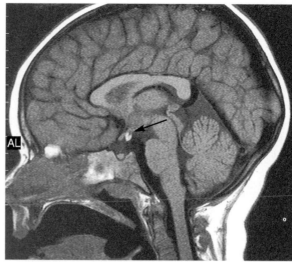

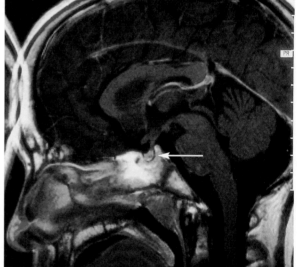

Figs 2.78 (top) and **2.79** (bottom) Ectopic bright spot and normal MRI scan for comparison showing pituitary stalk, posterior pituitary bright spot.

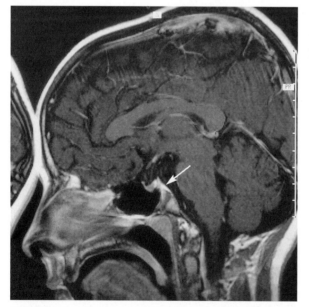

Fig. 2.77 Ectopic posterior pituitary bright spot (arrow) and absent pituitary stalk following head injury.

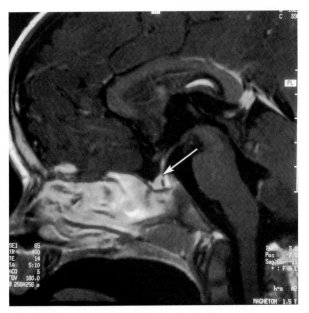

Fig. 2.80 Cyst of Rathke's cleft.

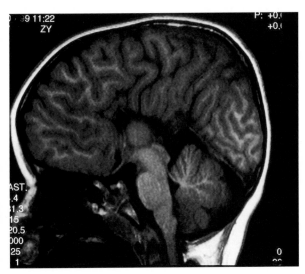

Fig. 2.81 Agenesis of the corpus callosum (with septo-optic dysplasia).

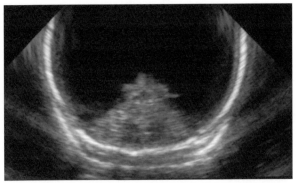

Fig. 2.82 Hydranencephaly with neonatal hypopituitarism and adipsic diabetes insipidus, ultrasound scan of brain.

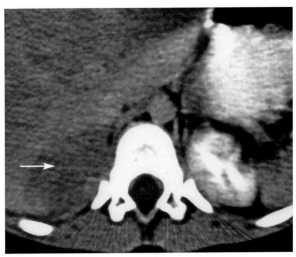

Fig. 2.83 CT scan of right-sided adrenal adenoma producing Cushing's syndrome (same patient as in Fig. 2.43). The hypodense tumor has displaced the right kidney downwards; the left kidney is outlined with contrast medium.

followed by a serum cortisol rhythm (early morning (0700–0900 hours) and late evening (2200–2400 hours)) and a simultaneous measurement of adreno-corticotropic hormone (ACTH) concentration. Suppression of ACTH implies an adrenal cause. Raised cortisol levels, UFC and loss of diurnal variation should prompt referral to a specialist center for further evaluation with dexamethasone testing (see Appendix) and localization of the source by MRI of the pituitary or CT of the abdomen and chest (**Figs 1.94 & 2.83**). Sampling for ACTH from the inferior petrosal sinus can help lateralize pituitary adenomas in 60–70% of cases where scanning is equivocal, in experienced units.

THERAPY OF SHORT STATURE

Idiopathic and primary short stature

Treatment of idiopathic short stature remains both experimental and controversial, and should remain in the realm of specialist centers. There may be early acceleration of growth rate but a shortened duration of growth, and there is currently little evidence to suggest that adult height is markedly increased. Growth hormone treatment should probably still be offered only as part of a formal clinical trial.

In the Ullrich–Turner syndrome there is current-ly convincing evidence for benefit on adult height

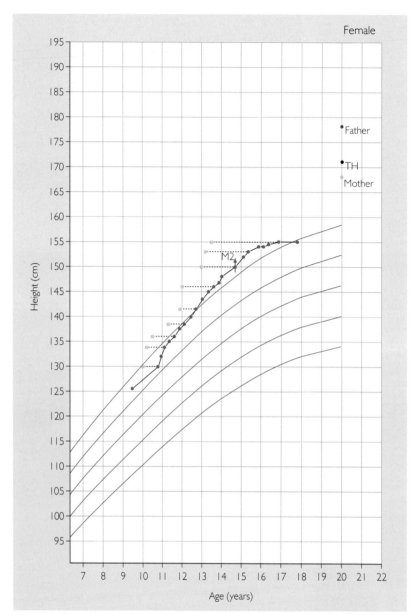

Fig. 2.84 Ullrich–Turner syndrome. Growth hormone therapy initiated at 11.8 years. There is an improvement in height from −3 to −2 SDS for normal Dutch girls, or from +1.5 to +2 SDS on the Turner chart shown.

(**Fig. 2.84**). The GH dose is 0.05 mg/kg daily, given as a daily subcutaneous injection. Anabolic steroids such as oxandrolone (dose 0.06 mg/kg daily) may have an added benefit.

Therapy with GH (up to 0.06 mg/kg daily) for 2–3 years has been used in patients with IUGR who have not shown catch-up after the age of 5 years, to promote growth to the normal centile range, although data on adult height are not available. Occasionally longer treatment regimens may be used in trial settings, with anecdotal benefit (**Fig. 2.85**).

GH therapy in Prader–Labhart–Willi syndrome has been shown to improve body composition as well as growth rate at a dose of 0.035 mg/kg daily.

In the skeletal dysplasias, surgical leg-lengthening techniques in specialist units (**Figs 2.27, 2.86–2.88**) offer the possibility of height gain in the order of 10–25 cm (4–10 inches). The use of medical growth-promoting therapies is being explored, but is likely to be of lesser importance than surgery.

In the storage disorders there may be a role for bone marrow transplantation to reduce the metabolic and skeletal consequences of the underlying defect. There is some evidence that the skeletal, if not many

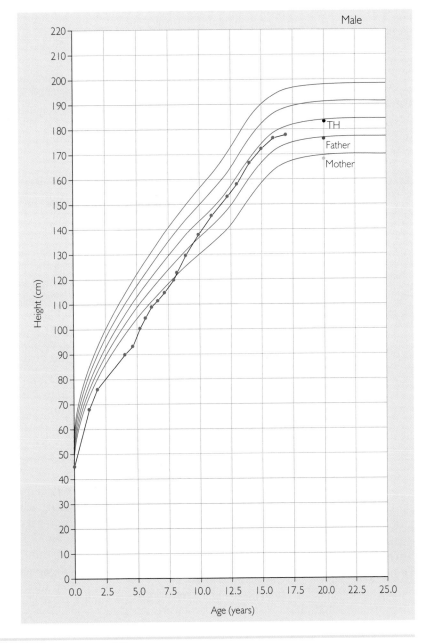

Fig. 2.85 IUGR with GH therapy given between 5 and 16 years. Height on starting therapy −4 SDS; adult height −0.44 SDS. Compare with Fig. 2.20.

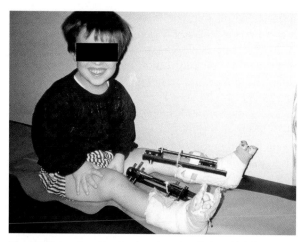

Fig. 2.86 Leg lengthening in achondroplasia with bilateral tibial fixators.

Fig. 2.87 Results of leg lengthening in achondroplasia after 2-year program of tibial and femoral lengthening. Before surgery unable to reach light switch.

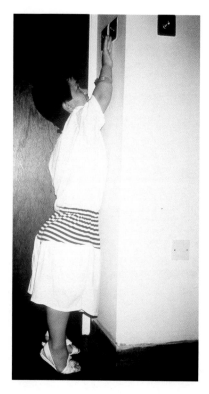

Fig. 2.88 Same patient as in Fig. 2.87 after surgery, with a height gain of 28 cm.

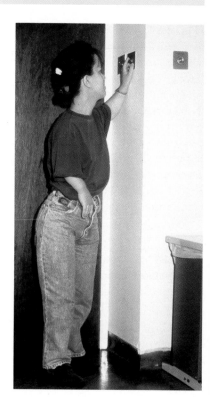

of the other, symptoms of these conditions can at least be stabilized by this procedure.

Secondary growth failure

If the growth failure is due to a systemic illness, successful treatment of the specific systemic disorder may produce catch-up growth. This is particularly true of disorders that are active in late childhood and early teenage life, where even a relatively brief period of amelioration of a disease process may allow for a more normal pubertal growth and an increased height prognosis.

GHD is treated with daily subcutaneous administration of synthetic growth hormone at a dose of 0.025–0.05 mg/kg daily (**Figs 2.89 & 2.90**). Laron syndrome may be treated with recombinant IGF-1 in specialized centers.

Hypothyroidism is easily treated with L-thyroxine tablets at a dose tailored to suppress the TSH level, usually between 50 and 150 µg/day. The catch-up growth that might be expected from the degree of skeletal immaturity present at diagnosis may not occur, especially if the growth failure is long-standing or occurs during puberty (**Fig. 2.91**).

Treatment of Cushing syndrome is always highly specialized. If due to an adrenal adenoma, it is treated by unilateral adrenalectomy. Adrenal carcinomas are highly aggressive, and combined medical and surgical treatment is required for any hope of success. Pituitary adenomas causing Cushing disease may be treated with trans-sphenoidal adenomectomy followed by temporary adrenal replacement therapy until adrenal function recovers. If resection of the pituitary adenoma is not possible, and in cases of the syndrome

Fig. 2.89 Growth hormone deficiency presenting at 6 years of age (height −4.7 SDS). Human GH treatment until 8.5 years (height −3.3 SDS) when withdrawn for 6 months because of possible contamination of pituitary-derived hGH with the Creutzfeldt–Jakob disease (CJD) prion, during which time growth almost ceased. Recommenced recombinant GH at 9.2 years. Central hypothyroidism diagnosed at 12.4 years and hypoadrenalism at 17.4 years. Spontaneous normal puberty at 14 years with adult height −0.9 SDS, at target height.

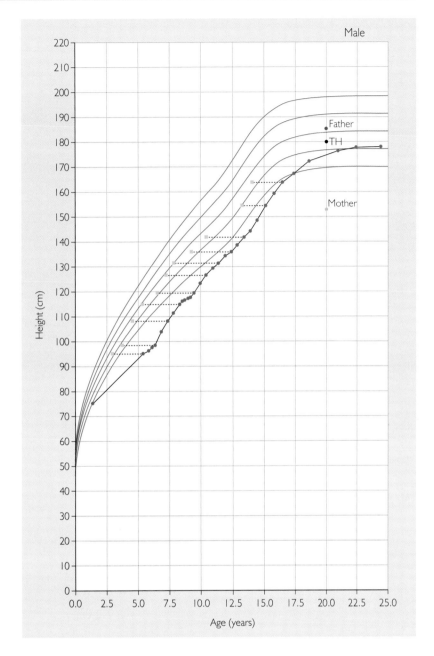

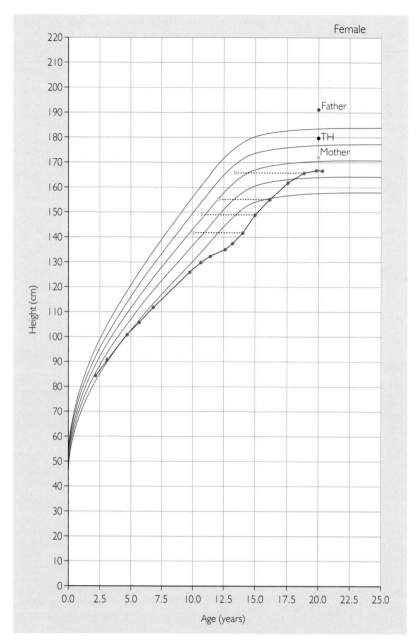

Fig. 2.90 Panhypopituitarism presenting late because the discrepancy between the subject's actual height (−2 to −4 SDS in mid-childhood) had not been interpreted in the context of the tall parents (target height + 1.7 SDS). Thyroxine and hydrocortisone started at 13.2 years, recombinant GH at 14 years and ethinylestradiol at 16 years. Adult height −0.6 SDS, below target height but within normal range.

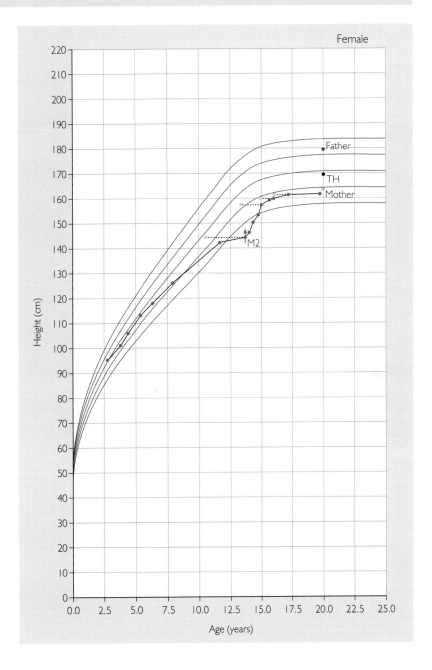

Fig. 2.91 Hypothyroidism presenting at 13.8 years (−2.9 SDS) with incomplete catch-up (adult height −1.4 SDS − below target range; previous height prior to hypothyroid state −0.4 SDS).

caused by bilateral nodular adrenal hyperplasia, then bilateral adrenalectomy may be required (but at the risk of causing the Nelson syndrome (see **Fig. 1.138**), followed by life-long replacement therapy with glucocorticoids and mineralocorticoids.

The growth failure and obesity due to systemic glucocorticoid administration are usually reversible in the early stages if remission is achieved. If vertebral collapse occurs, and if treatment is continued through pubertal years, then stunting is permanent. GH trials are ongoing, indicating that growth can be partially restored.

Psychosocial deprivation dwarfism may show impressive catch-up if it is possible to change the circumstances of care. Recovery of height and weight gain whilst separated from the usual carers can be used as retrospective evidence of the nature of the problem.

Chapter 3

The Tall Child

The classification of causes of tall stature is more straightforward than that of short stature. Idiopathic or genetic tall stature is by far the commonest cause. There are a relatively small number of primary syndromes of large size and secondary causes of increased adult height are rare. Some secondary conditions produce largeness for a period of the child's growth span, then a normal or even reduced adult height due to early fusion of the epiphyses. There are also primary disorders of blood supply or intrinsic to the growth plate that can produce areas of localized overgrowth.

NORMAL-VARIANT TALL STATURE

Normal-variant tall stature is defined by the absence of abnormalities in the history and physical examination. It can be subdivided similarly to short stature, described in Chapter 2.

Familial tall stature

This is characterized by:

- tall stature during the growth period and an increased adult height.
- a normal height velocity (varying around the 75th centile. As the height centile lines diverge with increasing age, a tall child on the 97th height centile will show a velocity that varies around the 75th velocity centile.)
- a height within the range defined by parental size, although doubtful paternity may sometimes cause confusion.
- bone age consistent with chronological age (±2 SD).
- a normal age of onset of puberty.
- often relatively long legs compared with sitting height.

Constitutional tall stature with advance in growth and adolescence

This type is characterized by:

- normal to tall stature during childhood.
- adult stature within the range defined by parental size.
- a moderately advanced bone age (not more than +2 SD above chronological age).

- an increased height velocity (>75%) in the later childhood years.
- early onset and cessation of puberty, often following the same pattern as one or both of the parents.

Combination

A combination of familial and constitutional conditions is often seen.

GROWTH HORMONE EXCESS

Pituitary gigantism (**Figs 3.1 & 3.2**) is extremely rare. It is usually produced by growth hormone (GH)

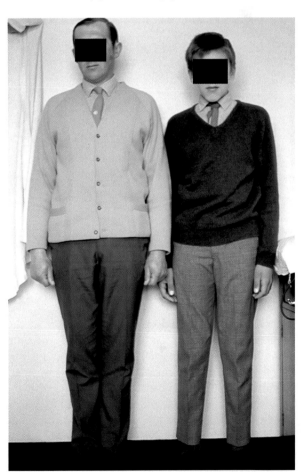

Fig. 3.1 Pituitary gigantism, age 9 years, in comparison to father.

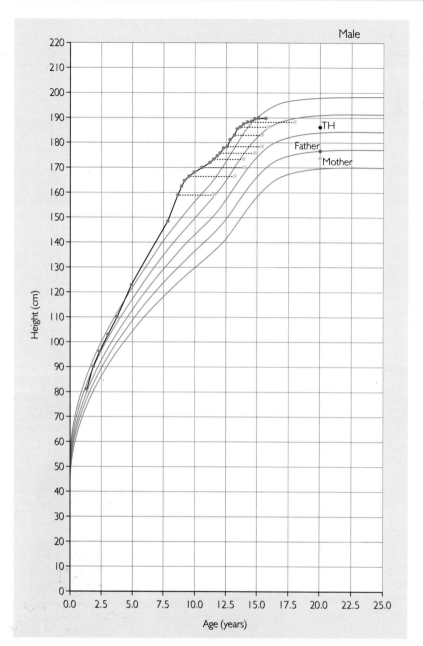

Fig. 3.2 Pituitary gigantism presenting as tall stature (+4.1 SDS) at 9 years of age with evidence of previous accelerating height velocity. Adenoma resected at 9.2 years with fall in SDS to an adult height of +1.6 SDS.

excess caused by a GH-producing adenoma in the pituitary. This may be seen as part of the McCune–Albright syndrome. Even more rarely, growth hormone releasing hormone (GHRH) excess, from tumorous sources, produces excessive growth. Proportionate, worsening tall stature with an increased height velocity is seen and, if no treatment is given, can produce heights in excess of 200 cm up to 247 cm in the female and 274 cm in the male. The same disease process produces acromegaly in adulthood after the fusion of the epiphyses, and a number of patients with a late childhood onset share many features of both

conditions. There may be prognathism, and signs and symptoms of optic chiasm compression. There may be increased sweating and a yellowish discoloration of the palms (see **Fig. 1.44**).

DYSMORPHIC SYNDROMES

Sex chromosome abnormalities (including aneuploidy)

Many abnormalities involving duplication of the X or Y chromosomes can occur, but only two are commonly associated with disproportionate tall stature, the

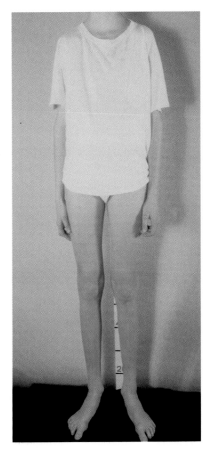

Fig. 3.3 XXY, final height (with treatment) 208 cm.

acceptability of tall stature mean that they often present in late childhood or early adult life.

XXX females have few external phenotypic features, but tend to be slender and tall with a proportion showing late puberty, amenorrhea or infertility. The mean IQ is 85.

Dysmorphic syndromes due to metabolic or connective tissue abnormality

The Marfan syndrome is a relatively common dominantly inherited disorder of one of the copies of a fibrillin gene on chromosome 17q. It is characterized externally by disproportionate tall stature (**Figs 3.4 & 3.5**) with relatively long legs (**Fig. 3.6**), arachnodactyly (**Fig. 3.7**), joint laxity (see **Figs 1.18–1.21**), hernias, scoliosis and chest deformities (see **Fig. 1.87**), myopia, dislocation or poor fixation of the lens (see **Fig. 1.119**) and a high arched palate (see **Fig. 1.70**). Internally there may be weakness of the collagenous structures, especially on the left side of the heart, producing mitral and aortic valve incompetence, aortic dilatation and dissection. Spontaneous pneumothorax may occur. Lumbosacral dural ectasia may be seen on magnetic resonance imaging (MRI) (see **Fig. 3.35**).

Beals contractural arachnodactyly (**Fig. 3.8**) is a rare, dominantly inherited, disorder of another copy of a fibrillin gene on chromosome 15q, and has some similarities with the Marfan syndrome. There are contractures at the knees, elbows and hands, and micrognathia. The ears may be 'crumpled' and there may be kyphoscoliosis.

Homocystinuria is an aminoaciduria that is associated with marfanoid tall stature (**Fig. 3.9**) but that presents more frequently because of the ocular complications such as ectopia lentis and severe myopia. Intellect is usually impaired and complications associated with thromboembolism occur.

Total lipodystrophy (see Ch. 4) produces extreme leanness and relative tall stature.

Dysmorphic syndromes with symmetrical overgrowth

Most of these syndromes are associated with intellectual impairment:

- Sotos syndrome (**Figs 3.10–3.14**).
- Weaver syndrome (**Figs 3.15 & 3.16**).
- Marshall–Smith syndrome.
- Beckwith–Wiedemann syndrome (**Figs 3.17–3.19**), which includes macrosomia (often more marked on one side of the body), with other dysmorphic features and hypoglycemia. There may be associated intellectual deficit as a result of the

Klinefelter (XXY, XXYY, XXXY and mosaic forms) and the XYY syndromes. In both the legs are relatively long compared with the back (**Fig. 3.3**).

Klinefelter syndrome is most commonly associated with the XXY karyotype, but variants with XXYY and mosaic forms can occur. (An XXXY form is more likely to be associated with slow growth.) There tends to be minor intellectual deficit, often exacerbated by behavioral problems and hypergonadotrophic hypogonadism. In later life there is a high incidence of diabetes mellitus. Infertility is usual but there are descriptions of successful intracytoplasmic sperm injection.

XYY males have a mild intellectual deficit and specific motor coordination problems. In the past it was said that there was an increase in antisocial behavior, but this is not now thought to be commonly the case. Cryptorchidism occurs but is not as universal as in the Klinefelter syndrome.

Both conditions are relatively common, occurring more than twice as frequently as the Ullrich–Turner syndrome in birth karyotype surveys; however, the relatively mild learning difficulties and the social

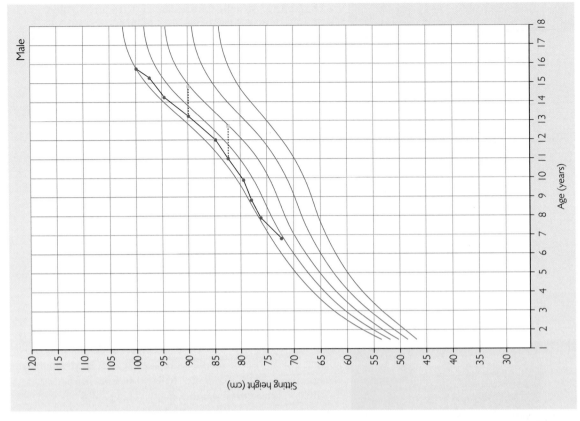

Fig. 3.5 Sitting height chart (+2 SDS) of the patient in Fig. 3.4.

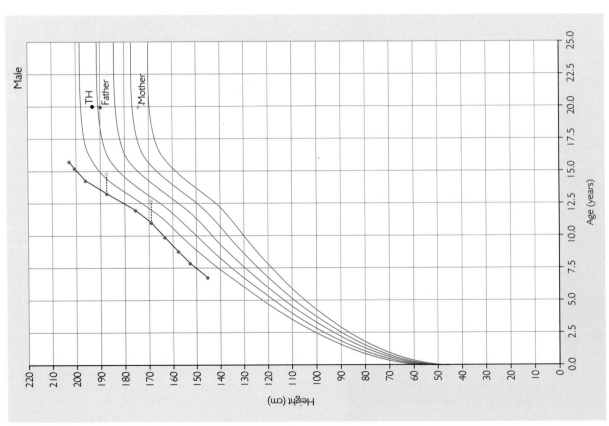

Fig. 3.4 Marfan syndrome occurring as a new mutation (note the normal parental heights). Moderate tall stature, +3.8 SDS; the disproportion is evident from

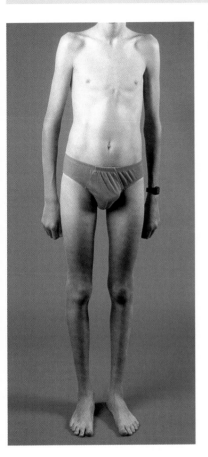

Fig. 3.6 Marfan syndrome.

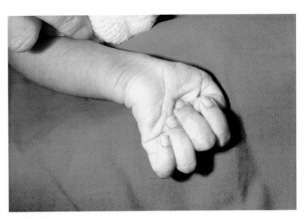

Fig. 3.8 Beals contractural arachnodactyly.

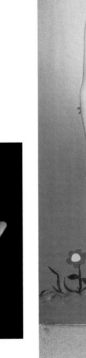

Fig. 3.9 Homocystinuria, 190.5 cm at 13.5 years.

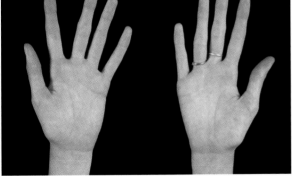

Fig. 3.7 Arachnodactyly in the Marfan syndrome.

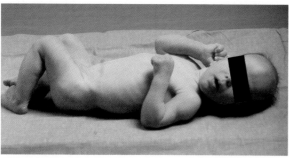

Fig. 3.10 Sotos syndrome as baby.

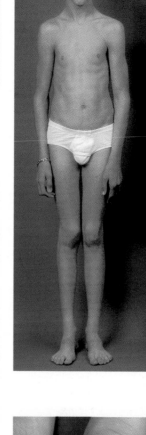

Fig. 3.12 Sotos syndrome as young adult (185 cm).

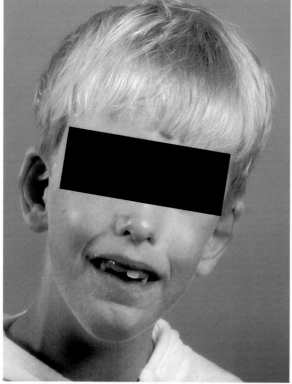

Fig. 3.11 Sotos syndrome as child.

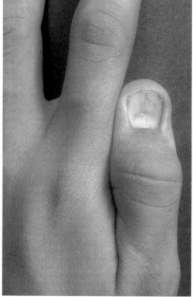

Fig. 3.13 Deep-set concave nails in Sotos syndrome.

Fig. 3.14 Sotos syndrome, height at 1 year +2.4 SDS with a final height of +2.68 SDS, but +3.6 SDS in mid-childhood. Target height was −0.2 SDS.

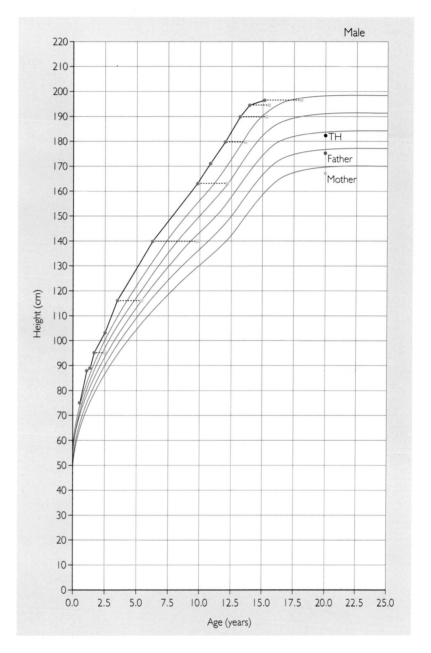

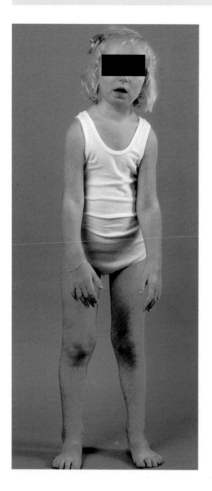

Fig. 3.15 Weaver syndrome, height >97%.

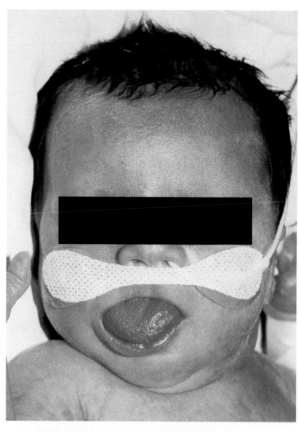

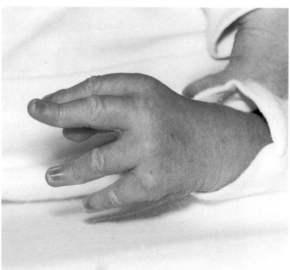

Fig. 3.16 Weaver syndrome, camptodactyly, broad middle phalanges and narrow nails.

Figs 3.17 (Top right), **3.18** (Bottom right) Beckwith–Wiedemann syndrome, face and demonstration of ear crease.

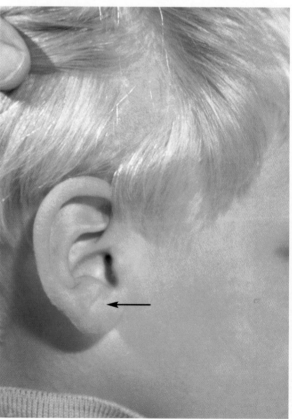

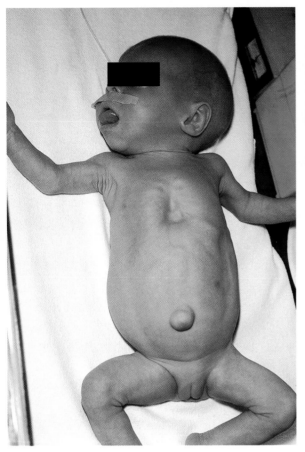

Fig. 3.19 Beckwith–Wiedemann syndrome, showing umbilical hernia and abdominal distension from organomegaly.

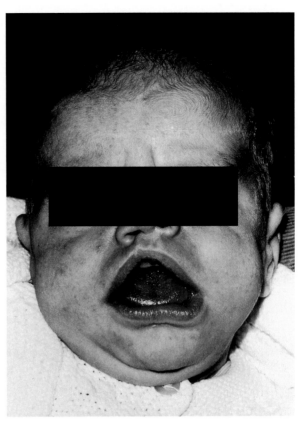

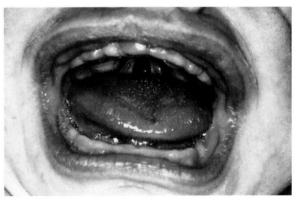

Figs 3.20 (Top), **3.21** (Bottom) Simpson–Golabi–Behmel syndrome with macrostomia and cleft palate with neonatal dental eruption.

hypoglycemia. There is evidence of relative overexpression *in utero* of the growth factor, insulin-like growth factor (IGF-2) and a tendency to Wilms tumor as a result of this. Simpson–Golabi–Behmel syndrome ('bulldog' syndrome; **Figs 3.20 & 3.21**) has overlapping features and is due to a deleting mutation of glypican 3, a membrane-bound proteoglycan that usually sequesters IGF-2 to make it unavailable to its receptor.

The main distinguishing features of these conditions are given in **Table 3.1**.

Fragile X syndrome, Bannayan–Riley–Ruvacalba, Elejade and Nevo syndromes may be associated with overgrowth.

Dysmorphic syndromes with partial or asymmetric overgrowth

The overgrowth in Beckwith–Wiedemann syndrome may be asymmetric, producing hemihypertrophy. Klippel–Trenaunay–Weber syndrome is tissue over-growth in association with cutaneous vascular nevi (**Fig. 3.22**). Proteus syndrome (**Figs 3.23–3.25**) is due to a chimeric tissue abnormality resulting in progressive overgrowth, lipomas and deformity.

SECONDARY CAUSES OF LARGE SIZE

Hyperinsulinism

Intrauterine hyperinsulinemia secondary to maternal diabetes (**Figs 3.26 & 3.27**) or persistent hyper-

	Beckwith–Wiedemann	Sotos	Weaver	Marshall–Smith
Head and face	Big at birth. Large muscle mass till teens Prominent occiput Facial hemangiomas Ear lobe crease Small mid-face Macroglossia	Big at birth. Growth rate slows after 4 years Prominent forehead Macrocephaly Hypertelorism, squint Prognathism Early teeth, narrow palate	Variable Flat occiput Macrocephaly Large ears Micrognathia Thin head hair, hypertrichosis	Ht > Wt. Bone age very advanced Prominent forehead Long head Big nose Shallow orbits Hypertrichosis
IQ, CNS	Hypoglycemia – may cause secondary IQ reduction	Abnormal glucose tolerance test. Mild/moderate primary IQ reduction	Primary IQ reduction	Primary IQ reduction. Myopathy
Other	Organomegaly Hemihypertrophy Cardiac defects	Deep-set nails – Cardiac defects	Hoarse voice. Nail hypoplasia. Hernias Stiff joints, camptodactyly Cardiac defects	Blue sclerae Immunity reduced Cardiac defects
Tumors	Wilms tumor. Hepato-, neuro-, gonado-blastomas	Wilms tumor. Vaginal, hepatic, parotid, neuro-ectodermal carcinomas	Neuroblastoma	?

Table 3.1 Features of the major syndromes associated with large size

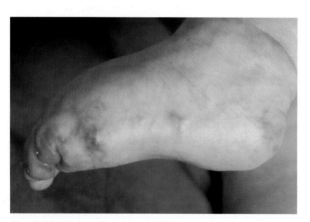

Fig. 3.22 Klippel–Trenaunay–Weber syndrome causing overgrowth of foot.

insulinemic hypoglycemia of infancy (PHHI) (previously called pancreatic endocrine dysregulation syndrome or nesidioblastosis) (**Fig. 3.28**) (see Ch. 11) both cause early macrosomia because insulin is a potent fetal growth factor. This increase in size is usually transient and followed by 'catch-down' growth once the abnormal insulin-secreting environment has been removed.

Hyperinsulinism may occur secondary to obesity (see Ch. 5). In childhood excess calorie intake is available for growth and may provoke hyperinsulinism, so producing a relatively tall stature characterized by: tall stature (at upper end of predicted target range), with weight ≥ height centile (**Fig. 3.29**), relatively early puberty, striae and high cheek color mimicking mild Cushing syndrome (**Fig. 3.30**), but with the contrasting rapid growth compared with the universal growth failure of steroid excess. There is frequently a similar habitus in one or both parents and siblings. If the hyperinsulinism is severe there may be coexisting acanthosis, and in the HAIR-AN (hyperandrogenization, acrochordons, insulin resistance and acanthosis nigricans) syndrome (see Ch. 10, **Fig. 10.18**) the facial features are described as 'acromegaloid'. Hypothalamic tumors and dysfunction

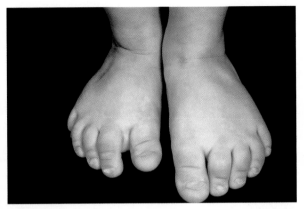

Fig. 3.23 Proteus syndrome, isolated areas of overgrowth.

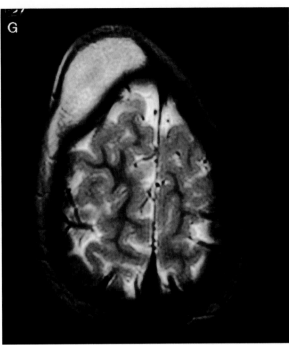

Fig. 3.25 Proteus syndrome with lipomata.

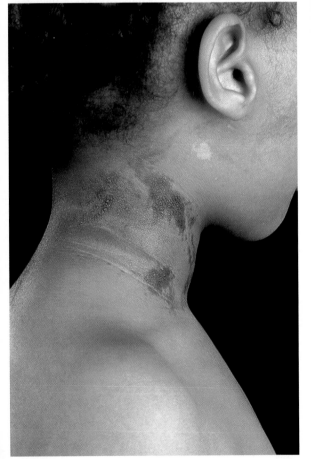

Fig. 3.24 Proteus syndrome with linear nevi.

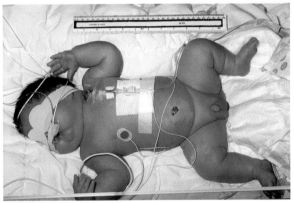

Fig. 3.26 Infant of a diabetic mother – macrosomia, plethora and jaundice requiring exchange transfusion.

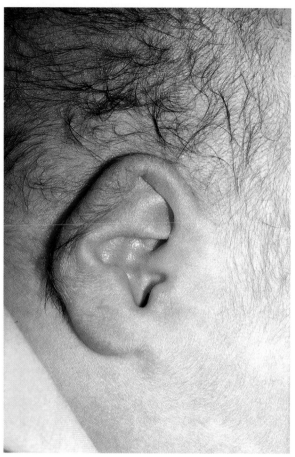

Fig. 3.27 Hairy ears in the infant of a diabetic mother, an unexplained but common finding.

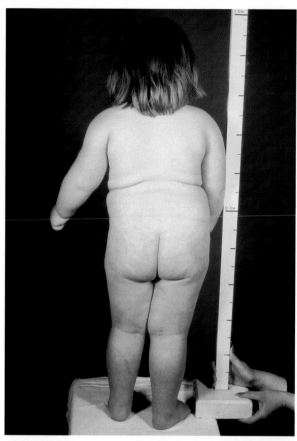

Fig. 3.29 Nutritional obesity, height >97%, target height 75%; 15 kg (33 lb) overweight for height at age 3 years.

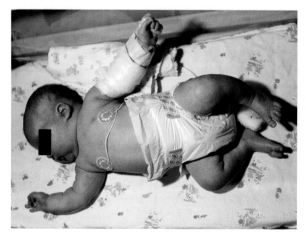

Fig. 3.28 Neonatal hyperinsulinism secondary to persistent hyperinsulinemic hypoglycemia of infancy (PHHI).

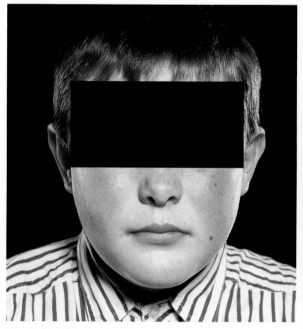

Fig. 3.30 High cheek color mimicking Cushing syndrome in nutritional obesity.

may produce overeating, obesity and overgrowth as a secondary phenomena (see **Figs 5.14 & 5.15**).

Thyrotoxicosis

If mild and hence unrecognized and untreated, thyrotoxicosis produces an acceleration of growth rate and relative tall stature in mid-childhood, although there is advanced osseous maturation and the eventual height is likely to be in the genetic range (**Figs 3.31 & 3.32**) (see also Ch. 9).

Precocious puberty

Precocious puberty is discussed in detail in Chapter 6; it leads to tall stature in childhood but not a tall adult height. Untreated, the increasingly advanced bone age leading to early epiphyseal fusion means that adult height is usually short.

OTHER CONDITIONS ASSOCIATED WITH DISPROPORTION AND RELATIVE TALL STATURE

Multiple endocrine adenomatosis or neoplasia (MEA or MEN) type IIb is a familial condition in which the occurrence of medullary carcinoma of the thyroid and pheochromocytoma is associated with mildly tall stature and a marfanoid habitus along with neuromas of the mucous membranes (see **Fig. 1.72**), bowel and conjunctiva (**Fig. 3.33**).

Hypogonadism can cause a modestly increased adult height with long legs (the so-called 'eunuchoid body habitus'), on the basis of late closure of the epiphyses and prolonged childhood growth of the legs coupled with failure of the sex hormone-mediated growth of the spine. The causes and work-up of hypogonadism are discussed in Chapter 7.

Similarly, but more severely, aromatase deficiency prevents the conversion of testosterone to estrogen in the male (as do estrogen receptor defects), and hence there is no stimulus for epiphyseal fusion. These rare individuals continue growing into adulthood; they have osteoporosis and infertility in association with massively raised follicle stimulating hormone (FSH) levels.

Familial glucocorticoid resistance may be associated with tall stature.

DIAGNOSTIC WORK-UP OF TALL STATURE

MEDICAL HISTORY AND PHYSICAL EXAMINATION

The following are the most relevant points to explore when taking a history of a child presenting with large size:

- Birth size, mother's health and gestational history, mode of delivery. Was mother virilized during pregnancy? (= aromatase deficiency in the offspring).
- Parental size and timing of puberty.
- Any family history of early heart disease or eye problems. Family history of endocrine malignancy, adrenal abnormalities (MEN-IIb, familial glucocorticoid resistance).
- Any symptoms suggestive of early sexual development.
- Any symptoms of sweating, tremor, frequent stool habit, anxiety or heat intolerance.
- Dietary intake.
- Neurologic symptoms including headache and visual disturbance. Is the sense of smell normal?

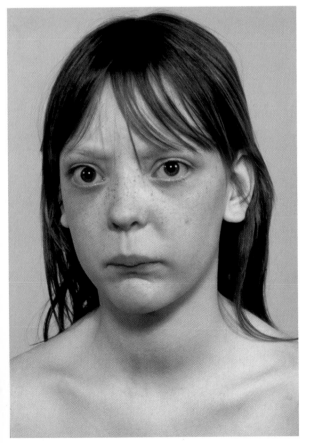

Fig. 3.31 Thyrotoxicosis.

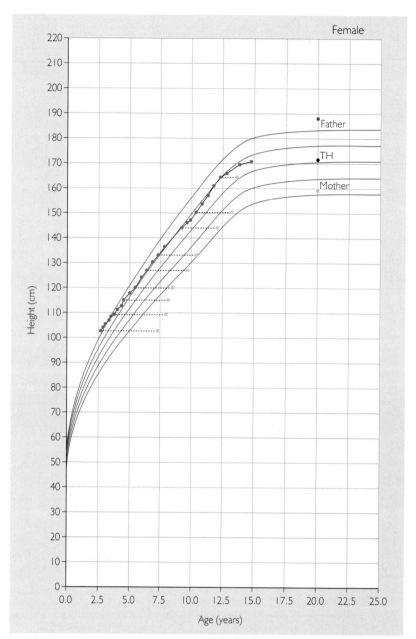

Fig. 3.32 Thyrotoxicosis presenting at 2.8 years with a bone age of 7.4 years and height of +2.4 SDS. Subsequent growth on antithyroid therapy for 4 years, followed by eventual remission, was normal (adult height + 0.6 SDS).

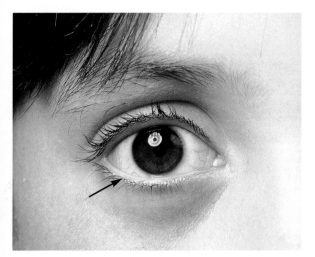

Fig. 3.33 Multiple endocrine adenomatosis type IIb, neuroma on right lower conjunctiva (arrow).

Fig. 3.34
Horizontal striae in idiopathic tall stature.

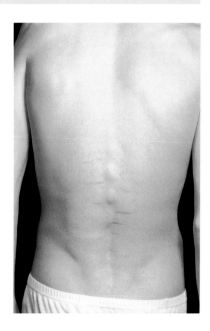

(Anosmia is associated with hypogonadism in the Kallmann syndrome; see Ch. 7.)
- Developmental or educational level. Any specific motor or behavioral defects?

On examination, look especially for:

- The pattern of growth of height, sitting height, weight and head circumference. The presence or absence of disproportion is an important feature. Head circumference is large in Sotos syndrome and, because the height standard deviation score (SDS) stabilizes after 2 years of age, these individuals become less noticeably tall.
- Horizontal skin striae on the back are often seen in rapidly growing tall individuals, for whatever cause (**Fig. 3.34**).
- Dysmorphic features as outlined in **Table 3.1**.
- Neuromas, enlarged thyroid or hypertension (paroxysmal initially), in MEN-IIb.
- Any evidence of hypogonadism or cryptorchidism; macro-orchidism (seen in fragile X syndrome, aromatase deficiency).
- Plethora and hairy ears are seen in infants of diabetic mothers.
- Discoloration of the palms, (in gigantism).
- Visual field deficit, optic disk appearance and the position of the lens.
- Goiter, tremor, exophthalmos or other signs of thyrotoxicosis.

INTERPRETATION OF THE CLUES

The absence of any physical abnormalities or disproportion with no evidence of sexual precocity indicates:

- If weight ≤ height centile = familial tall stature.
- If weight > height centile (or abnormal (>97%) weight-for-height plot) = nutritional.

Large size with specific dysmorphic features and intellectual defect:

- = one of the overgrowth syndromes.

Disproportion with normal intellect:

- With arachnodactyly = Marfan or Beals syndromes. There may be no family history if a new mutation has occurred.
- With only moderate tallness, neuromas on lips, tongue or eyelids and a positive family history (although new mutations occur frequently) = MEN type IIb.
- With moderate tall stature, hypogonadism and anosmia = Kallmann syndrome.
- With moderate tall stature and hypogonadism = isolated or iatrogenic (i.e. following irradiation), hypogonadism; aromatase deficiency.

Disproportion with intellectual defect:

- If hypogonadism or cryptorchidism = X chromosome duplication.
- If ocular and neurologic problems predominate = homocystinuria; fragile X syndrome.

Enlargement of one side of body or one limb:

- If associated with dysmorphic features as shown in **Table 3.1** = Beckwith–Wiedemann syndrome.

- If associated with
  hemangioma = Klippel–Trenaunay–Weber
  syndrome.
- If associated with linear nevi and
  lipomas = Proteus syndrome.

Large size with no disproportion:

- If present at birth = neonatal hyperinsulinism.
- If accelerating height velocity, neurologic signs of
  optic chiasm compression, sweatiness,
  prognathism or skin signs = pituitary
  gigantism.
- If goiter, exophthalmos, tremor,
  tachycardia = thyrotoxicosis.
- If early sexual development (less than 8 years in a
  girl, less than 9 years in a boy) = precocious
  puberty.

RADIOLOGICAL AND LABORATORY INVESTIGATIONS

These are less commonly required than in the investigation of short stature.

A hand and wrist radiograph for bone age will serve the dual purpose of providing an estimation of physiologic maturity and allow quantification of arachnodactyly. Lumbosacral dural ectasia in Marfan syndrome requires MRI, although this investigation is rarely indicated in the absence of lower-limb neurologic abnormalities (**Fig. 3.35**).

The bone age is mildly advanced in familial tall stature/early puberty, and more so in precocious puberty and thyrotoxicosis. The bone age is very advanced in the Marshall–Smith syndrome and less so in the other dysmorphic overgrowth syndromes. In the Weaver syndrome only the maturation of the carpal bones is in advance of the small bones of the hand.

A metacarpal index compares the average length:width ratios of the 2nd and 5th metacarpal bones in an attempt to define arachnodactyly as a value of more than 8.5. In practice, it adds little to an external clinical assessment.

In the presence of genital abnormalities the karyotype should be checked.

If there is any possibility of MEN-IIb, either because of a positive family history or the presence of mucosal neuromas in a child with a marfanoid habitus, it is essential rapidly to check the calcitonin level and urinary vanillylmandelic acid (VMA) level, and confirm the diagnosis by analysis of the *ret* proto-oncogene on chromosome 10q, because the implications for missing an early diagnosis of medullary cell carcinoma of the thyroid are so severe.

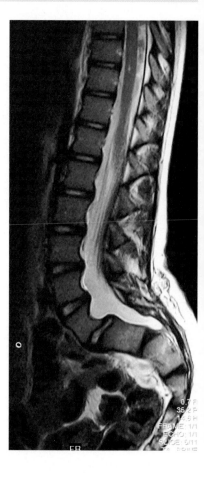

Fig. 3.35
Lumbosacral dural ectasia in Marfan syndrome.

Neonatal hyperinsulinism in infants born to non-diabetic mothers can be confirmed by the demonstration of inappropriately high insulin levels at the time of hypoglycemia.

If suspicion exists then thyroid function tests, to demonstrate a suppressed thyroid stimulating hormone (TSH) level, or urine estimation of homocystine levels are indicated.

The assessment of sexual precocity is described in Chapter 6 and hypogonadism in Chapter 7.

If pituitary gigantism is a possibility, a raised IGF-1 level may be a useful screening test, followed by either a physiologic GH profile (**Fig. 3.36**) or the demonstration of a failure of suppression of GH levels to a glucose load (see Appendix).

Uniparental isodisomy (producing failure of IGF-2 imprinting on 11p) may be demonstrated in 80% of those with Beckwith–Wiedemann syndrome.

THERAPY

The treatment of children to limit their adult height is a highly specialized area that should be confined to experienced centers.

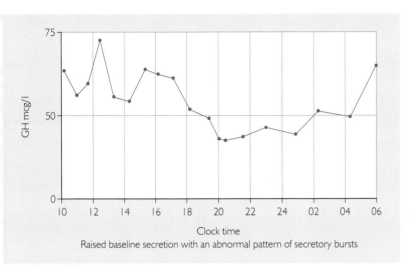

Fig. 3.36 GH profile in pituitary gigantism.

Raised baseline secretion with an abnormal pattern of secretory bursts

In idiopathic tall stature, a likely adult height of more than 185 cm (6 ft 1 inch) in a girl or 200 cm (6 ft 61/2 inches) in a boy may be arbitrarily defined as 'excessive', although much depends on the psychologic adjustment of the child and support from parents and peers. It is a mistake to treat children because of abnormal perceptions of tallness or past adverse experiences of one or both parents.

Artificial induction of an accelerated puberty will serve to limit adult height to a degree. This is usually performed by administering high daily doses of oral ethinylestradiol (100–200 µg) to girls and depot injections of testosterone (up to 500 mg every 2 weeks) to boys. Associated with this therapy are the psychologic problems of a sudden entry into sexual maturity and the physical ones of tender breasts and genitalia, a sudden onset of acne, etc. Priapism in boys on depot testosterone and thromboembolism in girls on estrogen treatment have been described. The future risks of long-term side effects, especially in girls of families with a strong history of breast cancer, are unknown but of concern.

Trials of recombinant long-acting somatostatin analog treatment are in progress and offer a more physiologic approach to therapy, but the late results of this treatment are still unknown.

There is probably no justification for treating the majority of those affected by the primary overgrowth syndromes as adult height is seldom a problem cosmetically.

It is often stated that sex hormone treatment of the Marfan syndrome should be approached with caution,

as there may be theoretical risks of increasing the likelihood of early cardiovascular disease, although published data to support this contention are lacking.

If a diagnosis of MEN-IIb is made, there should be urgent referral for prophylactic thyroidectomy, followed by thyroxine, vitamin D and calcium replacement therapy, and life-long surveillance for the development of pheochromocytoma.

Most boys with X duplication will need testosterone replacement therapy in order to undergo secondary sexual development and minimize disproportion. Conventionally this is performed with depot testosterone injections (50–100–250 mg sequentially; for details see Ch. 7), although patches and oral preparations may be used in some centers. All these treatments may worsen behavioral problems.

Surgical resection of long bone segments has been attempted to reduce height in various tall stature syndromes, but with limited success and a high morbidity due to resulting asymmetry. Drilling out the epiphyses at the upper tibia and lower femur may produce better results in experienced centers.

The treatments of sexual precocity, hypogonadism and thyrotoxicosis are discussed in Chapters 6, 7 and 9 respectively.

Basal brain tumors causing obesity should be referred to a specialist pediatric neurosurgeon for assessment and treatment. Likewise the trans-sphenoidal resection of a pituitary adenoma requires great expertise.

Chapter 4

The Thin Child

PHYSIOLOGY

Leanness can only be the result of an imbalance of energy intake, absorption, metabolism and output such that:

$$\text{Absorbed intake} \leq (\text{Output} + \text{Utilization})$$

If intake were greater in childhood, the extra calories would be used first for growth and then for fat deposition.

The commonest cause of thinness is failure of intake either from protein/calorie malnutrition endemic in many nations, or for psychosocial reasons in areas where food excess is usually more of a problem.

Food may be malabsorbed for a variety of reasons, or lost through vomit, stool or urine. Excess utilization may occur from chronic illness in any system and there are a few specific syndromes in which the endocrinologist may play a role.

Leptin levels will be low in the thin individual and this, plus other central factors, usually provides a drive to increase intake if food is made available. For unknown reasons this may not occur in anorexia nervosa and in the child with persistent growth failure secondary to intrauterine growth retardation (IUGR). Leptin also acts as a signal to initiate and maintain puberty, so there will be central hypogonadism. Insulin levels will also be low (except in cases associated with lipodystrophy and insulin resistance) and this acts to increase growth hormone (GH) and insulin-like growth factor (IGF-1) binding as an adaptive response to lack of energy. Hence prolonged calorie deficit is usually accompanied by growth failure and failure to enter or maintain puberty. The basal metabolic rate falls and there is a decreased conversion of thyroxine (T_4) to triiodothyronine (T_3).

Children normally grow in bursts. Over-frequent weighing will produce periods of zero weight gain, or even brief weight loss, in *normal* children. Therefore, a reasonable time interval should elapse between each measurement, and parental size should always be taken into account. It should also be remembered that 'catch-down growth' may be a normal phenomenon in the first 2 years if there has been an abnormal *in utero* environment producing overgrowth, or in the

situation of a tall mother and a short father. Finally, because of the definition of full-term delivery, cross-sectional standards for weight/length on the charts are based on data obtained from a population of between 37 and 42 weeks' gestation and may account for early centile crossing in some individuals.

There is evidence from many studies that IUGR or poor growth in infancy followed by catch-up growth can lead to the later development of adverse cardiovascular risk factors and insulin resistance (the 'Barker hypothesis'). It is unclear how this statistical effect relates to the management of individuals with pathologies described in this chapter, whereas the short-term effects of malnutrition have an obvious impact on the individual.

FAILURE OF INTAKE

MALNUTRITION

Protein-energy malnutrition can be subdivided into marasmus, which is usually seen between 6 and 12 months of age and is characterized by wasting and growth failure (**Figs 4.1 & 4.2**). If dietary protein is the main deficiency (kwashiorkor), there may be edema, apathy, skin and hair changes, and a swollen abdomen secondary to hepatomegaly (**Fig. 4.3**). There is a tendency to immunodeficiency (**Fig. 4.4**); in many countries with a high rate of malnutrition, a large proportion of the childhood population is also HIV positive, worsening the situation.

There may be associated vitamin deficiency states such as rickets (**Figs 4.5 & 4.6**) and pellagra (**Fig. 4.7**).

FAILURE TO THRIVE

This is a label describing a young child who is not gaining weight at an adequate rate. Inadequacy may be defined by weight–centile channel crossing over a stated period, as long as the reference standard is specified. Charts that allow for normal regression to the mean and variations in weight gain have been produced as conditional standards for weight gain and may be used in population screening. Similarly formulae using regression equations to calculate expected weight gain over a specified period can be derived from population studies and applied locally.

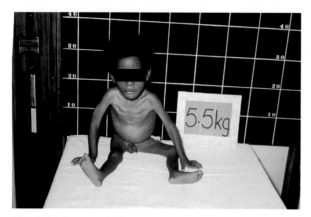

Fig. 4.1 Marasmus before nutritional rehabilitation.

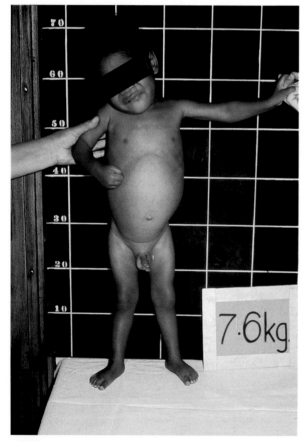

Fig. 4.2 Same patient as in Fig. 4.1 after nutritional rehabilitation.

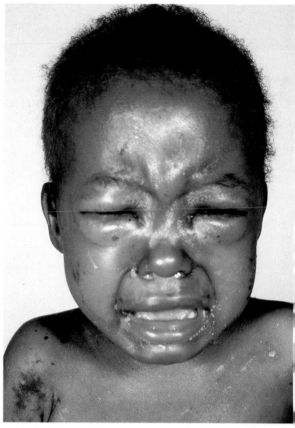

Fig. 4.3 Kwashiorkor.

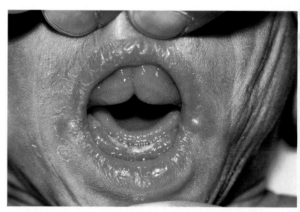

Fig. 4.4 Oral thrush and with angular stomatitis in B$_6$ riboflavin and niacin deficiency complicating severe malnutrition.

Each of these methods has different sensitivity and specificity at different ages and hence it is important to define the problem locally with appropriate referral guidelines. Parental (or medical) concern about poor weight gain may prompt referral. Intake is modified by psychosocial influences, and so maternal age and parity, extended family support, income and education should be taken into account. A family history of previous children with failure to thrive, explained or unexplained, especially if associated with consanguinity is important, as are previous infant deaths. Most cases of failure to thrive will be non-organic in nature, and the

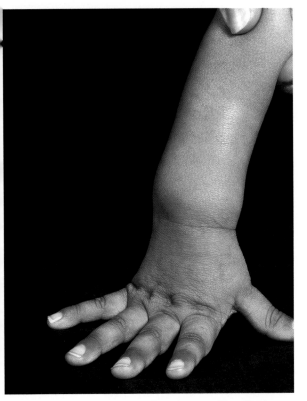

Fig. 4.5 Nutritional rickets with expansion of the distal forearm epiphyses.

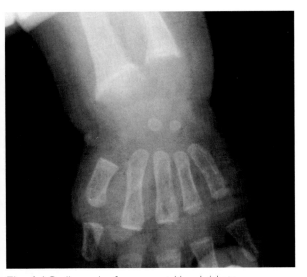

Fig. 4.6 Radiograph of severe nutritional rickets.

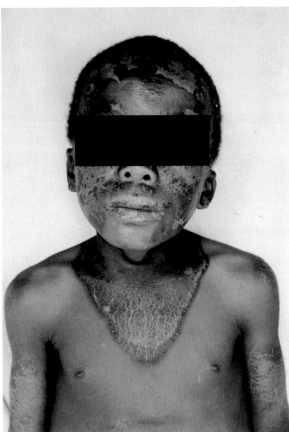

Fig. 4.7 Pellagra with 'Casal's necklace'.

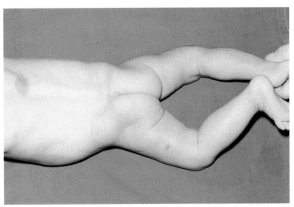

Fig. 4.8 Failure to thrive secondary to neglect, with bruise on upper back.

interaction between child and carer should be observed, as well as checking for neglect (**Fig. 4.8**). Cupping marks or scarification may be signs of use of traditional medicine and practices (**Fig. 4.9**). There is a recognized pattern of hyperphagic failure to thrive with growth failure that may be difficult to distinguish from GH deficiency.

ANOREXIA NERVOSA

This condition is commonest in adolescent females and consists of weight loss, amenorrhea and behavioral

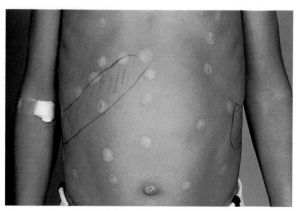

Fig. 4.9 Cupping marks. Reliance on traditional healing practices may delay referral for investigation and treatment.

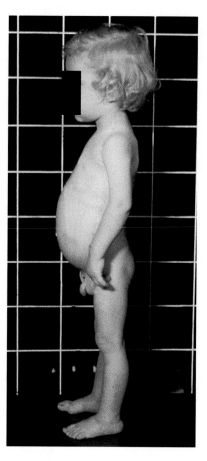

Fig. 4.10 Early-onset celiac disease.

changes related to food. Bulimia is a related disorder; sometimes occurring sequentially in the same individual where episodes of hyperphagia are interspersed with unusual means of weight reduction such as induced vomiting and laxative abuse. Luteinizing hormone (LH) and follicle stimulating hormone (FSH) levels are low and estrogen is usually undetectable. Even after recovery there may be a prolonged interval before normal hormone secretion is restored (see Ch. 7). Adaptive hormonal changes, including reduced T_3 levels, also occur. Osteoporosis and later fractures may be a consequence of the prolonged estrogen deficiency.

OTHER CAUSES OF FAILED INTAKE

Mechanical problems caused by cleft palate or neuromuscular abnormalities may prevent efficient feeding. If the 'critical window' for establishing enteral intake is missed in the first year, it may be difficult to teach to an older child who may require percutaneous gastrostomy PEG feeding. Breast-feeding failure is usually an early acute problem in some Western cultures, and can be overcome by support and education. Orange juice malnutrition is a specific recognized syndrome caused by the ingestion of large amounts of dilute orange squash; the child is thin with a distended abdomen and sloppy stools. Narcotic withdrawal and the fetal alcohol syndrome may produce early failure of weight gain.

FAILED ABSORPTION

Lactose intolerance usually is acquired following gastroenteritis with a loss of lactase in damaged microvilli in the small intestine. Severe congenital alactasia and other rare disaccharide deficiencies (amaltasia, asucrasia) are inherited as single-gene disorders. There are many non-caucasian populations with a high incidence of hypolactasia after infancy, and these individuals can tolerate only small amounts of dairy produce before suffering malabsorption and abdominal discomfort, but rarely fail to gain weight because of the aversive effects of lactose ingestion. However, lactose-containing feeds are inappropriate in famine-relief situations if the condition is common in the population.

Malabsorption may be secondary to the pancreatic exocrine failure seen in cystic fibrosis and the Schwachman–Diamond syndrome of growth failure, steatorrhea, metaphyseal dysplasia and neutropenia.

Celiac disease (**Figs 4.10 & 2.38**) and cow's milk protein intolerance (CMPI) may produce steatorrhea along with microcytic anemia and villus atrophy. Lymphangiectasia of the small intestine may also produce a protein-losing state.

Giardiasis (**Fig. 4.11**) and enteropathogenic *Escherichia coli* overgrowth may prevent nutrient absorption, as may the blind-loop syndrome and biliary problems.

Inflammatory bowel disease usually presents with abdominal pain and blood/mucus-containing stools,

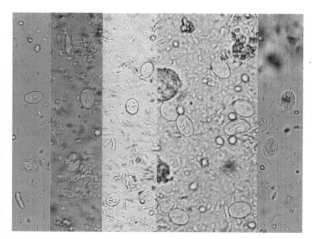

Fig. 4.11 Giardiasis showing birefringent 10-μm cysts in stool.

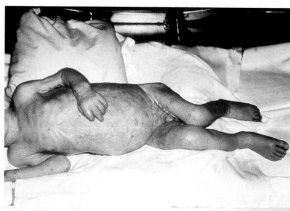

Fig. 4.12 Severe wasting in immunodeficiency.

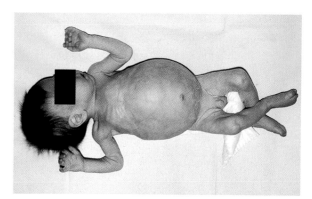

Fig. 4.13 Congenital cytomegalovirus infection, subsequent failure to thrive.

although it may occasionally present with failure to thrive, especially in the infantile form of ulcerative colitis. Failure to grow is a prominent feature of Crohn's disease, especially encompassing the pubertal years (**Fig. 2.33**), and these individuals are usually very underweight unless cushingoid secondary to treatment.

CALORIE LOSS

Vomiting from whatever cause will reduce calorie supply if it accounts for a significant portion of intake. Rumination (regurgitation of feeds as a habit comforting behavior in severe developmental delay) can cause significant calorie loss and dental erosion. The aminoacidurias (see below) often have vomiting as a presenting component.

Diarrhea produces intestinal hurry and a degree of malabsorption. Both can be due to numerous pathologies and also be induced factitiously by carers.

INCREASED UTILIZATION

Chronic infections, especially due to immunodeficiency and HIV, may produce severe wasting (**Fig. 4.12**). Congenital infections may produce IUGR with subsequent failure to thrive (**Fig. 4.13**). Overactivity may be secondary to attention deficit disorder or self-induced in athletes and gymnasts, sometimes coupled with anabolic steroid or laxative abuse. Malignancy, severe cardiac disease (especially in conjunction with chronic hypoxia) and liver disease can result in thinness or wasting. Chronic eczema, especially with nocturnal sleep disturbance from itching, can produce profound

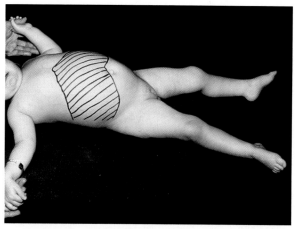

Fig. 4.14 Niemann–Pick disease.

thinness. Renal failure with metabolic acidosis may cause weight loss and there are specific syndromes of renal tubular acidosis that are accompanied by vomiting,

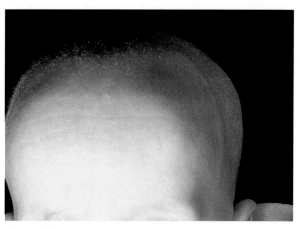

Fig. 4.15 Menke kinky hair disease.

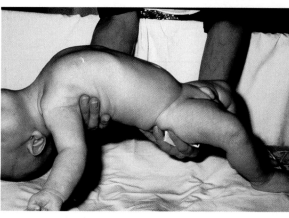

Fig. 4.16 Extreme hypotonia in biotinidase deficiency (completely reversed by subsequent biotin treatment).

rickets and growth failure. Bartter syndrome is caused by a failure of chloride reabsorption in the loop of Henle and a compensatory increase in plasma renin activity and hence hyperaldosteronism. It is characterized by hypochloremic alkalosis, hypokalemia, vomiting and failure to thrive. The de Toni–Fanconi syndrome of aminoaciduria, organic aciduria, glycosuria and hypophosphatemia may be due to cystinosis and heavy metal poisoning. A large number of other metabolic disorders may produce failure to thrive (**Table 4.1**).

Williams syndrome and other causes of hypercalcemia (see Ch. 11) produce weight loss and failure to thrive.

Diagnosis	Biochemistry	Additional effects
Urea cycle disorders	Branched-chain amino acid and organic acidurias	Vomiting, acidotic breathing and apneas, CNS features. Odd smell
Storage disorders	Glycogenoses, Wolman disease, infantile Gaucher and Niemann–Pick disease	CNS features, hepato(spleno)megaly (**Fig. 4.14**). Calcified adrenals in Wolman disease
Galactosemia	Galactose-1-phosphate uridyl transferase deficiency. Positive reducing sugars in urine	Lethargy, vomiting, liver failure, infections. Late cataracts and CNS features.
Hypophosphatasia	Early (recessive) and late (dominant) forms. Abnormality on 1p34-36. Low alkaline phosphatase level	Skin dimpling (see **Fig. 1.152**), CNS features, vomiting, fever. Poor bone mineralization
Menke disease	X-linked defect of copper transport	Lethargy, CNS features, abnormal temperature control. Abnormal hair (**Fig. 4.15**)
Fructose intolerance	1-Phosphofructaldolase deficiency	Vomiting, hypoglycemia, hepatomegaly
Biotin metabolic defects	Pyruvate carboxylase or biotinidase deficiency	Alopecia, floppiness (**Fig. 4.16**) rashes, lactic acidosis
Carnitine deficiencies	Fatty acid transport defect	Hypoglycemia, CNS features
Tyrosinemia type I	Fumarylacetoacetate hydrolase deficiency	CNS features, hepatomegaly and liver dysfunction, cabbage smell

Table 4.1 Some metabolic causes of failure to thrive (list not exhaustive)

Diabetes mellitus (see Ch. 10) produces catabolism due to failure of glucose uptake, as well as increased loss from glycosuria. Rarely, chronic poor regulation of blood sugar in a diabetic child can lead to short stature, wasting and hepatomegaly (the Mauriac syndrome) (**Figs 4.17 & 4.18**).

OTHER CAUSES OF EXTREME THINNESS

Russell–Silver syndrome (see **Table 2.2**) is characterized by IUGR, short stature, dysmorphic features and thinness. Leprechaunism (Donohue syndrome) (**Figs 4.19 & 4.20**) is characterized by IUGR, elfin facies, micrognathia with full lips, and hirsutism. The female may show clitoral hypertrophy, and both males and females may have sexual precocity. There is often hyperinsulinemia and acanthosis nigricans, and insulin receptor mutations have been described (see Ch. 10).

Partial lipodystrophies produce a muscular appearance and may again be associated with insulin resistance and cirrhosis in the autosomal recessive Berardinelli form (**Fig. 4.21**) or be acquired after infections when there is an associated abnormality of complement levels.

Progeria (**Fig. 4.22**), acrogeria and Werner syndromes are characterized by the appearance of early aging and cardiovascular disease with extreme thinness.

Diencephalic syndrome is a rare association of anterior hypothalamic tumors and extreme cachexia, usually presenting in early childhood (**Figs 4.23–4.26**). There is often hyperkinesia and later there may be associated endocrine abnormalities.

WORK-UP OF THE THIN CHILD

HISTORY AND EXAMINATION

- Most children will have non-organic failure to thrive and be pale, miserable and possibly show signs of overt neglect.
- Abdominal distension is seen in celiac disease and excess orange juice ingestion.
- Pigmentary changes = kwashiorkor.
- Edema and hepatomegaly = kwashiorkor.
- Opportunistic infections = severe malnutrition, diabetes, immunodeficiency.
- Lanugo hair (see **Fig. 1.147**) = anorexia.
- Excoriated eczema = nocturnal itching, atopy.
- Scratches on roof of mouth = bulimia.
- Dental erosion = bulimia and rumination.
- Weakness, developmental delay = neuromuscular

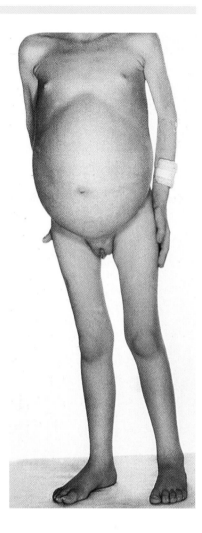

Fig. 4.17 Mauriac syndrome showing limb wasting and distended abdomen secondary to hepatomegaly.

problems, metabolic abnormalities.
- Focal CNS signs, café-au-lait spots = diencephalic syndrome.
- Respiratory signs = cystic fibrosis.
- Anal signs (skin tags and fissures) = inflammatory bowel disease (see **Fig. 1.95**).
- Anemia = severe nutritional lack, celiac disease and CMPI.
- Smelly wind = malabsorption, giardiasis ('purple burps').
- Abnormal smell = amino and organic acidurias (maple syrup = maple syrup urine disease; mousy = phenylketonuria; dried malt = oast-house urine disease; rancid butter = isovaleric acidemia; cat urine = β-methylcrotonyl coenzyme A carboxylase deficiency; dead fish = trimethylaminuria).
- Extreme thinness = malnutrition in endemic areas or secondary to severe neglect; anorexia, the lipodystrophies and premature aging syndromes.

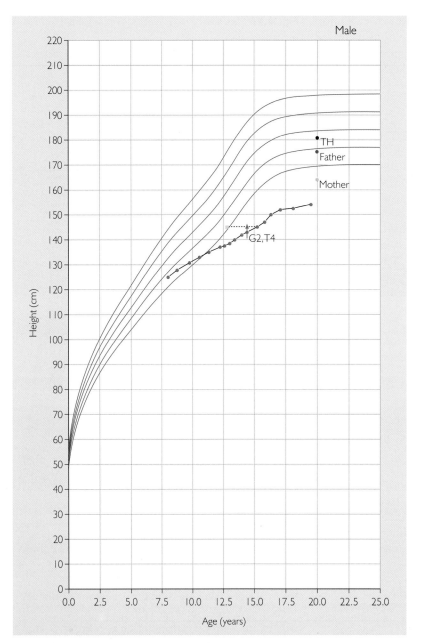

Fig. 4.18 Mauriac syndrome: height SDS −4 with delayed puberty and loss of final height secondary to long-standing poor diabetic control.

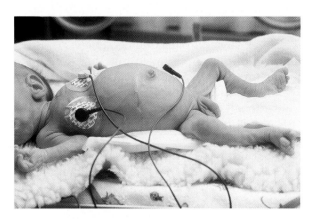

Fig. 4.19 Leprechaunism with severe IUGR.

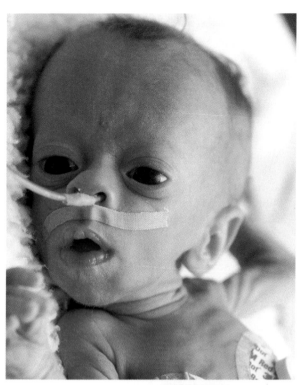

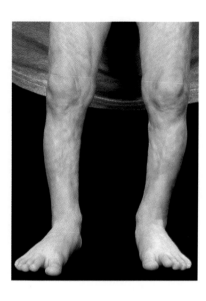

Fig. 4.20 Leprechaunism with lack of facial fat and full lips.

Fig. 4.22
Progeria with lipoatrophy and sceloderma-like changes of skin.

Fig. 4.21
Berardinelli form of lipodystrophy.

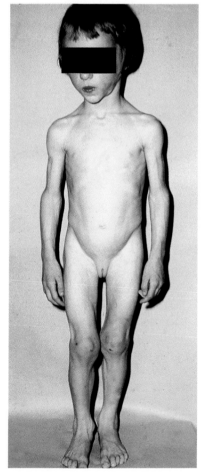

Fig. 4.23
Diencephalic syndrome with severe wasting.

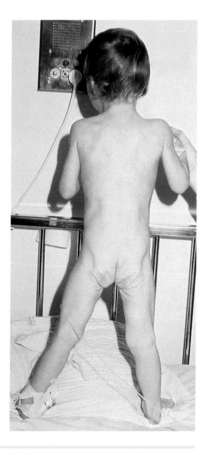

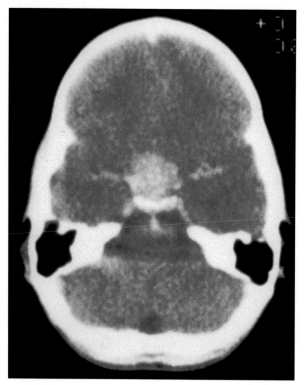

Fig. 4.24 Optic glioma in the patient shown in Fig. 4.23.

INVESTIGATIONS

Stool

- Macroscopic inspection for steatorrhea, blood, mucus.
- Microscopy for red blood cells (indicative of celiac disease, CMPI), *Giardia* cysts and fat globules – giardiasis; fat alone in cystic fibrosis and Schwachman syndrome.
- Culture for enteropathogenic *Escherichia coli*.
- Reducing substances are positive in lactose intolerance, alactasia and hypolactasia. Amaltasia and asucrasia also produce an acidic frothy stool positive for reducing substances; sugar chromatography will confirm the diagnosis in these rare cases.
- Stool pH is often reduced in presence of bacterial fermentation of undigested sugars.

Urine

- Microscopy and culture because unrecognized urinary tract infections and even renal failure from, for instance, posterior urethral valves, can cause failure to thrive (**Fig. 4.27**).
- Reducing substances for diabetes and galactosemia – further biochemical testing is then indicated.

Simple blood tests

- Full blood count for hemoglobin (Hb) and mean corpuscular volume (MCV) in particular. Microcytic anemia is a non-specific finding that may be secondary to inadequate iron intake or microscopic blood loss, and is present in renal failure and chronic ill health.
- Macrocytic anemia may be secondary to vitamin B_{12} or folate malabsorption with steatorrhea.
- Urea, creatinine and electrolytes to exclude hidden renal failure and rare metabolic disorders causing failure to thrive (i.e. Bartter syndrome of hyperchloremic alkalosis).

After these simple screening tests, further investigations may be indicated depending on the results, for instance anti-gliadin or cow's milk antibodies and jejunal biopsy; sweat tests or immunoreactive trypsin and genetic tests for cystic fibrosis. Chromosome analysis is indicated if there are any dysmorphic features (ring chromosome abnormalities have a predisposition to cause failure to thrive, sometimes with relatively mild dysmorphic features). Organic and amino acids and other metabolic tests may be indicated.

Chest radiography and ultrasonography may be indicated to exclude rare non-cyanotic and murmurless cardiac lesions, such as aberrant coronary arteries (**Fig. 4.28**) or fibroelastosis.

Lymphangiectasia of the small intestine may be demonstrated by a small bowel enema. Early cystic fibrosis may be indicated by multifocal consolidation (**Fig. 4.29**). Toxicological examination of blood, vomit, urine and stool should be undertaken if factitious illness induced by the carer is suspected.

TREATMENT

Dietary

Monitored increased intake at a therapeutic feeding station, along with vitamin supplementation as necessary, is ideal in populations with endemic malnutrition.

To treat non-organic failure to thrive it may be necessary to plan a period of in-patient observation and increasing social worker or medical/health visitor surveillance and support in the community setting. A dietitian can advise on regularizing food intake and cutting back dilute drink consumption.

Anorexia requires input from a multidisciplinary team of psychiatrists, nurses and dietitians in a supervised setting, and may necessitate nasogastric or even parenteral nutrition to stabilize body weight.

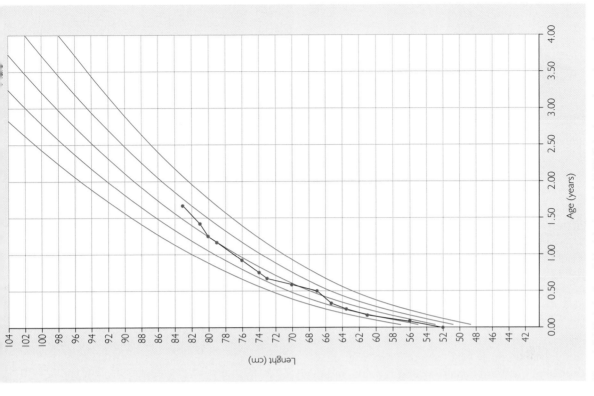

Fig. 4.26 Relatively mild height loss (–0.7 SDS) in the patient shown in Fig. 4.23.

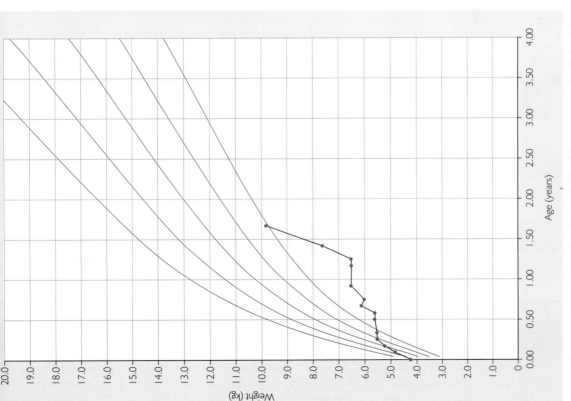

Fig. 4.25 Growth chart of the patient in Fig. 4.23 with extreme cachexia (weight SDS –4.5). Dramatic weight gain at 1.5 years following 4 weeks of radiotherapy.

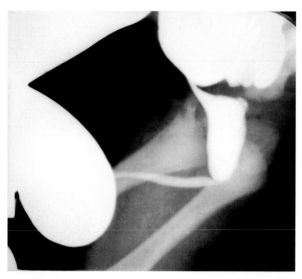

Fig. 4.27 Posterior urethral valves in 6-month-old male presenting with failure to thrive. Note distended posterior urethra and coexisting reflux.

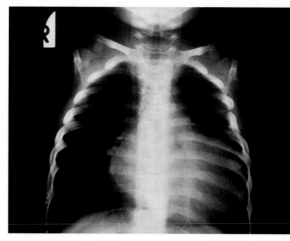

Fig. 4.28 Aberrant left coronary artery causing silent ischemia and failure to thrive.

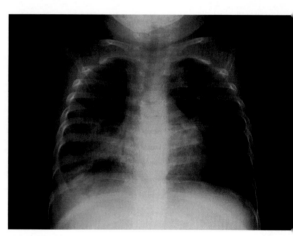

Fig. 4.29 Early cystic fibrosis not detected on neonatal screening; multifocal changes.

Other

Chronic vomiting may be a component of anatomical abnormalities of bowel anatomy and require surgical correction. It may also be seen in association with neurodevelopmental abnormalities. In these cases simple feed thickening and antireflux measures may suffice, but sometimes pro-kinetic agents are used. PEG feeds are often used for long-term management. Rumination may respond to phenothiazines.

Short-bowel syndrome may result from surgical resection or congenital abnormalities. If the absorptive surface is insufficient to allow normal growth even with dietary supplementation, then chronic intravenous nutrition may be required. There is some experimental evidence that GH may induce bowel lengthening.

Pancreatic exocrine failure can be treated with enzyme supplements with each meal, along with fat-soluble vitamins. Biliary abnormalities may respond to bile salt administration to emulsify feeds.

CMPI and celiac disease are treated by milk- and gluten-free diets respectively (initially there may be additional lactose intolerance in celiac disease until the villi have regrown, requiring a gluten- and milk-free diet), followed by re-biopsy to confirm response. Gluten enteropathy is life-long, but CMPI may remit after dietary intervention. Intestinal lymphangiectasia requires surgical resection as long as sufficient bowel length can be preserved for later successful feeding.

Temporary lactose intolerance requires 3–6 months of lactose-free diet to allow regeneration of the lactase-containing microvilli. Alactasia and the other autosomal recessive disaccharidase deficiencies require specific sugar-free diets life-long.

Poor weight gain secondary to immunodeficiency will improve with anti-retroviral or other immuno therapy, but relapses when infection recurs. There is some evidence that GH may have a useful anabolic role to play in these cases.

The insulin resistance in lipodystrophy is un responsive to exogenous insulin but may be improved by recombinant leptin and IGF-1 administration.

Treatment of specific metabolic or organ disease may reverse the failure to thrive. In particular in young children with renal tract abnormalities, antibiotic prophylaxis and investigation of the renal tract with surgical intervention, if required, are mandatory.

Bartter syndrome may be treated with a combination of salt supplements, potassium-sparing diuretics and indometacin.

Chapter 5

The Overweight Child

DEFINITION

Obesity implies the presence of excess body fat, and any increase in adipose mass is the result of increased storage of triglycerides. Thus, ideally, the diagnosis of obesity should be based on a direct demonstration of an increased amount of body fat. This is possible directly, for example with imaging techniques – computed tomography (CT), magnetic resonance imaging (MRI) and dual-energy X-ray absortptiometry (DEXA) scanning – and underwater weighing, and indirectly with ultrasonography, bioelectrical impedance analysis or skinfold thickness measurements. However, these technical measurements of body composition are not suitable for routine practice, and are limited to research protocols.

The use of skinfold thickness requires an experienced technician who knows how to use skinfold callipers appropriately (see **Figs 1.10–1.13**). Equations have been published to estimate fat mass from skinfold measurements, but their accuracy is limited, especially in individuals with very small or very large amounts of body fat.

Therefore, for clinical purposes, body weight is the usual proxy parameter for defining a child being thin (underweight), normal or fat (overweight). Overweight can also, by analogy to short or tall stature, be defined as a weight above the normal range, but in this case the situation is somewhat more complex. However, the cut-off limits for overweight and more extreme overweight (which is then labeled 'obesity') should be determined along with the reference data used to define the chosen cut-off limits for all age groups. It should be remembered that overweight can be caused not only by excess fat, but also by increased fat-free mass (e.g. muscle in well-trained athletes), and skinfold thickness measurements can help to differentiate in these cases.

There is a general consensus that body mass index (BMI, or Quetelet's index), calculated as weight (kg) divided by height (m) squared (weight/height^2), is the most suitable parameter to define overweight. It has a high correlation with fatness, is largely independent of height, and is the standard measure used in adulthood. Age- and sex-related references are available from many countries. In several of these references the strongly skewed distribution of BMI for age has been transformed into a Gaussian distribution, so that an individual BMI can be expressed as a standard deviation score (SDS) for age. Age reference values for BMI from the 1997 nationwide growth study in the Netherlands are shown in **Figs 5.1 & 5.2**.

Alternatively, weight can be plotted (on a logarithmic scale) versus height (on a linear scale) and compared with references for weight-for-height. An individual weight can then be expressed as a percentage of median weight for height. As the 90th centile is close to 110% of median weight-for-height, this percentage has also been used as cut-off for overweight. A comparison of weight-for-age percentile position with height-for-age percentile position has also been used in various countries, but this procedure systematically overestimates the target weight of adolescents.

With respect to the cut-off limits used to define underweight, overweight and obesity, an international task force of the World Health Organization and the European Childhood Obesity Group suggested pediatric centiles derived from the extrapolation of a BMI of 20, 25 and 30 kg/m^2 in young adults as the respective cut-off values. To establish the centiles, an analysis of six large population studies (from Brazil, the UK, Hong Kong, Netherlands, Singapore and the USA) resulted in two curves for each sex corresponding to 25 and 30 kg/m^2 in young adults (see **Figs 5.1 & 5.2**). These can now be used as the standard definitions for child overweight and obesity.

Although BMI SDS is the most practical index of overweight, it is still not a very accurate parameter of obesity for any given individual. In the absence of increased fat mass, body weight and hence BMI can be high due to a relatively high fat-free mass. On the other hand, excess fat mass will not be detected by increased BMI in cases of severe muscle wasting and osteoporosis.

BMI also gives no information about the distribution of body fat. In adults the regional distribution of body fat appears to be an important factor in determining

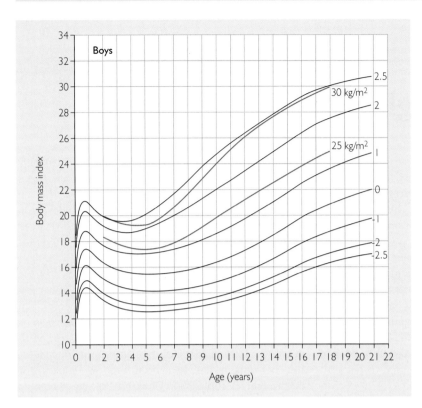

Fig. 5.1 Body mass index for age in Dutch boys compared with cut-off lines for overweight (extrapolated from 25 kg/m² at 18 years) and obesity (extrapolated from 30 kg/m²) according to international growth references (Cole et al. *BMJ* 2000; 320: 1240–3). Lines indicate 0, ±1, ±2 and ±2.5 SDS. From Fredriks et al. Fourth Dutch growth study. *Arch Dis Child* 2000; 82: 107–12.

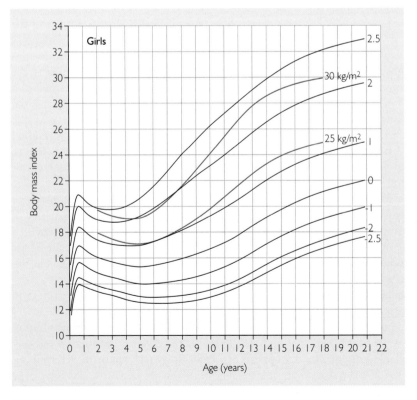

Fig. 5.2 Body mass index for age in Dutch girls, as in Fig. 5.1. From Fredriks et al. Fourth Dutch growth study. *Arch Dis Child* 2000; 82: 107–12.

the risk profile for various diseases (i.e. the components of the metabolic syndrome or syndrome X). Abdominal obesity, which generates an 'apple' form of the body habitus (android obesity), is associated with insulin resistance, cardiovascular disease, non-insulin-dependent diabetes mellitus, stroke and hyperlipidemia. In the case of a body habitus with a peripheral fat distribution in the femoral area, called the 'pear' shape (gynoid obesity), these risks are much lower. Body fat distribution can be assessed by measuring the waist and hip circumferences, and calculating the waist : hip ratio. However, while in adults a ratio greater than 0.9 in males and 0.8 in females is associated with increased risk of insulin resistance and associated diseases, such standards have not been established in childhood obesity. Recent Dutch references for waist and hip circumferences, and the waist : hip ratio are presented in **Figs 5.3–5.8**.

EPIDEMIOLOGY

In all industrialized countries the percentage of overweight children has increased spectacularly in the past few decades. Percentages obviously depend on the definition used. Using the international definition described above, in the Netherlands the mean prevalence of overweight increased from 9.4% in 1980 to 13.4% in 1997, and in many other industrialized countries higher percentages have been reported. In children of Moroccan and Turkish origin, the percentages were close to 20%. The main reasons for this increase are probably changes in diet and activity patterns. The amount of fat and other calorie-rich food components in the diet of children has increased tremendously, together with the growing consumption of fast food and sweetened soft drinks. At the same time, children and adolescents nowadays spend much time watching television and playing computer games, so that physical activity has decreased. There is also an interaction effect, as children consume many snacks while watching television, and at the same time they are bombarded by TV commercials advertising fast food. Physical activity is probably also decreased by the fact that many children and youngsters have few opportunities to play outdoors and by fewer facilities in school. It has been shown that the prevalence of overweight and obesity is associated with living in a city and with lower socioeconomic status. The increase in the percentage of overweight children can be considered a prelude to a great increase in the prevalence of obesity in adults, as many obese children will become obese adults. This will have grave consequences for public health, especially cardiovascular health.

As overweight causes earlier puberty, possibly through the influence of leptin on pulsatile gonadotropin secretion, the population trend toward a higher prevalence of overweight causes a shift in the age references for pubertal stages, especially for girls. In obese male adolescents gynecomastia is relatively common, probably due to aromatase activity in adipocytes producing estrone from androstenedione.

PHYSIOLOGY

A simplistic view of the control of body fat is that a control system of appetite and satiety, localized in the hypothalamus, regulates dietary intake, in order to balance energy expenditure. However, the precise regulatory mechanisms have not yet been clarified. Part of the controlling system is a negative feedback loop, in which leptin, produced by adipose tissue, provides a feedback signal to the hypothalamic centers. Serum leptin levels are age dependent and correlated with fat mass. Age references are available, but the clinical value of measurement of serum leptin levels is not yet clear. Leptin circulates bound to a specific carrier protein and is actively transported across the blood–brain barrier to act on specific receptors in the ventromedial nucleus of the hypothalamus, probably along with other signals from glucose and insulin. Subsequent interactions with neuropeptides (e.g. neuropeptide Y) and corticotropin releasing hormone (CRH) and pro-opiomelanocortin (POMC) in the arcuate and dorsomedial nucleus act to control feeding behavior mediated through the paraventricular nucleus. Recently, it has also become clear in animal studies that adipocytes produce a host of other specific proteins, one of which, resistin, may induce insulin resistance, thus linking diabetes to obesity, although there are few data in humans. Ghrelin, secreted by the gastrointestinal tract in response to gastric dilatation, may modulate central growth hormone (GH) release and hence peripheral lipolysis. Some undefined genetic factors may have had survival value when famine was common, but now lead to obesity in people living in affluent conditions.

Obesity causes alterations in endocrine physiology. The strongest effect is seen on the somatotropic axis, and includes low levels of serum GH (also in response to provocation), high levels of GH binding protein (GHBP), normal (or raised) levels of insulin-like growth factor (IGF-1) and IGF binding protein (IGFBP-3), and low levels of IGFBP-1. Serum triiodothyronine (T_3) concentration is slightly increased, probably as a result of increased conversion of thyroxine (T_4) to T_3. The prolactin response to thyrotropin releasing hormone (TRH) may be blunted. Cortisol secretion rate is increased, but

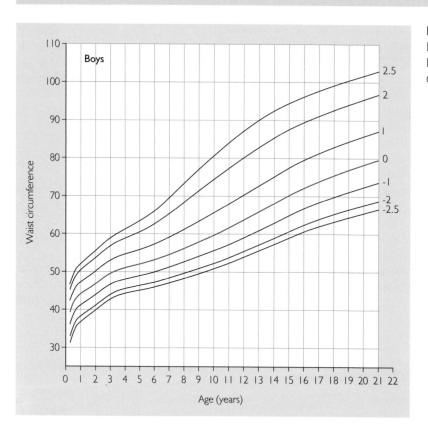

Fig. 5.3 Waist circumference in Dutch boys. From Fredriks et al. Fourth Dutch growth study. *Arch Dis Child* 2000; 82: 107–12.

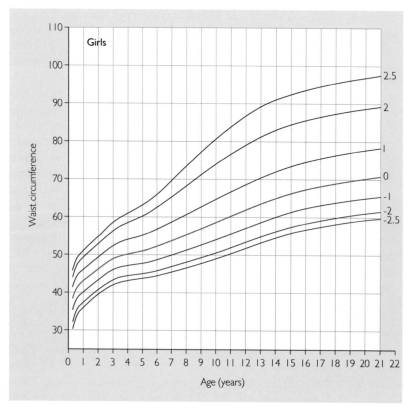

Fig. 5.4 Waist circumference in Dutch girls. From Fredriks et al. Fourth Dutch growth study. *Arch Dis Child* 2000; 82: 107–12.

Fig. 5.5 Hip circumference in Dutch boys. From Fredriks et al. Fourth Dutch growth study. *Arch Dis Child* 2000; 82: 107–12.

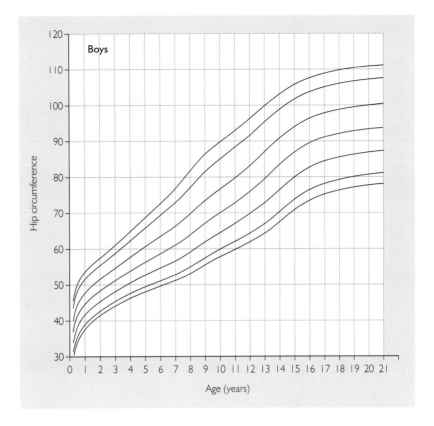

Fig. 5.6 Hip circumference in Dutch girls. From Fredriks et al. Fourth Dutch growth study. *Arch Dis Child* 2000; 82: 107–12.

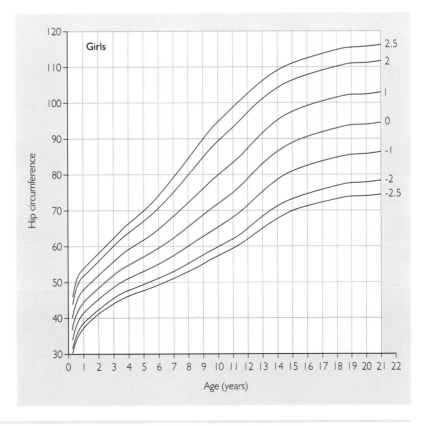

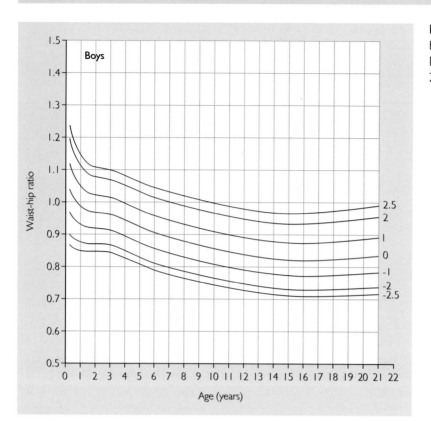

Fig. 5.7 Waist : hip ratio in Dutch boys. From Fredriks et al. Fourth Dutch growth study. *Arch Dis Child* 2000; 82: 107–12.

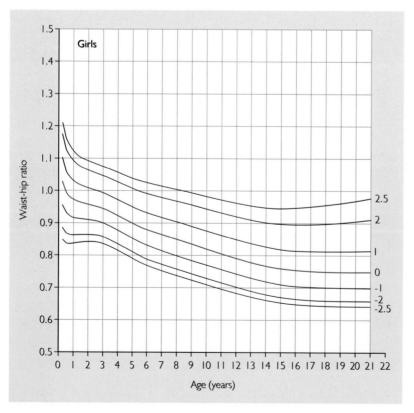

Fig. 5.8 Waist : hip ratio in Dutch girls. From Fredriks et al. Fourth Dutch growth study. *Arch Dis Child* 2000; 82: 107–12.

serum cortisol levels and urinary free cortisol excretion are normal. In boys serum testosterone and sex hormone binding globulin (SHBG) are decreased and estrogen (especially estrone) concentration is increased. In girls levels of both estrogens and androgens are increased, SHBG concentration is low, and puberty is advanced. Insulin resistance is usually present.

CAUSES

SIMPLE OBESITY

In most cases, obesity in childhood is caused by a combination of genetic and environmental factors. There is frequently a family history of overweight, which can be an expression of the genetic influences as well as the influence of family dietary practices. A dietary history usually indicates excessive calorie intake, although the actual intake is often underreported. This is usually called 'simple obesity', although its pathophysiology, as well as its treatment, is far from simple. Growth velocity is slightly increased, so that the majority of overweight and obese children have a height in the upper half of the population reference, and higher than the target height. Bone age is often slightly advanced, as well as the onset of puberty. Adult height is generally close to target height; however, those with the earliest progression into puberty may be several centimeters below their target height as adults. Psychologic disturbances are often present, and may play a role in the development of obesity. However, obesity also leads to psychologic problems and social stigmatization.

Examination

- The excess subcutaneous fat is often the only abnormality (**Figs 3.29 & 5.9**).
- Some children show high cheek color, mimicking Cushing syndrome (see **Fig. 3.30**). Striae (usually quite narrow) may also be present.
- Hypertension may be present (but a large sphygmomanometer cuff must be used).
- Hirsutism from polycystic ovary changes and the low SHBG levels secondary to insulin resistance (see **Figs 6.33–6.35**).
- Limited rotation of the hip may indicate slipped femoral epiphyses (**Fig. 5.10**).
- Acanthosis nigricans and skin tags may indicate insulin resistance (see **Fig. 1.140**).

Investigation

There may be a number of metabolic changes:

- Hyperinsulinemia and impaired fasting glucose, which can lead to glucose intolerance and type 2

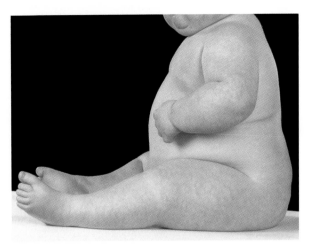

Fig. 5.9 Gross infantile obesity.

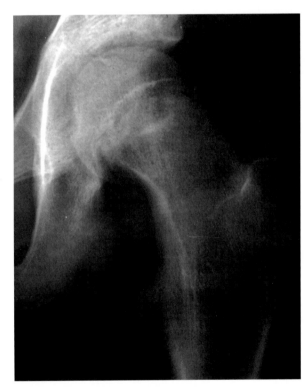

Fig. 5.10 Slipped capital femoral epiphysis.

diabetes mellitus. The incidence of this type of diabetes in childhood and adolescence has increased greatly in the past two decades (see Ch. 10).
- Hyperlipidemia is associated with obesity.
- Sleep apnea can occur with right heart failure in extreme cases (**Figs 5.11 & 5.12**).
- Non-alcoholic steatohepatitis (NASH) may result in progressive abnormalities of liver function (**Fig. 5.13**).

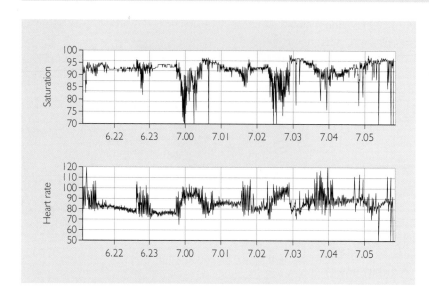

Fig. 5.11 Oximetry trace from the patient in Fig. 5.9 demonstrating sleep apnea with dips in oxygen saturation to less than 80%.

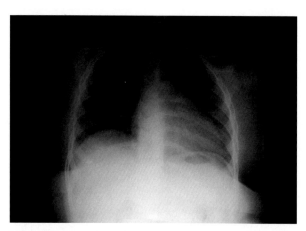

Fig. 5.12 Cor pulmonale with gross obesity (note subcutaneous fat thickness).

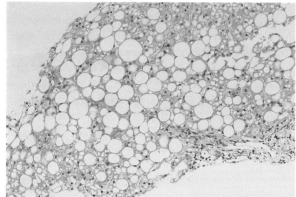

Fig. 5.13 Liver biopsy of non-alcoholic steatohepatitis (NASH) in simple dietary obesity. Note large fat-filled spaces. Liver function deranged with raised transaminases and γ-glycosyltransferase.

- In adulthood, persistent obesity can lead to the same disorders, as well as coronary heart disease, stroke, gallbladder disease, psychosocial disability and osteoarthritis.

ENDOCRINE CAUSES OF OVERWEIGHT

While simple obesity is associated with *increased* growth velocity, most endocrine causes of obesity are associated with a decreased growth rate. Although an endocrine cause can be found in only a small minority of obese children, it is important to perform additional investigations to diagnose or exclude an endocrine cause. The main clinical reason is for treatment but another, less medical, reason is that many parents know of the association between obesity and 'hormones or

glands' and expect endocrine causes to be investigated (see Ch. 2).

Juvenile hypothyroidism

This is characterized by slow growth, delayed bone maturation and (mostly mild) obesity (see Chs 2 & 9) (see **Fig. 9.5**). Substitution therapy with L-thyroxine normalizes the clinical picture completely, although adult height may be less than the target height (see **Fig. 2.91**).

Glucocorticoid excess

Glucocorticoid excess, due either to exogenous administration or to an increase in endogenous production, also causes slow growth and obesity. Even a small excess of steroids above physiologic substitution can cause obesity.

For the clinical characteristics of Cushing syndrome, see Chapter 2. The classic 'buffalo hump' and the centripetal fat distribution are not always seen in children. A 24-h urine free cortisol and a diurnal cortisol rhythm are probably the most sensitive screening tests. If clinical concern persists, an overnight dexamethasone suppression test is often performed followed by low- and high-dose dexamethasone suppression tests and imaging studies as appropriate (see Appendix). If Cushing syndrome or disease is treated successfully, BMI decreases, although often not completely (see **Figs 2.42 & 2.43**).

Growth hormone deficiency

GH deficiency is characterized primarily by slow growth, but in severe cases there may be truncal obesity (see **Fig. 2.9**). The truncal fat may have a dimpled appearance (see **Fig. 1.124**).

The BMI is usually in the normal range, except when a hypothalamic disorder (e.g. craniopharyngioma) is the cause of GH deficiency. GH treatment not only causes catch-up growth, but also normalization of body composition, with disappearance of truncal obesity.

Mauriac syndrome

This condition, which occurs when diabetes mellitus is poorly treated, is now rarely seen in industrialized countries (see **Figs 4.17 & 4.18**). Poor growth is combined with peripheral wasting and abdominal distension, leading to a superficial appearance of overweight.

Other conditions

There are also two endocrine conditions in which obesity is not associated with poor growth:

- Insulinoma, which is characterized primarily by hypoglycemia (see Ch. 11).
- Polycystic ovary syndrome (PCOS), a syndrome of dysregulation of the hypothalamo-pituitary–gonadal axis, of which the pathophysiology is still unclear (see Ch. 6). It is associated with obesity, insulin resistance, hypertension, hirsutism, menstrual irregularity and high serum levels of luteinizing hormone (LH). Its prevalence appears to have risen in adolescents along with the rising prevalence of obesity. A history of intrauterine growth retardation is said to be a risk factor.

CENTRAL NERVOUS SYSTEM CAUSES

Tumors, malformations, infiltration (histiocytosis) and damage by infections (meningitis, encephalitis) or

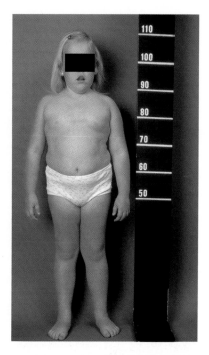

Fig. 5.14 Moderate obesity secondary to large arachnoid cyst, shown in Fig. 5.15.

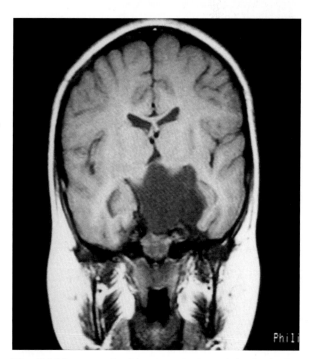

Fig. 5.15 Large arachnoid cyst causing hypothalamic obesity.

trauma (birth trauma or another causality) in the hypothalamus often result in abnormal weight gain. If a hypothalamic lesion is suspected, brain imaging (MRI) is indicated (**Figs 5.14–5.16**). Obesity may be extreme (morbid) in children with hypothalamic tumors, such as craniopharyngioma, particularly after

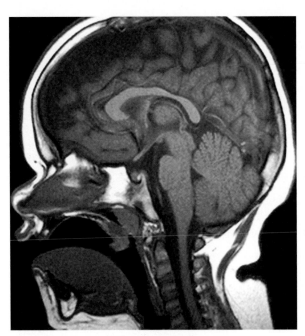

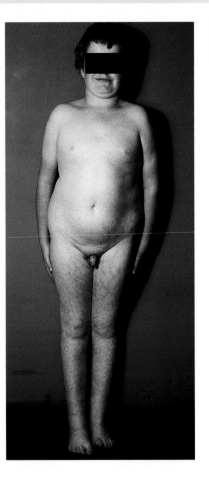

Fig. 5.17
Prader–Willi
syndrome.

Fig. 5.16 Normal MRI of pituitary and hypothalamus in suspected central disorder of eating behaviour in child with absent thyroid stimulating hormone (TSH) response to thyrotropin releasing hormone (TRH) and central hypothyroidism. Note the massive subcutaneous skinfold seen at the neck.

surgery. Compulsive eating and lack of satiety may be the most important etiologic factor, but it is likely that changes in energy expenditure are also involved. These forms of obesity are very difficult to treat.

CHROMOSOMAL DEFECTS

Chromosomal disorders with trisomy or deletion and duplication of the X chromosome are associated with mild obesity (such as Turner, Klinefelter and Down syndromes).

OTHER GENETIC DEFECTS

Prader–Willi syndrome

After a period of hypotonia and poor feeding in the first year, obesity typically develops between 1 and 4 years of age. There are a number of dysmorphic features, intellectual impairment, slow growth and hypogonadism (**Fig. 5.17**) (see also Ch. 2 – **Table 2.2, Figs 2.15 & 2.16**). The dietary treatment of obesity is usually very difficult, although with special behavior modification reasonable results can be obtained, particularly if started early. However, prevention of obesity in early childhood is most important.

Other

Other, less well known, syndromes associated with obesity are Beckwith–Wiedemann syndrome (see **Figs. 3.17–3.19**), Laurence–Moon–Biedl syndrome (see **Figs 1.117 & 5.18**), Alstrom syndrome, Cohen syndrome, Carpenter syndrome (see **Fig. 1.31**) and pseudohypoparathyroidism (see **Figs 1.28, 1.29, 1.81, 2.51**).

GENETIC DISORDERS OF CENTRAL APPETITE REGULATION

These abnormalities are rare, but potentially treatable. They offer some insights as to the genesis of obesity in the general population.

A few families with massive obesity due to leptin deficiency or leptin receptor defect have been described. There is often consanguinity and a family history of hypogonadism. Here, treatment with recombinant leptin can produce massive weight loss and restoration of pulsatile gonadotropin secretion (**Fig. 5.19**).

A small number of other rare abnormalities of hypothalamic signals of satiety have been described, including the red-haired human homolog of the Agouti

Fig. 5.18
Laurence–Moon
-Biedl syndrome.

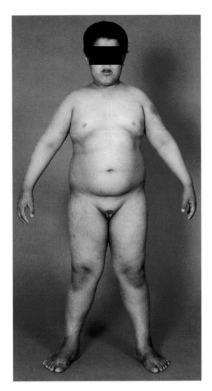

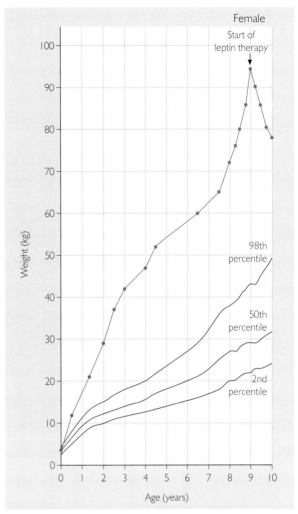

mouse due to POMC deficiency. More such rare defects will undoubtedly emerge with further research.

OBESITY ACCOMPANYING IMMOBILITY, MENTAL DISTURBANCE, SOCIAL AND CULTURAL PRESSURE

In children with muscular dystrophy, spina bifida, achondroplasia, immobilization after trauma and/or orthopedic surgery, and intellectual impairment, obesity is secondary to a combination of decreased energy expenses due to immobility, overprotection of parents, and abnormal food intake resulting from mental disturbance or social/cultural pressure. In such cases it may be useful to assess body composition, with auxological or technical means.

IATROGENIC OBESITY

Obesity can be caused by various medications:

- Corticosteroids (see endocrine causes).
- Overmedication with insulin in diabetes, which may lure adolescents into a vicious circle of insulin overdosage–hypoglycemia–overeating–obesity–insulin resistance and back to insulin overdosage.
- Sodium valproate, carbamazepine, phenothiazine, tricyclic antidepressants and cyproheptadine.

Fig. 5.19 Treatment of congenital leptin deficiency with recombinant leptin. In addition to weight loss there was a reversal of central hypogonadism. From Farooqi S et al. *N Engl J Med* 2000; 341: 879–84. Copyright © 2000 Massachusetts Medical Society. All rights reserved.

EVALUATION OF THE OVERWEIGHT CHILD

HISTORY AND EXAMINATION

Although in most obese children no pathologic cause can be found, to permit the label of 'simple obesity' to be given, a full history and physical examination have to be performed in all cases.

Growth should be plotted along with previous measurements of height and weight.

Data on height and weight of parents and siblings provide insight into possible genetic factors and familial dietary patterns.

A detailed history of diet (not forgetting non-diet soft drink use) and physical activity is essential, although

Fig. 5.20 Severe dietary obesity: weight +7.7 SDS.

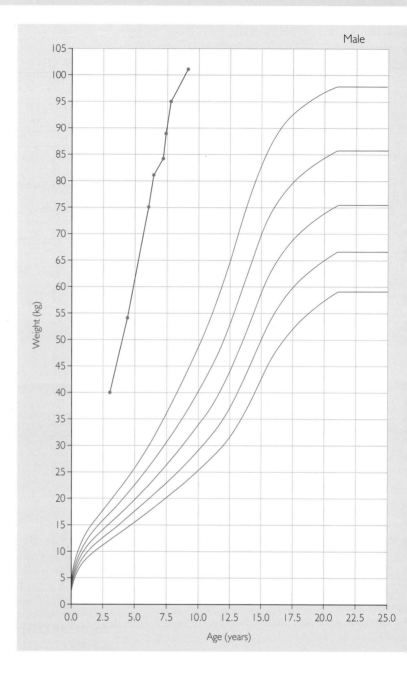

it may be difficult to get reliable information. More detailed and reliable information can be obtained by asking the child and family to fill a dietary diary and activity log, although compliance and accuracy may still be a problem.

A detailed psychosocial history is needed to understand the development of obesity, as well as the severity of the psychosocial consequences of obesity.

Interpretation of the clues

- Low height velocity points to hypothyroidism, Cushing syndrome or GH deficiency (see Ch. 2).

- A growth curve above the target height centile with mildly increased height velocity excludes these three endocrine causes and is compatible with 'simple' obesity (**Figs 5.20 & 5.21**).

- Calculating the weight gained in relation to height gained over a specified period can allow an estimation of the excess calorie intake; 1 kg fat is deposited by 9000 kilocalories (kcal) of excess intake (and releases 7000 kcal energy (28 MJ) when utilized). Therefore a gain in weight of 5 kg more than expected for the height gained over 1 year is equivalent to

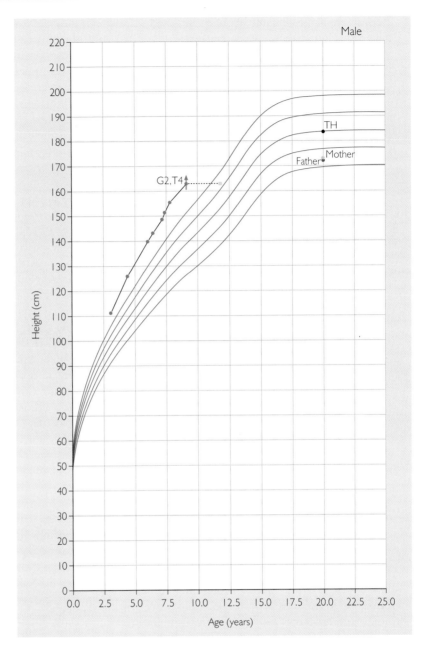

Fig. 5.21 Same patient as in Fig. 5.20 with height +3.5 SDS, compared with target height of 0 SDS. Advanced bone age and early pubertal changes at 9 years mean that final height is likely to be within the normal centile range but above target height.

5 × 9000 = 45 000/365 = 123 kcal per day excess to requirements, or about half a bag of potato chips.

- Polydipsia and polyuria = diabetes mellitus (type 2); rarely, diabetes insipidus.
- Headache, neurologic symptoms and signs = suspicion of CNS cause.
- Hypertension, plethora = Cushing syndrome.
- In female adolescents menstrual irregularities, hirsutism, acne, acanthosis nigricans = PCOS.
- Hirsutism = PCOS or Cushing syndrome.
- Fat distribution – a central (masculine, android) distribution is associated with an increased risk for cardiovascular morbidity and can be found in Cushing syndrome.
- A peripheral (feminine, gynoid) pattern is predominantly located in the lower body.
- Acanthosis nigricans = insulin resistance.
- Early hypotonia, small hands and feet, intellectual impairment, marked increase in energy intake after age 2 years = Prader–Willi syndrome.
- Polydactyly, retinitis pigmentosa = Laurence–Moon–Biedl syndrome.
- Hypogonadism = Prader–Willi syndrome, Laurence–Moon–Biedl syndrome, GH deficiency, leptin deficiency or CNS cause.

■ Neonatal hyperinsulinemic hypoglycemia and macrosomia in infancy, visceromegaly, macroglossia = Beckwith–Wiedemann syndrome.

■ Early onset of voracious appetite, parental consanguinity, a family history of hypogonadism and extreme obesity = leptin deficiency or receptor abnormality.

■ Red hair with early onset of voracious appetite, parental consanguinity and extreme obesity = POMC abnormality.

INVESTIGATIONS

If height is within the population and target ranges (particularly if it is in the upper range of the target range), and height velocity over the foregoing years is normal, an endocrine cause is virtually excluded and the likelihood of the diagnosis of simple obesity is very high. In the absence of other clues from the history and examination, except for clear indications that calorie and fat intake is too high in relation to energy expenditure, *further laboratory investigations are not strictly necessary*. Documentation of metabolic abnormalities associated with overweight may be helpful, as abnormal values may reinforce the wish of the child or adolescent and parents to work hard to lose weight. This can include liver function, fasting triglycerides, low and high density lipoproteins and total cholesterol, glucose, insulin and glycosylated hemoglobin levels. A bone age assessment does not provide much additional information, although it may be useful in predicting the age of pubertal onset.

Subclinical hypothyroidism can be excluded by measuring the level of thyroid stimulating hormone (TSH).

In the well growing, obese, adolescent female, if menstrual irregularities are reported, possibly combined with signs of hirsutism and/or acanthosis nigricans, investigation for PCOS may be required:

■ serum estrogens (E_1, E_2), androgens (testosterone, androstenedione, dehydroepiandrosterone sulfate (DHEAS)), SHBG and gonadotropins (LH, follicle stimulating hormone (FSH), either basal or stimulated). Classically, raised serum E_1, normal E_2, low SHBG, raised testosterone and free testosterone and/or androstenedione concentrations are found, as well as an LH level that is considerably higher than that of FSH. Abdominal sonography may show ovarian cysts but is not necessary for diagnosis in the presence of other features.

If the child is short, or the height velocity is low, then hypothyroidism, Cushing syndrome, GH deficiency and pseudohypoparathyroidism need exclusion (see Chs 2, 9 & 11, and Appendix).

If there are signs of Prader–Willi syndrome, specific genetic analysis is performed for deletion of the paternal allele at 15q11-13 or for a duplication of the maternal allele at this locus.

Serum leptin can be assayed in research protocols searching for rare genetic causes of obesity.

TREATMENT

The large increase of the prevalence of overweight and obesity in past decades would suggest that lifestyle changes, in particular diet and physical activity, should be the targets for preventive intervention at a population level. However, there are currently few societies where this action is being taken in a concerted manner.

At the same time, this suggests that treatment for simple obesity should consist of limiting calorie and fat intake, and stimulating physical activity. In practice, however, it appears very difficult for children and adolescents to lose weight successfully.

If the child or adolescent has hypertension, hepatitis, hyperlipidemia or glucose intolerance, an active approach toward weight reduction should be taken. This should ideally consist of a closely supervised diet and exercise plan in a family-based behavior modification program.

However, even in the absence of such abnormalities, treatment is indicated, as childhood obesity leads to approximately 30% of adult obesity and the obese child who becomes an obese adult will have more severe adult obesity than those whose obesity begins in adulthood. Long-term follow-up of obese adolescents has demonstrated that cardiovascular mortality and morbidity rates are increased compared with those in lean adolescents. The most effective treatment is a multidisciplinary, comprehensive and family-oriented approach. This includes a combination of behavioral modification procedures, education, dietary intervention with calorie restriction, and an activity and exercise program. However, such treatment programs are time consuming for patient, parent and health personnel, and unfortunately there is a considerable drop-out rate and a high rate of recidivism to obesity in the following years. For a more successful long-term outcome the child or adolescent, and if possible the parents, should change or modify attitudes, beliefs and behavior with respect to eating and physical activity.

Dietary therapy should focus on a calorie-restricted diet of normal foods that is balanced to provide the conventional distribution of carbohydrate (approximately 55% of total calories), fat (approximately 30%) and protein (approximately 15%). Intensive 'fad diets', as widely advertised for adults, should not be used in children and adolescents, because of health hazards. Moreover, such diets do nothing to modify the patient's eating habits so do not lead to sustained weight loss. While a decrease in physical activity is an important factor in the current increase of obesity, exercise is not an effective means of inducing weight loss unless combined with the reduction of calorie intake. Jogging for 2 km expends only as much energy as is contained in half a bar of chocolate. Exercise may have a greater impact on the maintenance of weight loss and fitness level.

Perversely, in societies where overweight is becoming more common the fear of obesity and the desire for a largely unattainable ideal body image is leading to unnecessary and potentially harmful dietary restriction in small growing children by well-meaning parents, and to a substantial increase in eating disorders amongst adolescents.

Fig. 5.22 Weight changes after resection of craniopharyngioma at age 7 years. Hypopituitarism treated with growth hormone, hydrocortisone and thyroxine, with induction of puberty at 13.5 years. Adult height –0.6 SDS. Relentless weight gain despite dietary intervention and introduction of orlistat at age 15.2 years for a 6-month trial. Patient is now being considered for gastric bypass surgery.

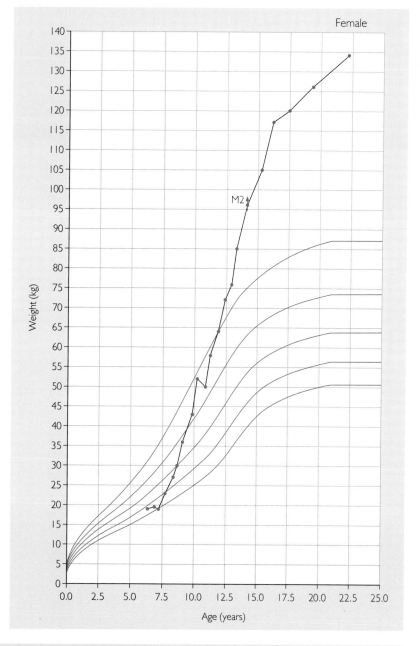

There is little experience of the use of pharmaceutical means of weight reduction in children. Orlistat is an intestinal lipase inhibitor that provokes malabsorption of ingested fat. It has been shown capable of helping adults to sustain dietary weight loss of as much as 10% in some studies, but provokes gastrointestinal symptoms unless fat intake is severely restricted, which may be unsafe in a growing child. Sibutramine is a centrally active appetite suppressant that is used as an adjunct to diet in adult obesity with some success. However, long-term safety is an issue and these agents should not currently be prescribed in childhood outside established research programs. Surgical management of obesity is common in adulthood in some centers and may be the best option for potentially life-saving treatment in extreme morbid obesity (i.e. adult BMI >40), despite the anesthetic risks; however, experience in children is very limited. The massive obesity seen after surgery for craniopharyngioma makes this and Prader–Willi syndrome the most likely pathology to require drug or surgical intervention in pediatric practice (**Fig. 5.22**).

Chapter 6

Early Sexual Development

HORMONAL CHANGES IN PUBERTY

The earliest biochemical event of puberty is the appearance of intermittent serum peaks of luteinizing hormone (LH) and follicle stimulating hormone (FSH) at night, caused by a pulsatile secretion of gonadotropin releasing hormone (GnRH) from the hypothalamus. The pituitary GnRH receptors are responsive only to pulsatile GnRH: continuous administration blocks the secretion of gonadotropins. The intermittent production of LH and FSH stimulates the gonads, leading to sex hormone secretion and the development of the germinal epithelium. Initially the sex hormone levels are raised for only part of the day.

In the male the enlargement of the testes from a prepubertal 3-mL volume to 4 mL heralds the onset of puberty as the Sertoli cell volume increases. It is possible to have functioning Leydig cells and testosterone secretion in damaged testes, for instance in the Klinefelter syndrome after irradiation, without a volume increase. Testicular testosterone (via target cell conversion to dihydrotestosterone; see Ch. 8) produces pubic hair and penile growth, and is slightly augmented by androgen secretion from the adrenal gland. Acne, mood swings, the breaking of the voice, attainment of an adult body odor and sweat pattern are all androgen-mediated events.

In the female the first external sign of puberty is an enlargement of the breast bud as estrogen is produced from the ovary. Some of the androgen-mediated effects seen in a girl, including pubic and axillary hair growth, are secondary to increased androgen secretion from a maturational change in the adrenal gland – adrenarche. Adrenarche is a separate event from puberty, with different regulation, and occurs in both sexes. Its androgenic features are usually subsumed in the male by testicular androgen production. In the female, along with some ovarian-derived androgens, adrenarche forms an important component of normal sexual development.

Leptin produced by white fat also acts as a peripheral signal to start hypothalamic activation of gonadotroph secretion once a certain fat mass has been attained (see Ch. 5). Cyclic LH and FSH production leads to ovarian enlargement, follicle production and ultimately to maturation of the uterus and endometrium, followed by menarche. These changes can be monitored by ultrasonography (**Figs 6.1–6.7**).

Peripheral aromatase conversion of testosterone to estrogen, especially by fatty tissue, is possible, and is

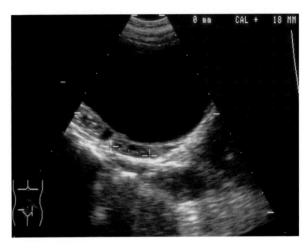

Fig. 6.1 After the neonatal period the ovaries are small (long axis 18 mm + – – – + in this section) and contain only one tiny follicle. Ovarian volume < 2 mL prepubertally.

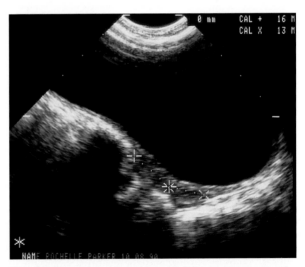

Fig. 6.2 Prepubertal uterus is small (16-mm long + — +) and tubular, and is not steeply angled in relation to the cervix (13-mm long × — ×). Uterine volume <2 mL prepubertally.

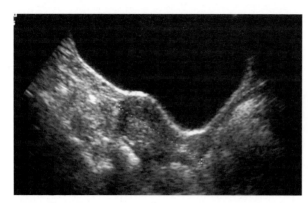

Fig. 6.3 In early puberty the uterus starts to enlarge (36 mm × — ×, 6 mL) and become pear shaped.

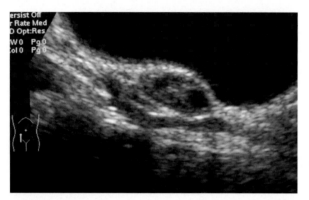

Fig. 6.4 In early puberty the ovaries become larger (here 2 mL) and contain one or two small cysts.

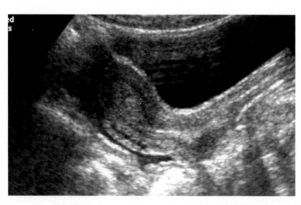

Fig. 6.5 In mid to late puberty a clear endometrial echo is seen and can be measured (× — × 30 mm).

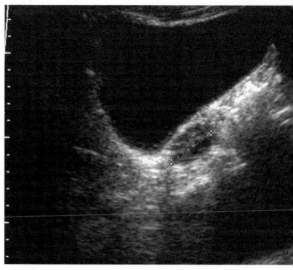

Fig. 6.6 In late puberty the ovaries enlarge (here 4-mL volume) and contain larger, peripheral follicles. During the menstrual cycle one such follicle will become dominant, enlarge until ovulation, then regress to form a corpus luteum.

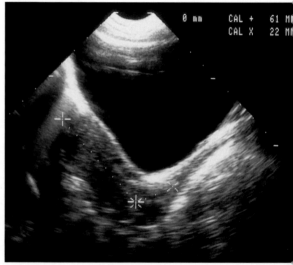

Fig. 6.7 The late pubertal uterus is clearly pear shaped (61-mm long + — +) and contains a midline endometrial echo. It is steeply angled in relation to the cervix (22-mm long × — ×) and the vagina can be clearly seen extending upwards to the right.

responsible for estrogen-mediated breast enlargement, gynecomastia, in some males. Estrogen in both sexes causes epiphyseal fusion and the eventual cessation of growth.

Neonates are exposed to the maternal hormone environment and may manifest changes secondary to natural or iatrogenic hormone exposure. Withdrawal bleeding in females (**Fig. 6.8**) and neonatal breast enlargement (see **Fig. 1.98**) in both sexes are a physiologic result of this process. Additionally there is a physiologic activation of the hypothalamic–pituitary–gonadal axis in the first months of life, especially in boys, which then subsides until puberty (**Figs 6.9–6.11**).

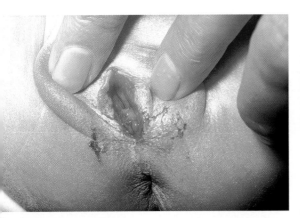

Fig. 6.8 Physiologic withdrawal bleeding in a neonate.

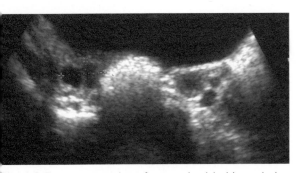

Fig. 6.9 Transverse section of neonatal pelvis. Uterus is the solid midline structure behind the bladder. Both ovaries contain large follicles secondary to physiologic neonatal activation of the hypothalamic–pituitary–ovarian axis.

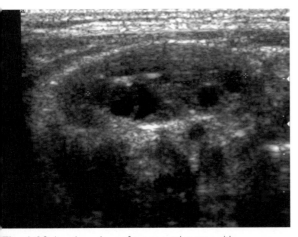

Fig. 6.10 Another view of a neonatal ovary with physiologic follicle formation and 2-mL volume.

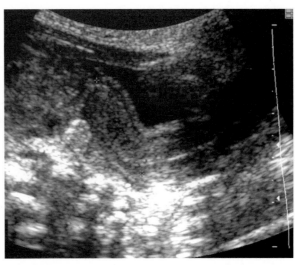

Fig. 6.11 The neonatal uterus can be quite bulky, with an endometrial echo, before settling down to the appearance shown in Fig. 6.1.

CLASSIFICATION OF EARLY PUBERTY

Early or precocious puberty (also called sexual precocity) is traditionally defined by the onset of puberty before the age of 8 years. In Europe this still seems a valid cut-off, but in the USA it has been proposed to use 7 years for white girls and 6.5 years for the African American population. The difference between Europe and the USA may be related to ethnic causes, a different prevalence of obesity or methodologic issues. This is earlier than in previous generations, although there is little evidence that menarche is occurring at a younger age, suggesting that the tempo of puberty in the early developers may be slower than previously. In boys 9 years remains the suggested cut-off for the start of normal sexual development. It can be subdivided into 'true' (or 'central') precocious puberty and 'pseudo' sexual precocity. True precocious puberty is all of the events of normal puberty occurring early, whereas in pseudo-precocious puberty only some aspects of sexual development occur, depending on whether androgens or estrogens are produced. Excess or early estrogen production in the female or testosterone in the male leads to iso-sexual development. Alternatively, excess or early estrogen production in the male or testosterone in the female leads to hetero-sexual development.

There are also two forms of partial development, which are usually considered as variations of normal: premature adrenarche or pubarche (early pubic hair) and premature thelarche (breast development). (Note that, as the first sign of true precocious puberty in a girl is breast development, the differentiation between early puberty and premature thelarche cannot be made only on the basis of a single physical examination: both growth pattern and bone age, which are normal in premature thelarche and accelerated in precocious puberty, must be considered.)

1 TRUE SEXUAL PRECOCITY (OR CENTRAL PRECOCIOUS PUBERTY)

This is characterized by:

- Concordant development of all structures usually involved in puberty: in a girl breast then pubic hair growth (**Fig. 6.12**), and uterine and ovarian maturation followed by menarche; in a boy testicular enlargement, and penile and pubic hair growth (**Fig. 6.13**).
- The simultaneous development of secondary effects such as mood swings, acne (**Fig. 6.14**), body odor.
- A pubertal height spurt (**Fig. 6.15**).
- Advanced bone age that continues to progress rapidly and leads to premature epiphyseal closure and hence reduced final height.

True sexual precocity may be idiopathic (in girls by far the most frequent form) or caused by abnormalities in the CNS (most commonly in boys). These can be congenital anomalies, hypothalamic hamartomas (**Figs 6.16–6.18**), raised intracranial pressure or tumors

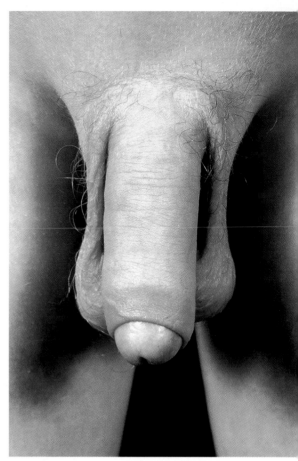

Fig. 6.13 Male genitalia in central precocious puberty showing concordant pubertal development.

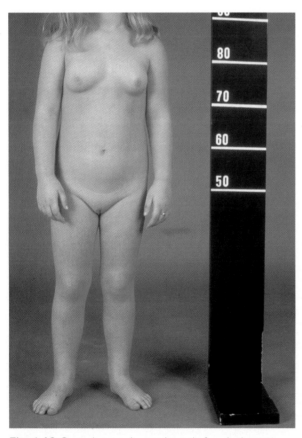

Fig. 6.12 Central precocious puberty in female, breasts stage 3, pubic hair stage 2, height 114 cm (3 ft 9 in or +1.3 SDS) at age 5.5 years.

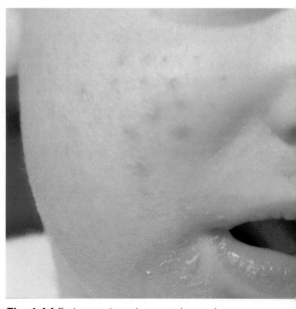

Fig. 6.14 Early acne in male precocious puberty.

Fig. 6.15 Precocious puberty presenting at 4.3 years with a bone age of 8.2 years. Treatment with intranasal gonadotropin analog therapy delayed menarche to 11.5 years and subsequent bony fusion to around 12 years, but with evidence of a reduced adult height of −2 SDS.

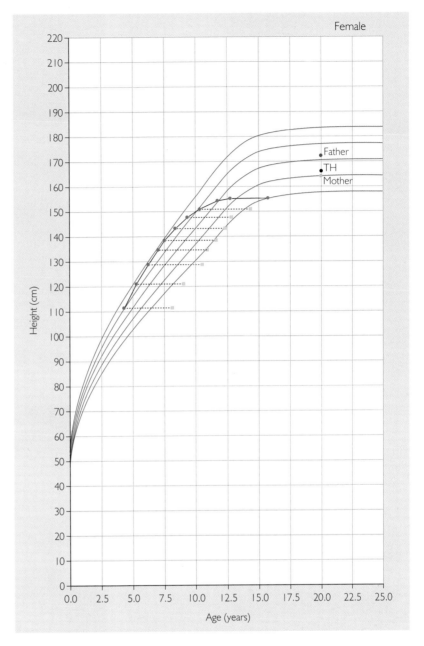

(**Fig. 6.19**), and may follow cranial irradiation, especially in girls (see Ch. 11). The intracranial lesions may arise *de novo* or be part of a predisposing condition such as neurofibromatosis (**Figs 6.20–6.22**). Sexual precocity can also rarely be seen with primary long-standing hypothyroidism due to a sequence homology between thyroid stimulating hormone (TSH) and human chorionic gonadotropin (hCG).

Girls adopted from developing countries to the developed world may demonstrate puberty that starts a little early but with rapid progression to menarche at 11+ (versus 12+) years and loss of adult stature.

Subacute torsion of the ovaries produces massive edema and maturation of stromal cells; there is often virilization from ovarian testosterone production followed by estrogenization and breast development. This can be very difficult to differentiate clinically from true central precocity other than the suppression of the LH–FSH axis and the typical ultrasonographic appearance (see below).

2 PSEUDO-SEXUAL PRECOCITY

This is characterized by:

■ Hypertrophy of the target tissue of the hormone being secreted in excess.

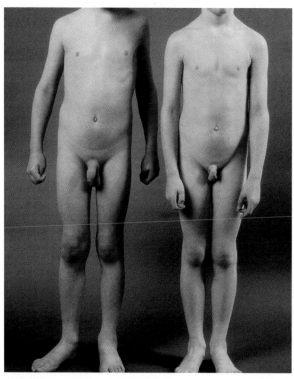

Fig. 6.16 Male precocious puberty due to hamartoma, with unaffected twin brother.

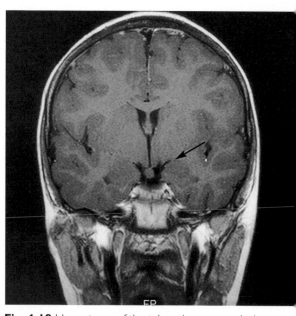

Fig. 6.18 Hamartoma of the tuber cinerum producing precocious puberty, transverse MRI.

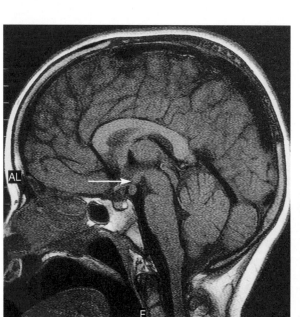

Fig. 6.17 Hamartoma of the tuber cinerum producing precocious puberty, lateral MRI.

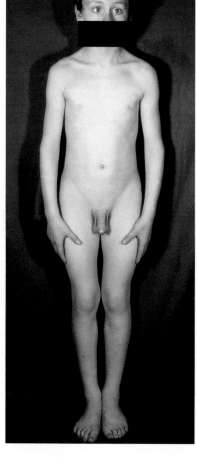

Fig. 6.19 Male central precocious puberty with sixth nerve palsy secondary to intracranial astrocytoma.

- Regression or inhibition of the structures that usually secrete the hormone at puberty.
- Advanced bone maturation.
- Accelerated growth rate.

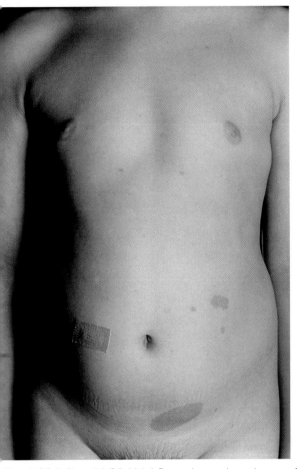 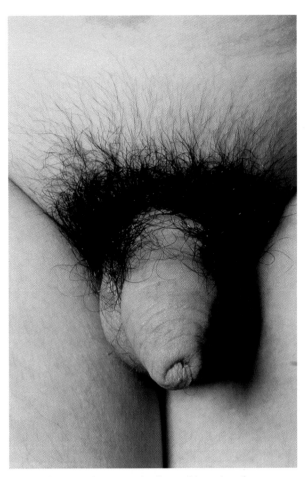

Figs 6.20 (left) and **6.21** (right) Precocious puberty in neurofibromatosis secondary to optic glioma. Note site of gonadotropin analog injection (with plaster), as well as enlargement of testes and penis with consonant pubic hair growth.

Fig. 6.22 Optic glioma in neurofibromatosis producing precocious puberty.

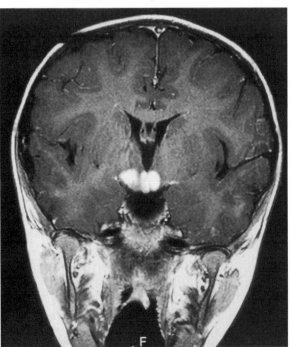

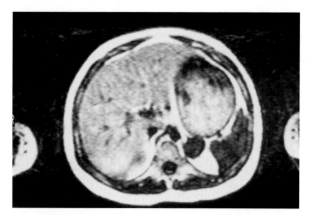

Fig. 6.23 Adrenal carcinoma producing virilization.

The development may be iso-sexual or less commonly hetero-sexual, and causes include adrenal tumors (**Fig. 6.23**) producing either testosterone or estrogen, non-salt-losing congenital virilizing adrenal hyperplasia (**Fig. 6.24**; see also Chs 8 & 11), exogenous gonadotropin or sex steroid administration, gonadal tumors producing estrogen or testosterone, gonadotropin- or hCG-producing tumors and estrogen-secreting ovarian cysts (**Figs 6.25 & 6.26**). Hetero-sexual pseudo-precocity in a female will often result in considerable clitoral hypertrophy (see Ch. 8), and this helps in the differentiation from premature adrenarche (see below).

Additionally the McCune–Albright syndrome produces discordant sexual development. The syndrome consists of irregular pigmented café-au-lait patches, usually unilateral and on the upper body (see **Fig. 1.135**). There are areas of bony dysplasia and cysts in the long bones (**Fig. 6.27**) and skull (**Fig. 6.28**). Pubertal signs are usually discordant with early bleeding in females and no evidence of gonadotropin cyclicity. It is much commoner in girls than boys and can also rarely cause thyrotoxicosis, gigantism and Cushing syndrome. It results from a generalized mutation of part of the G protein (a secondary messenger signaling receptor activation) in endocrine tissues, leading to overactivity.

Separate from the pathologic secretion from tumors described above, excess production of estrogen from peripheral aromatase conversion of testosterone in an often overweight male can cause pubertal gynecomastia (**Fig. 6.29**). Male breast development and lactorrhea from a prolactinoma is extremely uncommon (see below).

Testotoxicosis is a rare condition of familial male pseudo-precocious puberty leading to generally consonant changes of male puberty but with testes that are often small for the degree of virilization

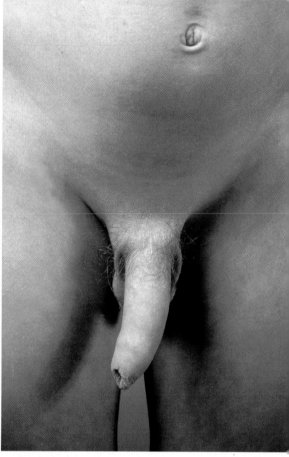

Fig. 6.24 Non-salt-losing 21-hydroxylase deficiency presenting late in a male with penile enlargement, pubic hair growth but small testes (indicating a non-testicular source of androgen).

present (**Figs 6.30 & 6.31**). There is an absence of cyclic gonadotropin activation, but a mutation causing a 'locking on' of the testicular LH receptor is present leading to early production of testosterone in the absence of circulating LH.

3(a) PREMATURE ADRENARCHE OR PUBARCHE

This is characterized by:

- Pubic and axillary hair growth (**Figs 1.108 & 6.32**).
- Acne, body odor and other androgen-mediated effects.
- A mildly advanced bone age.
- Usually no acceleration of height velocity.

The event termed 'adrenarche' is a normal age-related physiologic maturation of the adrenal cortex, probably under the influence of adrenocorticotropic

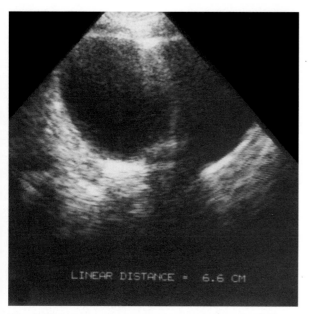

Fig. 6.25 Large estrogen-secreting ovarian cyst (on left), pushing bladder and uterus to the right.

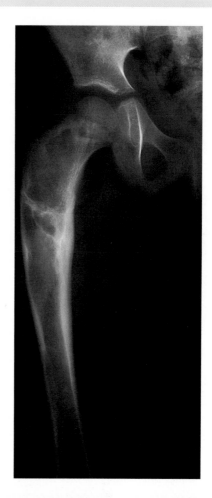

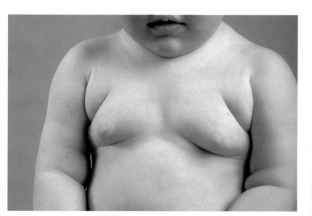

Fig. 6.26 Premature breast development secondary to an ovarian cyst.

hormone (ACTH) (or another postulated 'central adrenarche stimulating hormone' (CASH)), producing increased secretion of dehydroepiandrosterone (DHEA) and other androgenic precursors of testosterone. Its effects are usually incorporated into puberty. If early maturation occurs, the mild virilizing effects become cosmetically noticeable. Idiopathic dislocation of adrenarche from puberty is commoner in girls than in boys. There is some evidence that a genetically determined overactivity of one of the 17, 20-desmolase pathways for adrenal steroid production may result in familial adrenarche and in some cases of familial polycystic ovarian syndrome (PCOS). A large proportion of girls with premature adrenarche seem to go on to develop a

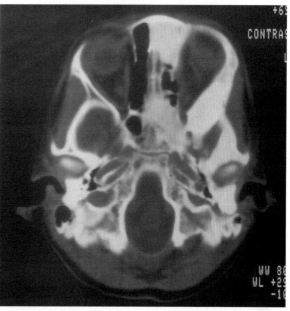

Figs 6.27 (top) **6.28** (bottom) Fibrous dysplasia of upper femur and fibrous dysplasia of base of skull and left orbit.

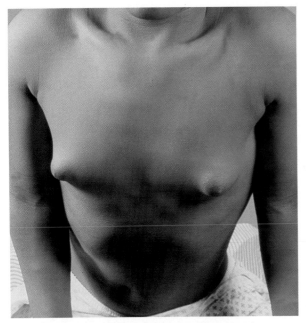

Fig. 6.29 Gynecomastia – required surgical resection.

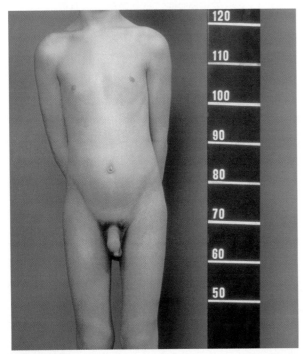

Fig. 6.30 Testotoxicosis – stage 4 penis and pubic hair growth but only 6-mL testes.

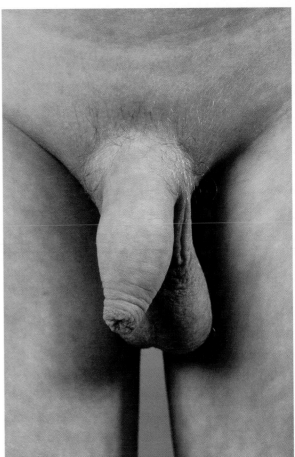

Fig. 6.31 Genitalia in another case of testotoxicosis. More concordant development but a family history of the condition.

are hydrocephalus and following meningitis (especially tubercular meningitis). Because it may occasionally be severe and a familial event, differentiation from late presenting atypical or non-classic congenital hyperplasia (CAH; see below) may be required.

3(b) HIRSUTISM

Other than adrenarche, excess hair production in the female (with or without later male-pattern baldness) may be due to other causes of excess adrenal activity or androgen production:

- Classic simple CAH.
- Late-onset CAH is common but often undiagnosed. The non-classic subtype is associated with human leukocyte antigen (HLA) types B14 and B35 (see Ch. 8).
- Cushing syndrome.
- Secondary to abnormal levels of testosterone produced by polycystic ovaries, which can

PCOS-like phenotype, including the 'metabolic syndrome X' (**Fig. 6.33**). Premature adrenarche may also be secondary to non-progressive intracranial lesions, presumably mediated by abnormal production of ACTH or CASH. The commonest intracranial causes

Fig. 6.32
Premature
adrenarche/
pubarche. No
breast
development and
stage 3 pubic hair
growth. There
was an adult
body odor and
mild acne but no
cliteromegaly.
Sibling illustrated
in Fig. 1.108.

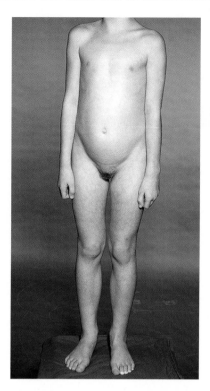

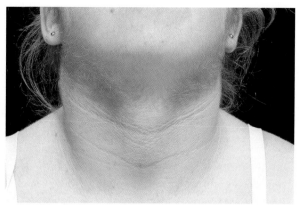

Fig. 6.34 Hirsutism secondary to insulin resistance, mild acanthosis seen in neck skin creases.

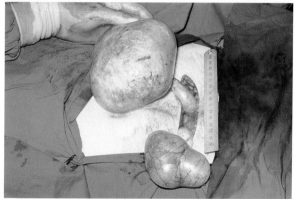

Fig. 6.35 Massive cystic ovarian changes in patient in Fig. 6.34.

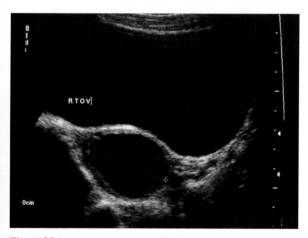

Fig. 6.33 Large ovarian cyst in CAH.

themselves be due to adrenal overactivity and hyperinsulinemia or occur as a primary event after puberty (**Figs 6.34 & 6.35**).

- Idiopathic hirsutism is possibly due to overactivity of skin 5α-reductase levels. This can be treated with enzyme blockers such as finasteride.
- Some girls or their parents perceive cosmetic problems that are due only to normal growth of dark hair.

It is said that hirsutism confined to the lower body is indicative of an adrenal source of androgens.

As well as treating any identified underlying cause it is also appropriate to advise cosmetic treatments such as bleaching, depilation and electrolysis.

4 PREMATURE THELARCHE

This benign condition is characterized by:

- Early breast enlargement (**Fig. 6.36**), usually in infancy, but which may occur throughout childhood and is often cyclic over periods of months.
- The absence of the subsequent appearance of any other pubertal changes.
- Normal growth and skeletal maturation.

In premature thelarche, waves of follicular development (above 3–4 mm) occur with FSH induction of aromatase. Low levels of estrogen can be detected by means of ultra-sensitive assays.

A variant condition with features intermediate between true central precocious puberty and thelarche

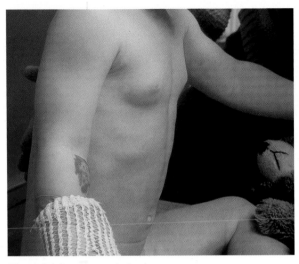

Fig. 6.36 Premature thelarche.

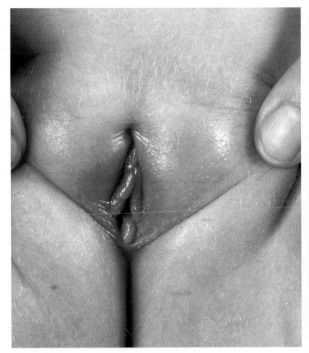

Fig. 6.37 Genitalia of patient shown in Fig. 6.26, showing early maturation of vulval mucosa.

has been described, in which FSH levels predominate (unlike true puberty, where LH > FSH levels).

5 ISOLATED PREMATURE MENARCHE

This is an ill-understood condition affecting prepubertal girls, often in the summer months. There may be cyclic bleeding every 4–6 weeks, for 3–4 days, for several months in a row. At no point are levels of gonadotropins raised, but there is a small endometrial echo visible on ultrasonography during the bleeding phase. The differential lies between sexual abuse, vaginal malignancy and cervical erosions, so examination under anesthesia may be required if the history and investigations are not typical.

DIAGNOSTIC WORK-UP

MEDICAL HISTORY AND EXAMINATION

The following items are of importance in the history:

- The exact timing of the onset of pubertal signs, including in a girl whether breast development occurred earlier or later than pubic hair growth.
- Vaginal discharge, which may be creamy or blood-stained.
- Growth pattern (any rapid growth recently? – this may be manifested by change relative to peers or changes in clothes and shoe size).
- Any symptoms suggestive of hypothyroidism.
- Any neurologic or visual symptoms.

- Any family history of precocity or suggestive of neurofibromatosis.
- Previous diseases leading to neurologic damage.
- Any exposure to drugs (estrogens, androgens, cimetidine). This can be iatrogenic, accidental (i.e. ingestion of the contraceptive pill) or factitious. There are also reports of traditional Chinese herbal remedies leading to both male and female precocity. Organochlorine pesticides related to DDT may cause sex steroid-like effects.
- Dietary exposure to contaminated poultry or beef where excessive veterinary administration may be a possibility.

The physical examination should concentrate on:

- A precise description of pubertal stage. (For longitudinal follow-up it is useful to measure breast diameter.)
- Height, sitting height and weight, and their evaluation versus age references and previous measurements. (As growth of the back is mediated partly by sex hormone secretion, early puberty will tend to produce a somewhat longer sitting height in relation to leg length.)
- Inspection of the color of the vulval mucosa; a pale color indicates estrogen activity (**Fig. 6.37**).
- Signs of hyperandrogenization (hirsutism, clitoral or penile enlargement, acne). Hirsutism may be

Score	1	2	3	4
Lip	Few outer hairs	Outer margin	>50%	Full
Chin	Few hairs	Scattered	Light cover	Heavy
Lower abdomen	Few, midline	Midline streak	Band	Inverted 'Y'
Thigh	Sparse, <25%	>25%	Complete, light	Heavy

Score each feature and add up the total. A score greater than 5 is indicative of significant hirsutism. The score can be used to document progression or regression of the signs.

Table 6.1 Simple grading of hirsutism

graded according to a simple scale (**Table 6.1**). Hirsutism exclusively on the lower body is most commonly due to an adrenal cause.

- Blood pressure (increased in the 11β-hydroxylase form of adrenal hyperplasia or with raised intracranial pressure).
- A search for pigmented birthmarks.
- Thyroid size and signs of hypothyroidism (see Ch. 9). (In the hypothyroid male the testicular volume may be increased to a greater extent than might be expected from the other pubertal signs. In the hypothyroid female periods may occur earlier than would be expected for the stage of breast development.)
- Hepatomegaly or abdominal mass.
- Pelvic mass (e.g. ovarian cyst or tumor) on abdominal or rectal examination.
- Neurologic examination (including fundoscopy).

INTERPRETATION OF THE CLUES

True precocity

- In a girl with no other signs or symptoms = likely to be idiopathic, but check with computed tomography (CT) or magnetic resonance imaging (MRI).
- With neurologic signs or symptoms = CNS lesion.
- With more than five café-au-lait spots and axillary freckles, with or without a positive family history = neurofibromatosis and optic glioma or other CNS tumor.
- Thyroid enlargement and/or typical symptoms and signs = hypothyroidism.

In tall boys and girls with a history of early pubic hair growth, sweatiness followed by other signs of puberty could be non-salt-losing CAH that has caused

massive advance of bone age and true puberty supervening on pseudo-precocity (**Fig. 6.38**).

Pseudo-precocity

- A positive family history = adrenarche or atypical 21-hydroxylase deficiency.
- Hypertension in a girl with virilization or a boy with pseudo-precocious puberty = 11β-hydroxylase deficiency.
- Cliteromegaly plus advanced bone age and accelerated growth = androgenization *not* secondary to adrenarche.
- Irregular café-au-lait spots and/or lytic bone lesions on radiography = McCune–Albright syndrome.
- Pelvic mass or mass felt per rectum = ovarian tumor.
- Hepatomegaly = hepatic tumor (producing hCG).
- Abdominal mass = adrenal tumor.
- Gynecomastia with unilateral testicular enlargement = germ cell tumor.
- Gynecomastia with no testicular enlargement = intra-abdominal tumor (often impalpable) or extraglandular aromatase conversion at puberty (commonest in, but not exclusive to, obese subjects).
- Previous diseases leading to neurologic damage = premature adrenarche.
- Early onset with cyclic breast enlargement = premature thelarche.
- Positive family history in a boy = familial testotoxicosis.

FURTHER INVESTIGATIONS

Evaluation of the growth pattern in the light of the pubertal stage is crucial for determining the number

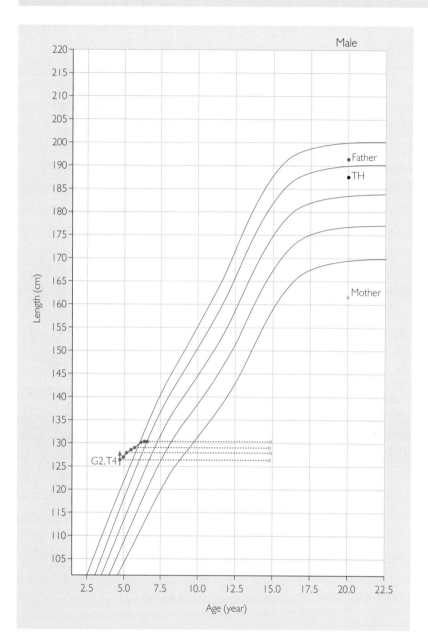

Fig. 6.38 Non-salt-losing CAH presenting as true central precocious puberty supervening on the massive advance in bone age due to adrenal testosterone. At presentation at 4.7 years of age, height +3.5 SDS with bone age of 14.8 years. Commenced treatment with hydrocortisone to suppress ACTH and LHRH agonists to suppress true puberty with no further progression of bone maturation.

of further investigations. The sex of the child is also relevant.

Girls

If there is only a minor degree of breast enlargement in a young girl, with no other signs of estrogen activity and a normal growth pattern, further investigations can be limited to a hand and wrist radiograph for bone age. If bone age is not accelerated, the child could be reviewed after some months to see whether the signs have subsided or progressed with pubic hair growth; height velocity could also be measured. If there is no progression of pubertal signs and a normal growth rate, the diagnosis is most likely to be premature thelarche or a temporary exposure to exogenous estrogens. Further review should be arranged and the care-giver instructed to return urgently if any more pubertal changes occur. Pelvic ultrasonography that showed one or two follicles in a low-volume ovary with no sign of uterine enlargement would give further reassurance (**Figs 6.39 & 6.40**).

If there are definite signs of estrogen activity (active breast development, pale mucosa of introitus, psychologic changes, growth acceleration and bone age acceleration), the following investigations are indicated:

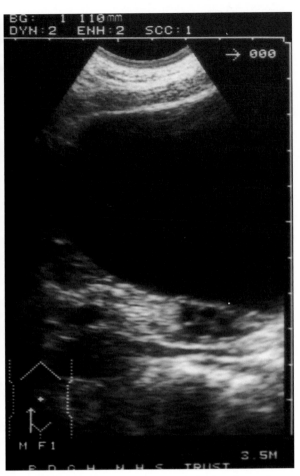

Fig. 6.39 The ovaries in premature thelarche show a few large cysts/follicles in small-volume glands. The uterus (not shown) is of prepubertal size (<2 mL) and shape.

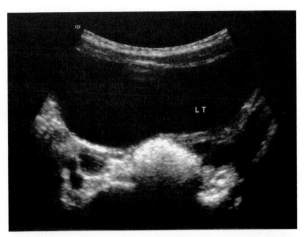

Fig. 6.40 Transverse section of both ovaries in thelarche.

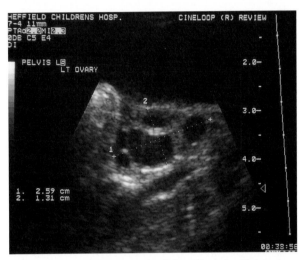

Fig. 6.41 Low-volume ovaries (26 × 13 mm) with large cysts in thelarche.

- Basal estradiol (E_2), LH, FSH.
- Thyroid function tests: (free) thyroxine (FT_4) and TSH.
- Abdominal ultrasonography (ovarian and uterine size) (**Figs 6.41–6.44**).
- Levels of inhibin B (a granulosa-derived glycoprotein that feeds back to the pituitary to inhibit FSH secretion) are raised in thelarche (but not inhibin A which comes from the corpus luteum) as opposed to true puberty where levels of both inhibin A and B levels are rasised.
- In case of doubt about the estrogen results, vaginal cytology can be considered (percentage of squamous cells).
- Luteinizing hormone releasing hormone (LHRH) test (see Appendix) in a specialized center. Before puberty, the increase in LH and FSH levels is low, with usually a greater rise of FSH than of LH concentration. During puberty, the increase in the levels of both gonadotropins is higher, with LH rising higher than FSH concentration in mid to late puberty. Therefore, the ratio of LH to FSH (>1) can be used as a marker of 'established' puberty.

If there is positive evidence for true precocious puberty (E_2 concentration greater than 50 pmol/L, LH/FSH ratio > 1, LH peak raised) and no hypothyroidism, further investigations to find the precise cause are needed with MRI or CT of the brain.

If there is positive evidence for pseudo-precocious puberty (raised E_2 concentration, depressed LH and FSH levels even after administration of LHRH), further investigations should be aimed at elucidating the precise cause. Sonography of the ovary, liver and adrenals should show the majority of tumors, although they may occasionally be intrathoracic. Occasionally CT

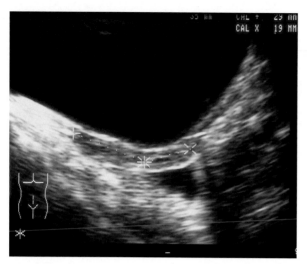

Fig. 6.42 Central precocious puberty demonstrated in girl presenting at 5 years with breast stage 2. There is enlargement of the uterus such that the body (+ — + 29 mm) is greater than the cervix (× — × 19 mm).

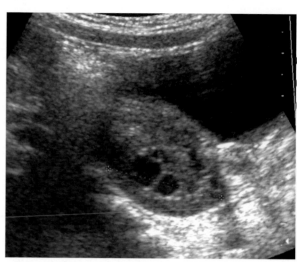

Fig. 6.44 Massively enlarged ovaries with peripheral follicles and central solid component. At laparoscopy to exclude tumor, bilateral twisting of the pedicles was observed and the diagnosis of massive ovarian edema secondary to chronic torsion confirmed on biopsy.

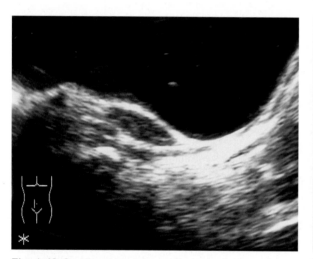

Fig. 6.43 Ovarian enlargement with the beginnings of peripheral follicle formation in the patient in Fig. 6.42. This can occur only as part of cyclical gonadotropin secretion.

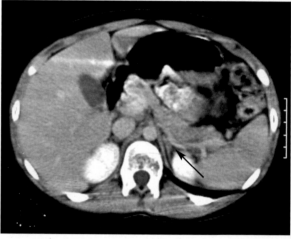

Fig. 6.45 Abdominal CT showing normal small tricorn adrenal.

of the adrenal may be required to look for small lesions (**Fig. 6.45**).

If there are mild signs of androgen excess and if growth and bone age are normal, the diagnosis is almost certainly benign precocious adrenarche and no further investigations are needed. (For documentation, plasma levels of DHEA sulfate (DHEAS), which is usually slightly elevated, can be measured, and a urinary steroid profile will show a mild increase in adrenal cortical metabolites.) In non-classical 21-hydroxylase deficiency, which may mimic precocious adrenarche, a short ACTH (Synacthen) test (see Appendix) to provide an estimate of

the basal levels and rise of 17α-hydroxyprogesterone may be required to confirm the diagnosis.

If there is more severe virilization with cliteromegaly, accelerated height velocity and bone maturation, a urinary steroid profile and measurement of plasma or salivary 17α-hydroxyprogesterone, dehydroepi-androsterone (DHA), DHEAS and androstenedione will allow the diagnosis of most forms of CAH and androgen-producing tumors. Tumors can be localized by means of ultrasonography or CT.

If there is abnormal pigmentation, radiography of the skeleton will help to confirm McCune–Albright syndrome, in which case thyroid and adrenal function should also be checked.

Boys

If there are definite signs of puberty with enlarging testes, basal serum testosterone, LH and FSH levels should be measured and an LHRH test performed in a specialist center. If the level of testosterone is increased (>1.0 nmol/L) and the LHRH test shows a pubertal pattern (see above), true precocious puberty is diagnosed. As the frequency of cerebral abnormalities in boys with true precocious puberty is relatively high, CT or MRI is mandatory (**Figs 6.46 & 6.47**).

If the testosterone level is increased, with small soft testes, pseudo-precocious puberty is likely and LH and FSH levels will remain suppressed during the LHRH test. Further determinations of other steroids in the urine and plasma (androstenedione, DHEAS, DHEA and 17α-hydroxyprogesterone) are indicated to determine the source of the androgens. It is possible to use the relative values to distinguish between premature adrenarche (relatively rare in the male), exogenous anabolic steroid administration, the various non-salt-losing forms of CAH and adrenal tumors.

If isolated gynecomastia is present then testosterone, prolactin, E_2, hCG and LH levels should be measured. hCG and/or E_2 concenetrations are raised in some estrogen-secreting tumors, which may be testicular (detected by ultrasonography) or extragonadal (detected by further ultrasonography or CT). Primary testicular damage with increased menopausal LH levels – and hypothalamic or pituitary hypogonadism with undetectable LH levels – also may present with gynecomastia (obviously in the absence of other signs of sexual maturation; see Chs 7 & 8). Prolactinomas in childhood (**Fig. 6.48**) are extremely rare and usually present with CNS signs, although this is the only cause, if seen, of lactorrhea (**Fig. 6.49**). If the estrogen level is only slightly raised or all the tests are normal, then extraglandular aromatase conversion of testosterone to estrogen is likely.

THERAPY

True precocious puberty will result in a reduced final height, and early pubertal development can lead to psychologic problems. For these reasons treatment is usually offered in specialist units. Current therapy uses depot slow-release LHRH analogs i.m. or s.c. (depending on the preparation) every 4–12 weeks.

To prevent initial hyperstimulation and worsening of the precocity it is usual to treat concurrently for the

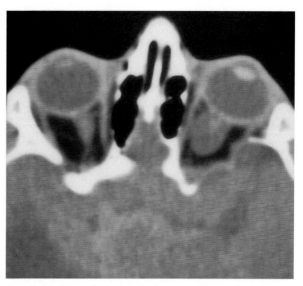

Fig. 6.46 Optic glioma producing sexual precocity in a male with neurofibromatosis. Thickened left optic nerve.

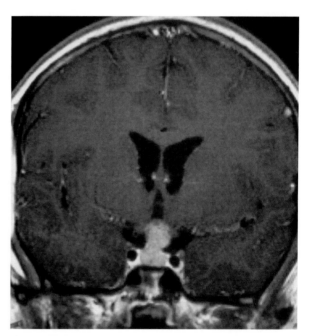

Fig. 6.47 Chiasmatic tumor in boy with precocious puberty.

first 6 weeks with the oral sex-steroid synthesis blocker, cyproterone acetate (100 mg/m² body surface per 24 h, divided into two or three doses). (Cyproterone acetate alone can be used as prolonged therapy for sexual precocity but, whilst effective in stopping the progress of pubertal development, it does not influence final height. It may have associated side effects such as fatigue, and biochemically it leads to hypocortisolism so that a stress regimen of glucocorticoids is necessary.)

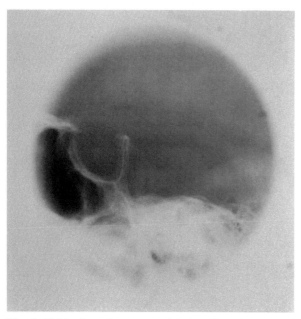

Fig. 6.48 Massive enlargement of pituitary fossa secondary to prolactinoma.

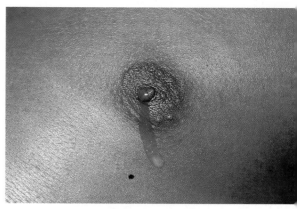

Fig. 6.49 Lactorrhea in a male with a prolactinoma.

GnRH analog treatment is continued until the final height prediction has become acceptable and the child's peer group is showing pubertal changes. Puberty will then continue from the point of initiation of therapy and there are currently no long-term recognized side effects.

Testotoxicosis and the McCune–Albright syndrome, both being gonadotropin independent, will not respond to LHRH analog treatment and hence cyproterone acetate or ketoconazole (which blocks several steps in adrenal steroid synthesis, including testosterone) represents the most reasonable choice of therapy. If the bone age has been pushed much past 12 years by these conditions, central puberty will supervene and additional GnRH treatment may be necessary.

Pseudo-precocity secondary to tumorous sources of sex steroids requires expert oncologic and surgical intervention. Any of the forms of CAH presenting with virilization with or without hypertension are treated with steroid replacement, as should late presenting non-classic 21-hydroxylase deficiency (see Chs 8 & 11). If true central precocity has supervened, LHRH analogs are additionally required.

Adrenarche is benign, although of cosmetic importance, as is isolated hirsutism. Later polycystic ovaries may require treatment to regularize periods. In the older patient anti-androgens combined with a contraceptive preparation could be considered under careful supervision. Excess hair can be treated with depilatory creams and electrolysis. Skin cleansers and topical antibiotic preparations may ameliorate acne.

Thelarche usually requires no intervention, although a progressive FSH dominant form ('thelarche variant') is sometimes treated with LHRH analogs, with limited success.

Idiopathic gynecomastia is best treated by an experienced plastic surgeon, because the results of medical therapy are disappointing.

Chapter 7

Late Sexual Development

If a delay or lack of pubertal development is defined as above the 97th centile for population references, a recent Dutch study showed that the 97th centile for B2 is 12.7 years and for G2 13.4 years. For practical purposes, however, delayed puberty can be diagnosed if breast stage 2 in girls has not started at 13 years of age, and if genital stage 2 (testicular volume ≥4 mL) has not started in boys at age 14 years. In practice, many children present because of concern about their appearance several years before these limits. Because of the lack of a pubertal growth spurt, many of these patients will present primarily with short stature (see Ch. 2).

CLASSIFICATION OF LATE PUBERTY

Delayed puberty is classified according to the serum gonadotropin levels: high concentrations indicate primary gonadal failure and low concentrations indicate disorders at the hypothalamic–pituitary level.

HYPERGONADOTROPIC HYPOGONADISM

Congenital primary gonadal failure

- Gonadal dysgenesis associated with sex chromosome abnormalities (e.g. Ullrich–Turner and Klinefelter syndromes).
- Idiopathic syndromic abnormalities. There are more than 20 named syndromes that are associated with hypergonadotrophic hypogonadism.
- Genetic disorders of enzyme production causing sex steroid deficiency.
- Pure gonadal dysgenesis (defective germ cell migration).
- Complete androgen insensitivity caused by receptor/post-receptor abnormalities. Here the gonads are functional but the tissues unresponsive (see Ch. 8). Complete forms that do not present as female infants with bilateral inguinal hernias usually present as primary amenorrhea.

Acquired primary gonadal failure

- Autoimmune disorders.
- Galactosemia.

- Infections.
- Irradiation to the gonad and some chemotherapy regimens (see Ch. 11).
- Trauma *in utero* or later torsion, 'vanishing testes', etc.

HYPOGONADOTROPIC HYPOGONADISM

Temporary deficiency, associated with delayed maturation

- Constitutional delay of growth and adolescence (physiologic).
- Chronic illnesses and systemic diseases.
- Hypothyroidism (also associated with sexual precocity).
- Anorexia nervosa.
- Excessive physical training.
- Excessive emotional and/or physical stress.
- Malnutrition.

Permanent pathological deficiency

- Isolated (with anosmia = Kallmann syndrome).
- As part of a syndromic malformation (Again there are a number of eponymous conditions associated with central gonadotropin lack.)
- In the context of multiple pituitary deficiencies, idiopathic or due to anatomic malformations and acquired lesions.

DIAGNOSTIC WORK-UP

MEDICAL HISTORY AND EXAMINATION

Features of importance in the history:

- Family history of delayed sexual development.
- Family history of autoimmune or endocrine disease.
- Family history of infertility.
- Parental size.
- Birth and pregnancy details.
- Any learning problems.
- Previous medical treatments and surgery, including 'minor' procedures such as orchidopexy or neonatal hernia repair.

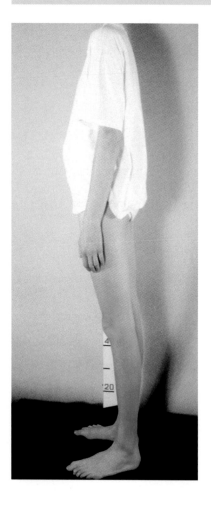

Fig. 7.1
Eunuchoid body habitus (47XXY).

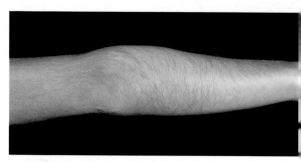

Fig. 7.2 Excess lanugo hair as may be seen in anorexia nervosa.

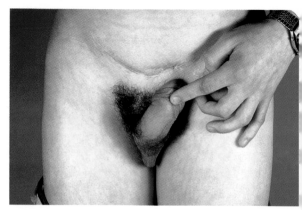

Fig. 7.3 Cryptorchidism, here with functioning intra-abdominal testes.

- Disordered eating behavior.
- Absent sense of smell. (A patient with anosmia may be able to detect the presence of an odor, especially of volatile substances, but be unable to differentiate between smells.)
- Social pressures – the sexual development of the close peer group.
- Levels of exercise.

The physical examination should concentrate on:

- Height, weight, adiposity (see **Fig. 2.10**).
- Body proportions. Because much of the growth of the back at puberty is mediated by sex hormone secretion, patients with delayed puberty, but no other endocrinopathy, will tend to have long legs compared with their backs – so-called eunuchoid body proportions (**Fig. 7.1**)
- Hirsutism (see Ch. 6).
- Lanugo hair (may be a sign of eating disorders) (**Fig. 7.2**).
- Hernia repairs or other operative scars.

- External genital appearance (measure gently stretched penis length; see Ch. 8). Anatomic abnormalities of the genital tract such as imperforate hymen or absent uterus, presenting as primary amenorrhea without delay of other sexual characteristics, may require ultrasonographic investigation, examination under anesthesia or laparoscopy.
- The presence of cryptorchidism (**Fig. 7.3**).
- Dysmorphic features.
- Signs of thyroid disease.
- Neurologic signs.
- Gynecomastia (see **Fig. 6.29**).
- Lactorrhea (see **Fig. 6.49**).
- Sense of smell.

Interpretation of the clues

- Typical dysmorphic features and short stature = Ullrich–Turner syndrome (see Ch. 2). Remember that up to 40% of girls with the Ullrich–Turner syndrome will have no external phenotypic abnormality (**Fig. 7.4**).

Fig. 7.4
Ullrich–Turner syndrome with few dysmorphic features except infantilism and a wide carrying angle.

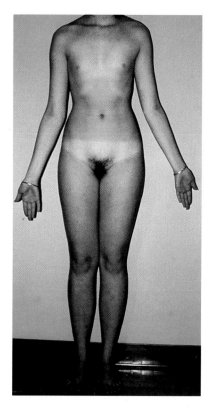

Fig. 7.5
Prader–Labhart–Willi syndrome.

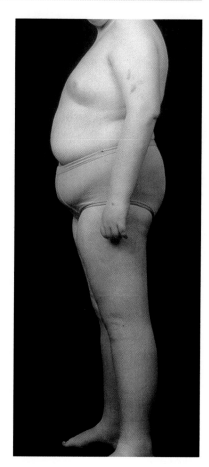

- Dysmorphic features, short stature and obesity = Prader–Labhart–Willi syndrome (**Figs 7.5 & 7.6**).
- Dysmorphic features, other abnormalities such as retinitis pigmentosa (see **Fig. 1.117**) = syndromic malformation such as the Bardet–Biedl or Laurence–Moon syndromes (see **Fig. 5.18**).
- Other specific dysmorphic syndromes and hypogonadism.
- Tall stature, disproportion and cryptorchidism or small firm testes = Klinefelter syndrome.
- Under-virilized male with gynecomastia and hypertension = late presenting 17α-hydroxylase deficiency.
- Under-virilized male or phenotypic 46XY female with late virilization = late presenting partial 17-ketosteroid reductase deficiency (or 17β-hydroxysteroid dehydrogenase deficiency); partial androgen insensitivity syndrome (see Ch. 8).
- Failure of breast development, often with some evidence of adrenal androgen activity = gonadal dysgenesis (**Fig. 7.7**).
- Hypogonadism with alopecia, vitiligo, candidiasis = autoimmune polyendocrinopathy IIIc (**Fig. 7.8**).
- Family history of delay (often in same-sex parent or sib) = constitutional delay of growth and adolescence.

Fig. 7.6 Close up of genitalia in Prader–Labhart–Willi syndrome.

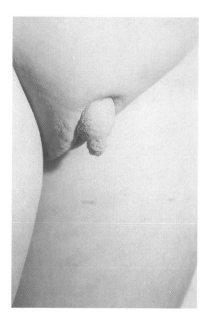

- Extreme thinness or falling weight, disordered eating and behavior in relation to food = anorexia nervosa (**Fig. 7.9**). Past anorexia can cause severe delay of puberty for many years after

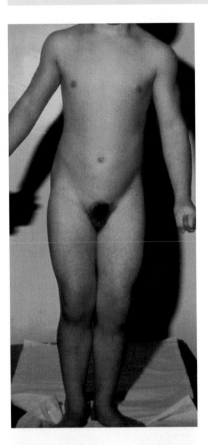

Fig. 7.7 Gonadal dysgenesis with adrenal source of pubic hair.

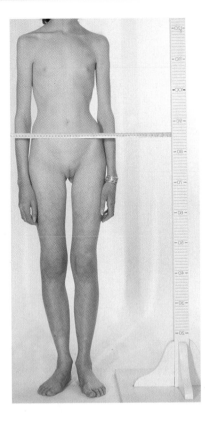

Fig. 7.9 Anorexia nervosa.

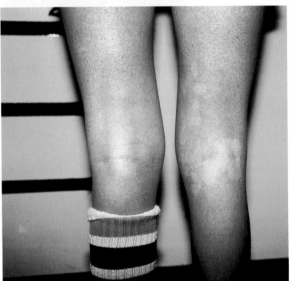

Fig. 7.8 Vitiligo.

successful restoration of adequate weight (**Fig. 7.10**). In addition to this psychiatric spectrum, simple fear of obesity with dieting is very common and can produce delay.

■ Anosmia, small penis and testes or cryptorchidism = Kallmann syndrome.

■ Hypogonadism and lactorrhea = prolactinoma (see **Figs 6.48 & 6.49**).
■ Hypogonadism with hypothyroidism and short stature = panhypopituitarism (**Fig. 7.11**).

FURTHER INVESTIGATIONS

On the basis of a proper history and physical examination, a tentative diagnosis can often be made. Thereafter, basal serum testosterone or estradiol and gonadotropin levels should be measured in specialized units, along with a bone age. Inhibin levels can be a useful marker of gonadal function. In permanent hyper- or hypogonadotropic hypogonadism, bone age can be higher than 11 (girls) or 13 (boys) years in the absence of pubertal signs, while this is unusual in temporary deficiency. Thereafter tests will depend on whether there is hyper- or hypogonadotropism.

Hypergonadotropic hypogonadism

By definition, the levels of gonadotropins are raised – often the follicle stimulating hormone (FSH) level to a greater extent than that of luteinizing hormone (LH).

Even in the absence of abnormal genitalia or dysmorphic features, karyotyping should be performed. It may be necessary to take both blood and fibroblast specimens to exclude tissue mosaicism.

Fig. 7.10 Past anorexia causing later extreme delay of puberty (menses at 20 years).

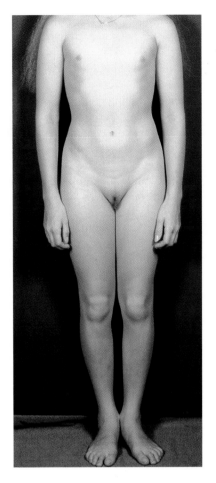

Fig. 7.11 Panhypopituitarism with infantilism, age 13.5 years.

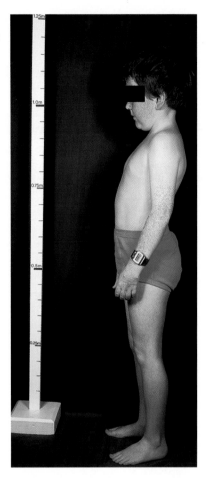

If there is hypertension, a urinary adrenal steroid profile will help diagnose variants of steroid synthesis disorders.

Pelvic ultrasonography will reveal the absence of even small prepubertal ovaries if streak gonads are present. When the testes in a male are impalpable, they may be localized with ultrasonography either in the inguinal canal or intra-abdominally (**Fig. 7.12**). To determine whether there is functioning gonadal tissue a short human chorionic gonadotropin (hCG) test can be performed (see Appendix). Administration of this LH-like compound will cause production of estrogen or testosterone, which can be measured as a rise from the basal values. Occasionally a prolonged test is required for absolute proof of lack of gonadal tissue.

In a male with impalpable gonads and a rise in testosterone concentration in response to hCG, but in whom ultrasonography fails to locate the tissue, laparoscopy is needed to assess the possibility of orchidopexy or the need for gonadectomy to prevent undetected malignant change.

Autoantibodies to the thyroid, adrenal and ovary

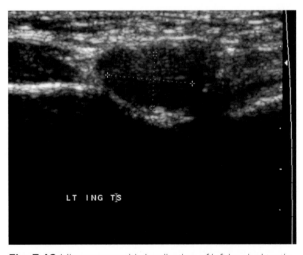

Fig. 7.12 Ultrasonographic localization of left inguinal testis.

can be estimated in the presence of a family history or suggestive physical signs.

Inhibin A (in the female) and inhibin B levels in both sexes can serve as useful markers of gonadal function. Inhibin A levels (produced from the corpus) fall before FSH levels rise in ovarian damage. Inhibin B (produced by granulosa cells in the female and Sertoli cells in the male) fall early in ovarian or testicular damage – for instance after radiotherapy – and levels rise if testicular function returns.

Hypogonadotropic hypogonadism

To differentiate between permanent and temporary gonadotropin deficiency, a luteinizing hormone releasing hormone (LHRH) test can be performed (see Appendix). The results may be equivocal because, although complete failure of a rise of gonadotropin concentration is suggestive of central hypogonadism, a blunted response can occur just before the onset of delayed puberty. Differentiation from partial central deficiency may thus be difficult without serial retesting before or after a period of treatment (see below).

If there is short stature or signs of hypothyroidism, a combined anterior pituitary function test with basal thyroid function (FT_4) is indicated (see Appendix), along with imaging of the central nervous system if multiple deficiencies are proven.

Occasionally the short stature and long legs in comparison to the back that is seen in delayed puberty can be mimicked by the milder forms of spondylo-epiphyseal dysplasia, and a limited skeletal survey may be needed.

THERAPY

HYPERGONADOTROPIC HYPOGONADISM

Males

In males, counseling is indicated regarding the need for treatment (long-term testosterone), infertility and the option of testicular prostheses. Testosterone treatment is started at about 12.5 years (50–100 mg once a month by depot i.m. injection, or oral testosterone undecanoate 40 mg on alternate days increasing to a daily dose after 6 months) to ensure normal physical and psychosocial development, normal sexual function and to protect the cardiovascular system and bone mineral density. Prostheses are usually placed at the end of pubertal development and the dose of testosterone is increased (250 mg by depot i.m. injection once every 3 weeks, or oral testosterone undecanoate 80–240 mg per day) to achieve a normal level of sexual activity.

Females

In females treatment is needed with estrogens to induce breast development, to prevent osteoporosis and to ensure a normal psychosocial development.

Ethinylestradiol is commonly used. The starting dosage is 0.05 μg per kg body weight given orally (usually about 2 μg per day or on alternate days). Alternatively matrix-based patches of 25 μg can be cut up into halves and quarters to provide similar low doses transdermally. An initial low dosage appears to improve final height by preventing early bony fusion and there is an improved cosmetic appearance of the breasts. The dosage is gradually increased over a period of 2–3 years to reach a substitution dosage of 20–30 μg, with progestagens at a dosage of 5–10 mg medroxy-progesterone per day for 10–14 days per month. When growth is completed, transcutaneous patches or a triphasic contraceptive pill can be conveniently used. Counseling regarding infertility is required, although the use of egg donation and gametocyte transfer allows the possible artificial induction of pregnancy in some individuals.

HYPOGONADOTROPIC HYPOGONADISM

Males

In males initially it may be difficult to separate constitutional delay from central hypogonadism. For psychologic reasons a pragmatic approach is to offer testosterone treatment. This may be given either in a depot dosage of 50–100 mg testosterone esters every 3–4 weeks intramuscularly or as oral testosterone undecanoate 20–40 mg per day. Testosterone is also available as a buccal pellet, a gel and as various designs of patch, but experience of these preparations in pediatric practice is limited. An alternative approach is to use the anabolic steroid oxandrolone in a dose of 1.25–2.5 mg per day orally.

Usually these treatments are discontinued after 3–4 months, and the development of testicular size is checked along with serum testosterone measurements. If puberty starts (testicular volume >4 mL), testosterone or oxandrolone treatment can be stopped to allow natural puberty to progress. If there is failure of subsequent development, a further 3-month course and re-evaluation of the possibility of permanent central hypogonadism may be necessary. In cases of a permanent gonadotropin deficiency, testosterone treatment is continued for life. Intermittent biosynthetic gonadotropin administration, human menopausal gonadotropin (hMG), hCG and pulsatile LHRH infusion have all been used to induce spermatogenesis; a rise in inhibin B levels can be used as a marker of successful treatment.

Females

In females pubertal delay requiring treatment is rare but may be treated with low dosages of ethinylestradiol as described above. In case of permanent central hypogonadism, estrogen substitution is indicated. The dosage is gradually increased over 2–3 years, for example from 4 to 10 to 20 and later 30 µg ethinylestradiol per day (either as tablets or a divided matrix patch), while medroxyprogesterone (for 10–14 days per month) is added to ensure regular menses. Patches or triphasic contraceptive preparations may again be used conveniently until menopausal age or hormone replacement therapy continued life-long.

Hypopituitary females often have sparse pubic hair growth (secondary to lack of adrenal maturation and androgen production). This cosmetic problem can be treated with topical, or low-dose oral or injected, testosterone, or with oral dehydroepiandrosterone sulfate (DHEAS), if required.

Chapter 8

Abnormal Genitalia

NORMAL DEVELOPMENT OF THE GENITALIA

For the purpose of this book, only a few aspects of genital development will be highlighted to facilitate understanding of the various disorders.

A crucial point is that the external genitalia develop 'automatically' in the female direction *unless* there is testosterone activity in a critical period between 4 and 12 weeks of gestation. Furthermore, the Müllerian ducts develop into the uterus and fallopian tubes *unless* Müllerian inhibiting factor (MIF) is produced and is effective. Both hormones are produced only by the testis. Therefore the testis and the two hormones it produces are essential for the development of the genitalia, while the ovary and estrogens do not appear essential in that period.

The primitive gonads condense from the genital ridges and are populated by germ cells that have migrated in from the yolk sac. Factors transcribed from autosomal chromosomes (chromosome 11, WT1; chromosome 9, SF1; chromosome 17, SOX9; chromosome 2, LHR) help control the early process of gonadal development. A gene on the X (short arm) chromosome, *DAX1*, acts as an anti-testis factor if present in a 'double dose'. Thereafter the presence of one gene, called testis determining gene (*TDG* or *SRY*), which usually resides on the Y chromosome, leads to the development of the undifferentiated gonad into a testis (**Fig. 8.1**). SRY is a 240 amino acid transcription factor active for only 36 hours of embryogenesis. A further gene, encoding spermatogenesis factor (SGF), is required for normal Sertoli cell function.

Therefore, several disorders at the chromosomal level can prevent the testis from differentiating. These disorders include duplication of *DAX1*, camptomelic dwarfism (*SOX9* mutation (**Fig. 8.2**), Leydig cell agenesis (LHR mutation), Drash syndrome (WT1 mutation) and mosaicisms of the sex chromosomes (e.g. 46XY/45X in mixed gonadal dysgenesis, and many others); also translocation of the *TDG* to another chromosome, for instance an X chromosome (XX males; **Fig. 8.3**), and deletion of the *TDG* (XY female). At a more subtle scale, abnormalities of *TDG* (deletions, mutations) also lead to insufficient differentiation of

the testis (XY females with gonadal dysgenesis). These disorders (which may be generalized, chimeric or localized to the gonads) can lead to either an undifferentiated gonad or a dysgenetic testis. A combination of testicular and ovarian tissue, as seen in true hermaphroditism, may have many complex causes including tissue mosaicism and chimerism, causing XX- and Y-containing tissue to be expressed simultaneously in the gonads.

After differentiation the normal testis produces testosterone, inhibin and MIF. Inhibin B is a glycoprotein that feeds back to the pituitary to inhibit the secretion of follicle stimulating hormone (FSH). Its presence can serve as a useful marker of the presence of gonadal tissue. The presence of MIF leads to regression of the Müllerian ducts. If MIF production does not occur in the presence of a normal testosterone secretion, for example due to agenesis of Sertoli cells or a mutation in the MIF gene, the Müllerian duct develops into a uterus while the external genitalia are those of a normal male (**Fig. 8.4**). As would be expected, MIF receptor abnormalities lead to a similar persistent Müllerian duct syndrome as is seen in MIF gene mutations or deletions.

The presence of testosterone normally leads to male differentiation of the external genitalia and development of the Wolffian ducts. If testosterone production does not occur, the external genitalia do not develop in the male direction and the Wolffian duct does not develop into the internal male duct (vas deferens). Lack of testosterone production may be due to agenesis of the Leydig cells, luteinizing hormone (LH) receptor mutations, an inability of Leydig cells to produce testosterone (SF1 mutations and enzyme deficiencies of testosterone biosynthesis, which are common to the testis and adrenal gland) or a lack of stimulation of testosterone secretion as a result of insufficient production or action of placental human chorionic gonadotropin (hCG) and pituitary gonadotropins.

Although directly active on embryonic Wolffian structures and muscle, testosterone can exert its effect on the external genitalia only if it is converted to dihydrotestosterone (DHT) within the target cells by 5α-reductase. DHT is subsequently bound to an

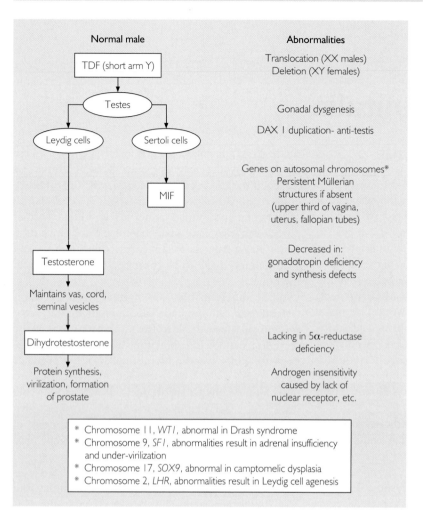

Normal male

TDF (short arm Y)

Testes

Leydig cells | Sertoli cells

MIF

Testosterone

Maintains vas, cord, seminal vesicles

Dihydrotestosterone

Protein synthesis, virilization, formation of prostate

Abnormalities

Translocation (XX males)
Deletion (XY females)

Gonadal dysgenesis

DAX I duplication- anti-testis

Genes on autosomal chromosomes*
Persistent Müllerian structures if absent
(upper third of vagina, uterus, fallopian tubes)

Decreased in:
gonadotropin deficiency and synthesis defects

Lacking in 5α-reductase deficiency

Androgen insensitivity caused by lack of nuclear receptor, etc.

* Chromosome 11, *WT1*, abnormal in Drash syndrome
* Chromosome 9, *SF1*, abnormalities result in adrenal insufficiency and under-virilization
* Chromosome 17, *SOX9*, abnormal in camptomelic dysplasia
* Chromosome 2, *LHR*, abnormalities result in Leydig cell agenesis

Fig. 8.1 The cascade of male genital development.

androgen receptor and acts on the nucleus to exert its effects on the synthesis of virilizing proteins. Therefore, even if testosterone is produced normally, there can be disorders at the enzymatic, receptor and post-receptor level causing complete or partial insensitivity to the hormone.

For instance, if the converting enzyme (5α-reductase) is absent or mutated there will be incomplete virilization, but because 5α-reductase is present in at least two isoforms, which are differentially expressed with age, an initially externally phenotypic female may undergo masculinization at puberty.

If the androgen receptor is absent or mutated, or if there are post-receptor disorders, the external genitalia will be either completely female or masculinized to an extent determined by the completeness of the defect – complete or partial androgen insensitivity syndrome (formerly called testicular feminization).

The commonest cause of excessive testosterone production leading to virilization in the female is con-

genital adrenal hyperplasia (CAH). Cortisol secretion is regulated in a classic feedback loop with adrenocorticotropic hormone (ACTH), and hence if cortisol secretion is blocked by any enzymatic deficiency in the adrenal there is no negative feedback, and increased ACTH secretion leads to an enlargement of the adrenal and over-secretion of steroid precursors and steroids not on the affected pathway (**Figs 8.5 & 8.6**).

Of all the possible adrenal enzyme deficiencies, 21-hydroxylase deficiency is by far the most frequent, with an incidence of between 1 in 5000 and 1 in 20 000 births, depending on the population. There are two clinical variants of the 'classic' condition: the simple virilizing form and the salt-wasting form. (There is also a late-onset 'non-classic' subtype with less prominent clinical features.) Copies of the gene *CYP21* and its inactive pseudogene *CYP21P* are carried on chromosome 6p and are closely linked to the human leukocyte antigen (HLA) type of the individual. The gene may

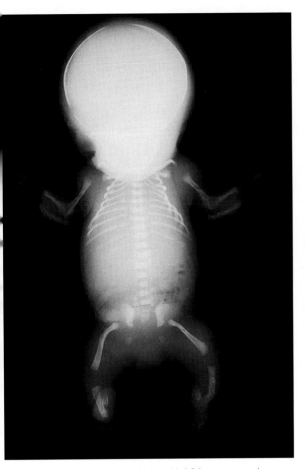

Fig. 8.2 Camptomelic dysplasia with XY sex reversal.

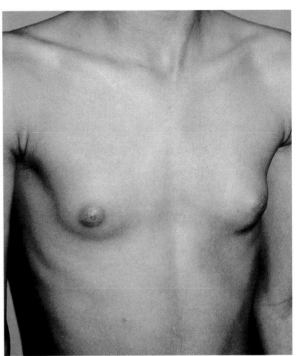

Fig. 8.3 XX male presenting at puberty with gynecomastia.

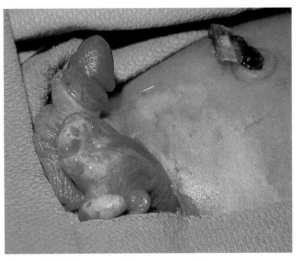

Fig. 8.4 MIF deficiency. The uterus and fallopian tubes can be seen externalized at operation in this phenotypic male (penis visible top left).

be deleted, inactivated by a point mutation or converted to a pseudogene during cross-over. The defect is expressed in only the zona fasciculata in the simple virilizing form, and in both the fasciculata and glomerulosa in the salt-wasting form. The salt-wasting form is strongly associated with HLA types BW47 and DR7. Similar variation in the expression of salt loss or the balance of over- or under-virilization seen, for instance, in 3β-hydroxysteroid dehydrogenase deficiency is presumably explained in a similar fashion.

The mechanism of synthesis of testosterone is the same in the adrenal and the testes. Enzyme deficiencies on this pathway leading to cortisol deficiency will thus lead to male pseudo-hermaphroditism with adrenal hyperplasia. Defects 'lower down' the pathway (after 17, 20-desmolase) will have no effect on cortisol production and present with simple under-virilization.

Dehydroepiandrosterone is relatively overproduced in adrenarche (see chapter 7) and in tumors. It is also metabolized by the placenta to estriol, which appears in the maternal urine and can serve as a surrogate marker for fetal adrenal function.

GENDER IDENTITY

Every individual, whatever the disturbance in the process of genital differentiation, develops a gender identity, i.e. feels himself or herself to be a male or female. This gender identity is based partly on the physical appearance of the external genitalia but also on the poorly understood effects of antenatal hormone exposure on the brain, and other unknown factors.

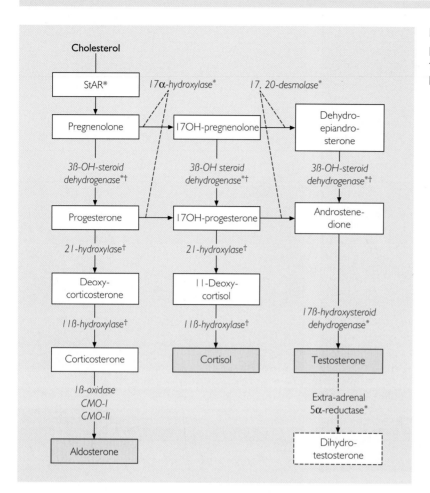

Fig. 8.5 Adrenal steroid synthesis pathway. *Undervirilized; †overvirilized; *†either, depending on level of expression.

The genital appearance largely determines the initial behavior of the parents and, to an extent, that of young children themselves. Gender-specific behavior may be observed during early childhood, for instance in the masculinized play behavior of girls with CAH. There may be subsequent readjustment of perceived gender identity and sexual behavior by the child at puberty, or later. A schematic picture of the development of gender identity is shown in **Fig. 8.7**.

In cases in which the physical appearance of the external genitalia is ambiguous, a decision about the sex of rearing has to be made by the parents and pediatrician in the best interests of the child. The diagnosis and the long-term need for surgery (which may be on several occasions) and medication should be discussed. The likelihood of testosterone responsiveness and the size of the phallus are important, although there are reports of good male sexual function with extremely small phallus size. A normal male phallus is very difficult to create surgically. It may be possible to predict later fertility, but current advances in fertility preservation and *in vitro* methods may make this advice less certain. The least predictable aspect relates to the likely gender identity of the child and future sexually functioning adult. There is a strong argument for doing as little irreversible as possible in the early years that is compatible with good health and social functioning, and to allow the competent older child to decide the issue. However, this may present practical difficulties at school, and some early surgical or medical intervention may still be required.

Clitoral reduction and later vaginoplasty can produce acceptable appearance and function in the severely masculinized XX individual (e.g. with CAH), who will be fertile. There are, however, increased problems with sexual identity, and some women request gender reassignment as adults.

Fig. 8.6 Schematic representation of the common form of congenital adrenal hyperplasia, 21-hydroxylase deficiency.

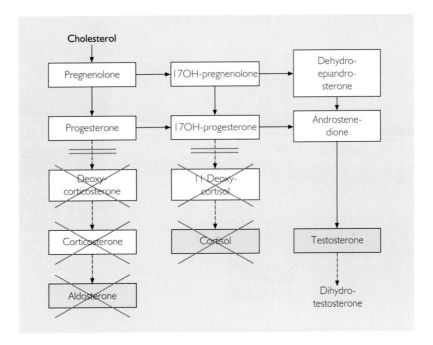

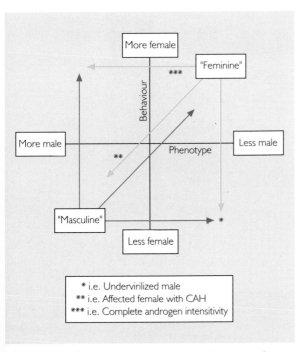

Fig. 8.7 'Gender' is defined by a complex interplay of chromosomal, phenotypic, genital, behavioral, sexual and legal components. It may be modified by fetal hormones, postnatal hormones, and peer or care-giver behavior. A heterosexual male in the bottom left quadrant, or a heterosexual female in the upper right quadrant, may be 'moved' in the three directions shown by the modifying influences of hormones and upbringing, as well as yet unknown influences that can be both transient and permanent.

CLASSIFICATION

There are four groups of intersex disorders based on the appearance of the gonads.

1. Undifferentiated or absent gonads

Abnormal gonadogenesis may occur with or without chromosomal abnormalities. There is some confusion about the classification if gonadal dysgenesis is associated with an XY chromosomal pattern: some authors classify these forms in the group of male pseudo-hermaphroditism and others in the group of undifferentiated gonads; in the present classification only the gross abnormalities of the gonads (XY pure gonadal dysgenesis, congenital anorchia (vanishing testes)) are included in this group. If all or part of the short arm of the X chromosome is duplicated, it is possible to have an XY karyotype but two doses of the *DAX1* gene. This acts to suppress testicular formation and leads to under-virilization and variable persistence of Müllerian structures (**Fig. 8.8**).

2. True hermaphroditism

This involves the presence of both ovarian and testicular tissue (**Figs 8.9–8.11**); any pattern of sex chromosomes can be found in these cases.

3. Male pseudo-hermaphroditism

This condition – insufficient masculinization in the presence of a testis – can be due to absent testes,

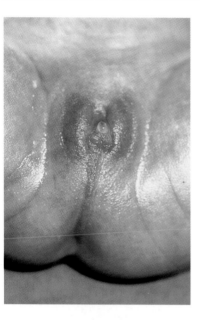

Fig. 8.8 *DAX1* duplication leading to severe undervirilization.

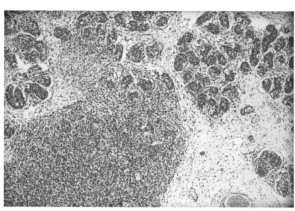

Fig. 8.10 Histology of gonad in true hermaphroditism showing ovo-testis. Ovarian tissue is shown as dense stroma with oocytes; testicular tissue shows tubule formation. Peripheral blood karyotype 46XX. Skin and gonad showed chimeric 46XX–69XXY karyotype.

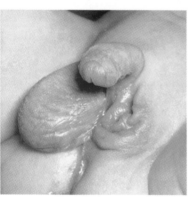

Fig. 8.9 True hermaphrodite. Right-sided descended testis, internal left ovo-testis, hypospadias.

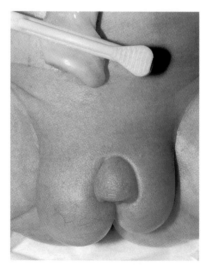

Fig. 8.11 External genitalia of same case as **8.10**.

absent biosynthesis, target organ resistance, or other effects.

Absent testes

- Insufficient stimulation by gonadotropins: hypopituitarism or isolated gonadotropin deficiency (**Fig. 8.12**), which may be part of a syndrome (**Fig. 8.13**). The association of isolated gonadotropin deficiency with anosmia is called the Kallmann syndrome. These defects present more commonly with isolated micropenis, but testicular development can sometimes be so poor that incomplete virilization occurs.
- Leydig cell agenesis and LH receptor mutations.
- Drash syndrome with nephritis and later Wilms tumor due to WT1 hemizygosity.

Absent biosynthesis

- Disturbed androgen synthesis, because of enzymatic disorders: StAR (steroid acute

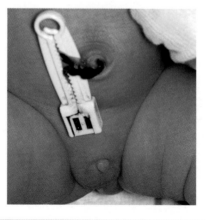

Fig. 8.12 Micropenis and cryptorchidism in panhypopituitarism. Infant had cleft palate and developed hypoglycemia.

Fig. 8.13
Micropenis and
cryptorchidism in
Prader–Labhart–
Willi syndrome.

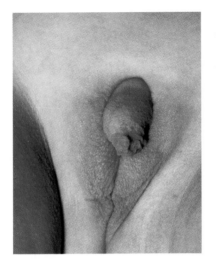

Fig. 8.16 Non-
salt-losing 3β-
hydroxysteroid
dehydrogenase
deficiency.

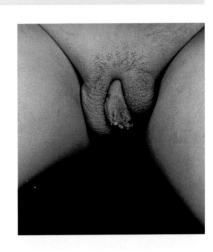

Fig. 8.14 StAR
deficiency
(congenital lipoid
hyperplasia),
external
appearance.

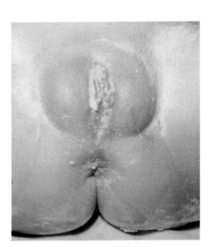

Fig. 8.17
Karyotypic male
with 17-
ketosteroid
reductase
deficiency (17β-
hydroxysteroid
dehydrogenase
deficiency).

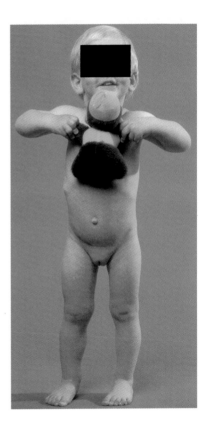

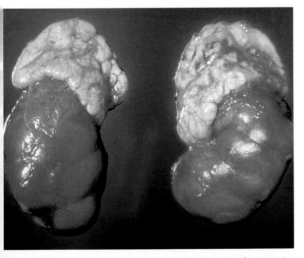

Fig. 8.15 Post-mortem appearance of adrenals of patient in
Fig. 8.14.

regulatory protein; **Figs 8.14 & 8.15**) deficiency
also called congenital lipoid hyperplasia, 17α-
hydroxylase, 3β-hydroxysteroid dehydrogenase
(**Fig. 8.16**), 17, 20-desmolase, 17-ketosteroid
reductase (**Figs 8.17–8.21**) (also called 17β-
hydroxysteroid dehydrogenase deficiency).

■ Smith–Lemli–Opitz syndrome with genital
ambiguity in the male, cleft palate and digital
abnormalities (see **Figs 1.30 & 1.69**).

■ Reduced 5α-reductase activity (**Fig. 8.22**).

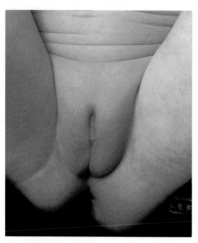

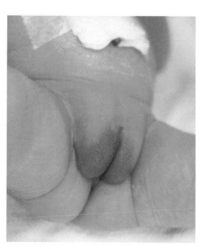

Figs 8.18–8.21 Karyotypic males with 17-ketosteroid reductase deficiency (17β-hydroxysteroid dehydrogenase deficiency) – close-up views of genital appearance to show variability. Note pigmentation in Fig. 8.19.

Fig. 8.19

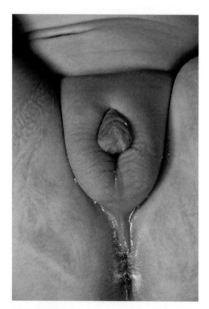

Fig. 8.20

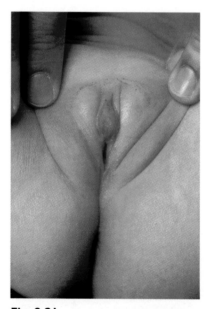

Fig. 8.21

Target organ resistance

- Androgen insensitivity syndrome (complete or partial): androgen receptor or post-receptor defect (**Figs 8.23–8.25**).

Other

- Timing defect (late hormonal secretion *in utero*).
- Isolated MIF deficiency.
- Maternal ingestion of anti-androgens.
- Idiopathic.

4. Female pseudo-hermaphroditism

Excessive masculinization in the presence of ovaries is by far the commonest cause of abnormal genitalia. It may be subclassified as:

- CAH; 21-hydroxylase (accounting for 90% of all intersex conditions), 11β-hydroxylase (approx. 5%) or 3β-hydroxysteroid dehydrogenase deficiency (approx. 1%).
- Excess of maternal androgens either as ingestion of androgens (or 19-nortestosterone-derived

Fig. 8.22
5α-Reductase
deficiency.

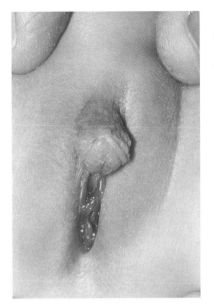

Fig. 8.23 Partial
androgen
insensitivity with
descended testes
in bifid labio-
scrotal folds.

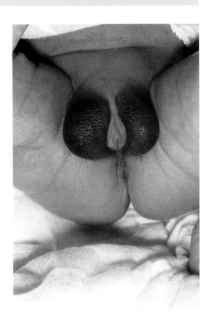

Fig. 8.24 Less
severe partial
androgen
insensitivity with
severe
hypospadias and
maldescent of
testes.

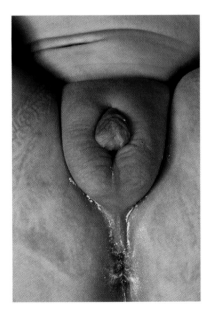

Fig. 8.25 Partial
androgen
insensitivity
syndrome at
adolescence, male
sex of rearing –
note gynecomastia
from peripheral
aromatase
conversion of
testosterone to
estrogen.
Abundant pubic
hair implies only
partial resistance.

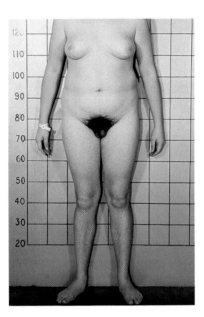

progestagens) or virilizing tumors, luteomas and
maternal CAH.

■ Non-specific, associated with other congenital
anomalies.

■ Idiopathic.

Additionally *isolated micropenis* and *cryptorchidism* are
considered in this chapter.

DIAGNOSTIC WORK-UP OF INTERSEX CONDITIONS

HISTORY AND CLINICAL EXAMINATION

As with most congenital defects, the history should
concentrate on maternal health, pregnancy details and
family history:

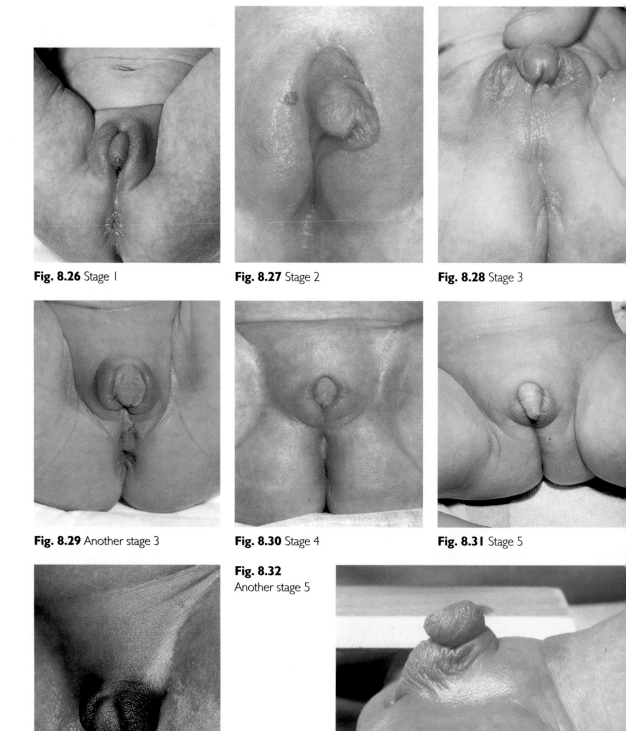

Fig. 8.26 Stage 1

Fig. 8.27 Stage 2

Fig. 8.28 Stage 3

Fig. 8.29 Another stage 3

Fig. 8.30 Stage 4

Fig. 8.31 Stage 5

Fig. 8.32
Another stage 5

Fig. 8.33 Complete masculinization in 46XX CAH.

Figs 8.26–8.33 Stages of masculinization in 21-hydroxylase deficiency from relatively minor to complete.

Fig. 8.34 Male genitalia in 21-hydroxylase deficiency.

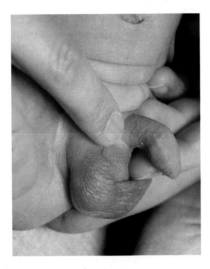

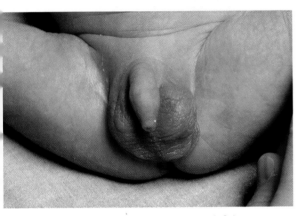

Fig. 8.35 Male genitalia in 21-hydroxylase deficiency.

- Symptoms of virilization in the mother.
- Drugs during pregnancy.
- Unexplained infant deaths.
- Genital ambiguity, short stature or pronounced hirsutism in the family.
- Parental consanguinity.

The physical examination should include a thorough inspection and palpation of the external genitalia, blood pressure (raised in 11β-hydroxylase deficiency) and a search for other congenital anomalies. Ambiguous genitalia include the whole spectrum from the normal male to normal female genitalia. Five intermediate stages have been distinguished by Prader (**Figs 8.26–8.33**). Any abnormality of the external genitalia should lead to further investigations, including apparently normal female genitalia with palpable gonads in the labia or inguinal area, females with bilateral inguinal hernias or apparently normal males with impalpable gonads. Male infants with CAH may show signs of excess testosterone production by an increase in scrotal pigmentation and a

slight increase in penis size (**Figs 8.34 & 8.35**); these signs are often missed, however, and then the presentation is as collapse with hyponatremia and acidosis or, in non-salt losers, as the 'infantile Hercules syndrome' (see Ch. 11).

In cases of female pseudo-hermaphroditism the mother should be examined for signs of virilization and hypertension that would indicate a maternal source of testosterone.

Interpretation of the clues

If gonads are palpable externally, there is at least a *TDG* (testis determining gene) present, usually on a Y chromosome. (A proportion of patients with complete androgen insensitivity syndrome will present with apparently normal female external genitalia but bilateral hernias that contain testes.)

Otherwise, in the absence of obvious maternal pathology or family history, *it is not wise to try to base a diagnosis on external appearance alone*. Further elucidation will come from investigation in specialist centers.

INVESTIGATIONS

Karyotype

Many laboratories can provide a result at least on the presence or absence of a Y chromosome within a few days. The final result of the karyotype may take several weeks. (Buccal smears can be taken and investigated for the presence of Barr bodies. If seen, at least two X chromosomes are present. This investigation should be abandoned if rapid chromosome testing is available.)

Further investigations are determined by the karyotype.

XX karyotype

- Biochemical assessment should include several estimations of serum sodium and potassium concentrations; some forms of CAH can lead to salt loss, which is not always present in the first weeks.
- Kidney function should be checked to detect any associated renal disorders and, if suspected, in addition to ultrasonography, a renogram or intravenous pyelogram (IVP) should be obtained.
- The anatomy of the internal genitalia is investigated by ultrasonography (to check for gonads, uterus and vagina) and a contrast examination of the urogenital sinus – a cervical imprint seen with a contrast examination proves

the presence of a uterus (**Figs 8.36 & 8.37**) that may not be apparent on ultrasonography.

- Cystoscopy may be performed to evaluate the urethra and bladder.
- Laparoscopy may allow for the further differentiation of internal anatomy and direct visualization of the gonads, along with possible gonadal biopsy.

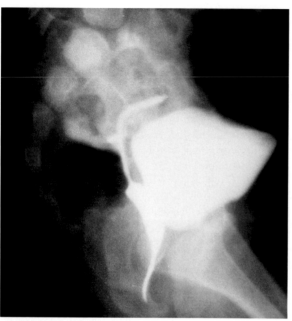

Fig. 8.36 Cloacagram showing filling of vagina, fistula to bladder, cervical imprint and uterine cavity.

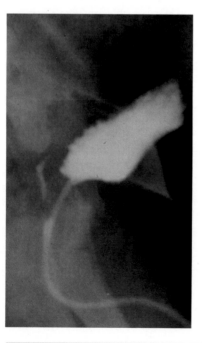

Fig. 8.37 Cloacagram showing high insertion of narrow utricle/vagina into male-appearing urethra – more severe virilization requiring more complex surgery than patient in Fig. 8.36.

- Plasma 17α-hydroxyprogesterone concentration is raised in the commonest form of CAH, 21-hydroxylase deficiency (see **Fig. 8.6**). Additionally levels of testosterone, androstenedione and dehydroepiandrosterone (DHEA) will be increased and are responsible for the virilization that occurs. Cortisol production will be diminished and in 80% of cases there will be salt losing secondary to aldosterone deficiency.
- In 11β-hydroxylase deficiency, plasma deoxycorticosterone (DOC) concentration will be raised in addition to the above androgens (and there will be hypertension due to the salt-retaining properties of DOC). Cortisol production will be diminished.
- In 3β-hydroxysteroid dehydrogenase deficiency there will be salt losing and cortisol deficiency with an increased DHEA concentration. The level of pregnenolone will be raised and a urinary steroid profile will show a characteristic increase in pregnenediol and pregnenetriol concentrations. This deficiency can cause both male and female pseudo-hermaphroditism, presumably depending on the activity of accessory pathways of testosterone synthesis from DHEA.
- Occasionally a urinary steroid profile, plasma steroid levels, ultrasonography and radiography will have to be performed on the mother to determine the source of androgens in an infant virilized secondary to a maternal cause.

XY karyotype

- Measurements of serum levels of testosterone, DHT and its steroid precursors androstenedione and DHEA should be performed, both before and after one hCG injection of 1500 units i.m (see Appendix). A normal testosterone rise excludes Leydig cell agenesis and enzymatic disorders of testosterone biosynthesis, and is more compatible with a partial androgen insensitivity syndrome (as an individual with the complete syndrome will have phenotypically normal female genitalia: **Fig. 8.38**). The ratio between testosterone and its precursors indicates the precise level of enzyme defect in disorders of testosterone biosynthesis (see **Fig. 8.5**): a high ratio (>1.25) between androstenedione and testosterone indicates 17β-hydroxysteroid dehydrogenase deficiency; a high DHEAS concentration indicates a 3β-hydroxysteroid dehydrogenase defect; very low levels of 17α-hydroxyprogesterone, androstenedione and testosterone in the

Fig. 8.38
Complete androgen insensitivity syndrome presenting at puberty with sparse pubic hair growth and amenorrhea.

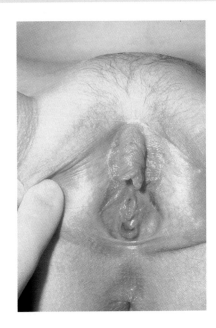

presence of high progesterone levels indicate 17α-hydroxylase deficiency; high progesterone and 17α-hydroxyprogesterone levels with low androstenedione and testosterone levels indicate a 17, 20-desmolase deficiency. Very low levels of all steroids are seen in Leydig cell aplasia and when the first set of proteins that transports cholesterol from the mitochondrion outer leaflet to the inner one to allow the desmolase enzyme system to cleave the side chain (StAR) is deficient. If the level of testosterone increases and there is little or no rise in DHT (T: DHT ratio >25) then the defect lies in the conversion of testosterone to DHT by 5α-reductase.

■ The sex hormone binding globulin (SHBG) response to the anabolic steroid stanazolol can be used to estimate the degree of androgen insensitivity (unfortunately the test is reliable only after 4 months of age). In normal individuals there is a 50% reduction in SHBG concentration from the baseline 4 days after a 3-day course of treatment (0.5 mg/kg). In complete androgen insensitivity syndrome there is no response or even a slight rise in the level. Those with a fall of less than 20% will probably not respond sufficiently to later treatment to be raised successfully as males.

■ It is possible to search for duplication of *DAX1*, and mutations of *WT1*, *SF1*, *SOX9* and the LH receptor (*LHR*) genes in cases where there has been an early failure of testicular development.

■ Genital skin fibroblasts can be obtained for assay of androgen receptor levels and elucidation of post-receptor defects in specialist units. Fibroblast

karyotyping should also be performed (preferably from the skin as well) to exclude tissue mosaicism.

■ Hematuria and proteinuria are seen as early as the first day of life in Drash syndrome.

■ 7-Dehydrocholesterol levels are raised in Smith–Lemli–Opitz syndrome.

■ Anti-Müllerian hormone (MIF) can be assayed in cases of persistent Müllerian duct syndrome and also gives a clue as to the presence of functioning testicular tissue.

True hermaphrodites

In true hermaphroditism, and in the presence of a Y chromosome with internal genitalia and female sex of rearing, laparoscopy is indicated to inspect the internal genitalia (gonads and uterus) and to biopsy or remove gonadal tissue incompatible with the assigned sex. Tissue karyotyping should again be performed.

THERAPY

From the outset the physician should explain to the parents that there is some doubt concerning the sex of the infant and that further investigations are needed. The parents must be told to delay registration of the child until there is a degree of certainty about the sex of rearing. Psychologic support and counseling are essential and much attention should be directed towards this neglected aspect of care. Preferably a psychologist or social worker should be involved.

FEMALE SEX OF REARING

Therapy is dependent on the precise diagnosis. If a female sex is assigned and the clitoris is enlarged, then cliteroplasty should be considered, preserving the venous and nervous supply to the glans (**Figs 8.39 & 8.40**). Alternatively, if a less permanent approach has been recommended, the clitoris may be 'buried'. If there is complete or partial fusion of the labial folds, either a one-stage or two-stage operation schedule can be designed. Highly specialized surgeons tend to perform vaginoplasty early in life, and to ensure connection to the uterus, if present (e.g. in CAH). A drawback is that regular dilatation may be needed in childhood. Others may perform initial cliteroplasty together with a separation of the fused labia, and at puberty perform vaginoplasty and connection to the uterus, if required. The vagina can be widened by regular use of dilators in collaboration with a gynecologist.

In all cases of CAH, treatment with hydrocortisone is indicated to suppress ACTH levels and to maintain normal growth rate and skeletal maturation. This

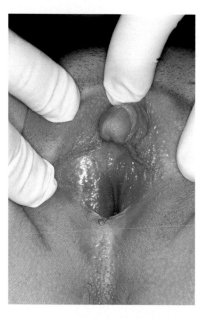

Fig. 8.39 Late presenting simple virilizing 21-hydroxylase deficiency (height +1.8 SDS, chronologic age 7.5 years, bone age 14.7 years) – before clitoroplasty.

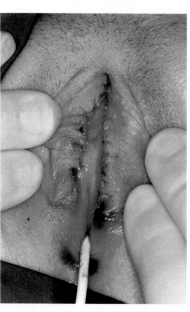

Fig. 8.40 Same patient as in Fig. 8.39 after clitoroplasty. In this case the vaginal orifice was adequate and no later surgery was required. (The stage 5 pubic hair has been shaved off.)

In neonates with 21-hydroxylase deficiency the hydrocortisone dosage is often close to 30 mg/m² daily. Later it can gradually be decreased to 15–25 mg/m² daily, and 12–15 mg/m² daily from 2 years onwards. Hydrocortisone should be divided as a three times a day dose, usually with 50% given on waking to mimic the normal diurnal secretion of cortisol.

In forms of CAH in which salt loss is present, either clinically or subclinically (i.e. detected only by raised plasma renin activity (PRA) levels; see Ch. 11), then 9α-fluorocortisone (fludrocortisone acetate) should be added at a dose of between 0.03 and 0.12 μg per day. The dose should be adjusted by measurement of blood pressure and PRA (raised PRA levels mean that the dosage should be increased; a low PRA concentration indicates over-treatment). At the time of diagnosis, in hot weather and in some severely affected individuals, sodium chloride, 1 g per 10 kg body weight, may also be needed. Adequate salt and mineralocorticoid replacement is necessary to achieve satisfactory overall control.

If there is presence of even a portion of a normal ovary then secondary sex characteristics should develop at puberty (although fertility will be less certain). In cases of prolonged exposure to high androgen levels, for instance in late-presenting CAH, a polycystic change may occur in the ovaries leading to dysmenorrhea and later hirsutism even in the presence of adequate replacement therapy (see **Fig. 6.33**). If no ovarian tissue is present, estrogen treatment is necessary from around 10 years of age (see Ch. 7).

In the more complete forms of androgen insensitivity syndrome, the testes are removed either in early life or after puberty, as there is an increased risk of later malignancy. The presence of testes at puberty allows for some normal female sexual development without medication as testosterone is converted by aromatase to estrogen. However, the risk of malignancy before puberty, although very low, may still be considered too high to accept, and gonadectomy is increasingly performed in early life. Estrogen treatment is then necessary for the development of female secondary characteristics (see Ch. 7).

MALE SEX OF REARING

To normalize the external genitalia initially, a hypospadias repair may need to be performed in one or several stages, depending on the severity of the defect (**Fig. 8.43**). Vaginal remnants and any internal female structures can also be removed. Three-month courses of gonadotropin releasing hormone (GnRH) analogs or hCG can be used to attempt to induce

treatment and its monitoring are highly specialized and should be confined to experienced centers. Some authorities recommend the use of regular multiple daily profiles of blood or salivary 17α-hydroxyprogesterone and androstenedione along with plasma renin activity to monitor control (by confirming day-long suppression). Others only use regular (at least 6-monthly) measurement of bone age coupled with accurate estimations of height velocity to monitor control: a raised height velocity (>50%) and rapidly advancing bone age (>chronological advance) demonstrate under-treatment; a low height velocity usually indicates over-treatment or other pathology (**Figs 8.41 & 8.42**).

Fig. 8.41 Simple congenital adrenal hyperplasia secondary to 21-hydroxylase deficiency in a male. Bone age 5.6 years at 4.7 years of age with height −2 SDS, within target range but with evidence of early virilization. With hydrocortisone replacement therapy there is an improvement in height to −0.9 SDS, within the target range and a gradual normalization of the bone age.

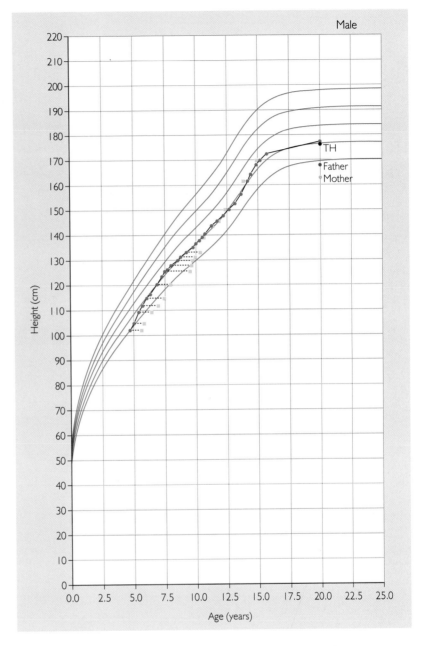

testicular decent; however, at least 80% will still require surgery. Orchidopexy, again in one or several stages, should bring the testes to the scrotum, if possible. If the testes are internal and there is no possibility of successful orchidopexy to bring them to a position where they can be examined externally, then careful consideration should be given to gonadectomy to remove the potential risk of later undetected malignant change.

Testosterone injections (25 mg testosterone esters i.m. every 3 weeks on three occasions) can be given to increase the infant's penile size. Topical testosterone cream, 2.5% for 3 months, may also prove effective (but if applied by female care-givers, they must wear gloves).

At puberty, in the absence of functioning testes, testosterone replacement treatment is required. A mixture of testosterone esters given as a depot intra-muscular injection is commonly used, which gives acceptable testosterone levels for about 3–4 weeks. This treatment is started at approximately 12–13 years of age, and the dosage is slowly increased from 50 to 250 mg every 3–4 weeks. Testosterone buccal lozenges, transdermal patches and gel are becoming available as alternative modalities of application. Even a relatively small, damaged testicular remnant may be able to

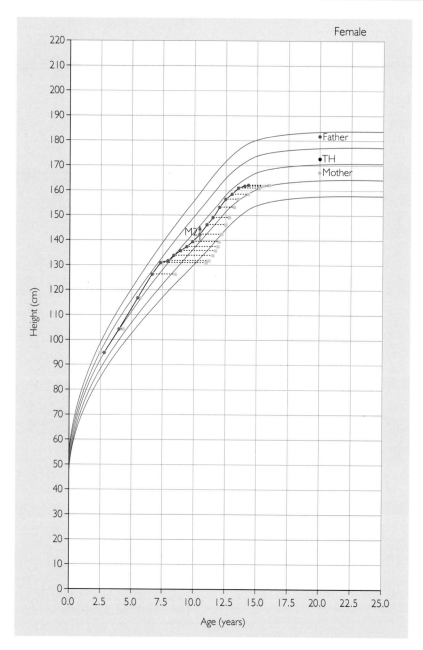

Fig. 8.42 Congenital adrenal hyperplasia in a female subject presenting with ambiguous genitalia. There is evidence of undertreatment between 5.5 and 7.4 years with an advancing bone age and increased height velocity indicating non-suppression of testosterone levels. There is subsequent regaining of control with gradual improvement of height prediction but a mildly reduced adult height (−0.5 SDS) in relation to the target range (+0.2 SDS).

produce sufficient testosterone to allow spontaneous (see **Fig. 7.3**) virilization, although fertility will be unlikely. Intracytoplasmic sperm injection (ICSI) is being used in some centers to allow fertilization from small damaged testes.

In cases due to forms of CAH, replacement therapy as outlined above should be commenced at diagnosis.

MICROPENIS

Micropenis is defined as a stretched penile length of more than 2 SD below the average for age. This equates

to less than 2 cm at birth and less than 4 cm before normal puberty. The stretched penile length is measured by taking a wooden spatula and pressing it alongside the penis on to the pubic bone. A mark is than made at the level of the top of the penile glans, and the length measured (**Fig. 8.44**). This procedure is to ensure that the part of the penis that is buried in the subcutaneous fat is being measured. A 'hidden' penis may be misdiagnosed as micropenis unless this technique is used.

Fig. 8.43 True hermaphrodite following penile repair. Spontaneous pubic hair growth from testicular remnant.

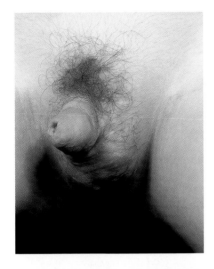

Fig. 8.44 Measurement of stretched penile shaft length.

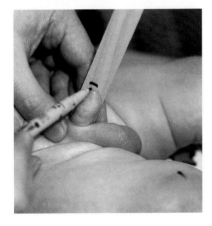

ETIOLOGY

Micropenis can be caused by hypogonadotropic hypogonadism, either isolated or in combination with other pituitary deficiencies, especially growth hormone (GH) deficiency. It is also seen in cases of primary hypogonadism and in incomplete forms of the androgen insensitivity syndrome.

DIAGNOSTIC WORK-UP

Initially exclude pituitary dysfunction. This can be done by measuring serum free thyroxine (T_4) and thyroid stimulating hormone (TSH), as well as the serum cortisol level at 0900 hours (before 3 months of age there is no circadian rhythm, and three or four random levels or a Synacthen test can be used as a substitute). Low basal values are suggestive of other pituitary problems. If hypoglycemia occurs (see Ch. 11), take blood for cortisol and GH estimation. If the cortisol value is abnormally low, the diagnosis is likely to be hypopituitarism without the need for further stimulation tests. A rise in GH concentration in response to

hypoglycemia may not always occur in the neonatal period and the GH axis should thus be re-evaluated if there is evidence of later faltering of growth.

If the infant is seen between birth and 4 months of age, a basal serum testosterone measurement is useful, as in this period there is a physiologic rise with a peak at 8 weeks. A normal testosterone level rules out a serious disorder of testicular androgen secretion. Also during the first 4 months (and in the pubertal age range), measurements of basal serum LH and FSH may be useful. Grossly increased values indicate primary gonadal failure, and undetectable levels indicate the need for further testing.

At any other age, or if the baseline testosterone level is low or inconclusive, a short hCG test is performed, measuring testosterone and DHT levels 3 days after the injection (see Appendix). A rise in testosterone and DHT indicates normal testicular function and 5α-reductase activity.

Outside the first 4 months basal levels of LH and FSH are also not very helpful and, although an LHRH test can be performed (see Appendix), the results often do not provide certainty about the differentiation between hypogonadotropic hypogonadism and normal function (see Ch. 7).

THERAPY

Micropenis should be treated by a series of three or four depot intramuscular injections of testosterone esters or topical testosterone, as described above. In infants and small children the injectable dosage is 25 mg (and larger doses can be given at puberty). If the micropenis is associated with cryptorchidism, it may be more appropriate to use hCG or gonadotropins for 2–3 months to try to achieve testicular descent and penile growth from endogenous secretion of testosterone (see below). If there is poor response in terms of growth of the penis, a form of androgen insensitivity is likely, and in extreme cases a lack of response in infancy may give rise to reconsideration of the decision about sex of rearing, although sexual function is often adequate. Late presenting cases who respond poorly have the unsatisfactory options of augmentative surgery or gender reassignment.

CRYPTORCHIDISM

ETIOLOGY

If the testes are impalpable in a phenotypic male, the possibility of an XX individual with severe female pseudo-hermaphroditism should always be considered

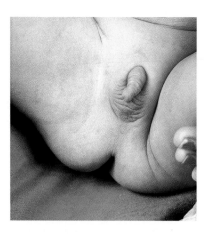

Fig. 8.45
Congenital anorchia. This may be due to torsion *in utero*, when laparoscopy will show a blind ending vas.

first. Congenital anorchia may occur after the production of MIF has occurred, presumably as a result of late *in utero* torsion (**Fig. 8.45**) or infarction.

Simple cryptorchidism is, however, common. In premature babies, the testes can still descend during the first year of life. Cryptorchidism may be caused by either mechanical factors or a failure of the normal hormonal environment. Rarely it may be due to mutations of a gene, *RLF* (relaxin-like factor), which controls gubernacular contraction.

Cryptorchidism is seen with increased frequency in:

- gonadotropin deficiency.
- testicular dysgenesis, including chromosomal abnormalities.
- association with other congenital malformations and syndromes.

DIAGNOSTIC WORK-UP

Medical history and physical examination

The history should concentrate on maternal health and treatment during pregnancy, mode and time of delivery, and family history of genital abnormalities. In later presenting cases enquiry should be made regarding the sense of smell and mental development (see Ch. 7).

The physical examination should exclude other dysmorphic features or malformations and be performed in both the supine and squatting positions. The maximal descent of the testes is noted, and the ease of retraction after manipulation. Highly retractile testes can mimic maldescent.

Interpretation of the clues

Impalpable testes:

- With no other abnormalities = simple cryptorchidism, anorchia, female pseudo-hermaphroditism.

- With micropenis, with or without hypospadias = partial androgen synthesis or insensitivity syndromes.
- With anosmia and micropenis = the Kallmann syndrome.
- With intelletual impairment or dysmorphic features = syndromic abnormality.
- With micropenis and/or midline defects = gonadotropin deficiency.
- Above features plus neonatal hypoglycemia = multiple pituitary hormone deficiency.
- With tall stature (testes may be high in the inguinal canal and small and firm) = Klinefelter syndrome.

THERAPY

Orchidopexy is performed if there is cryptorchidism with no possibility of descent when assessed by an experienced surgeon. The optimal time for operating is debated, but surgery is usually performed at around 2–3 years of age. If there is any doubt about the possibility of descent, and in cases of presumed central gonadotropin deficiency, a course of hCG can be given (500 units twice a week i.m. for 5 weeks at 1–6 years of age, and 1000 units twice a week in later childhood). If there is no satisfactory result, surgery is necessary.

MISCELLANEOUS GENITAL ABNORMALITIES

Many variations on normal anatomy exist in both sexes. They are usually spontaneous malformations, although they may be associated with other syndromic abnormalities.

Hernias are common in males but, occasionally, may unexpectedly contain Müllerian structures (**Fig. 8.46**).

The male may have a shawl scrotum of varying severity (**Figs 8.47 & 8.48**), with or without a bifid appearance (**Fig. 8.49**). The shaft of the penis may be completely within the scrotal skin and require operative release. These abnormalities may be isolated or exist as part of a chromosomal abnormality or eponymous syndrome.

Hypospadias and epispadias are usually isolated, but severe hypospadias (**Fig. 8.50**) may represent the incomplete form of androgen insensitivity syndrome. Other bizarre abnormalities, including reversed genitalia (**Fig. 8.51**) and trifid scrotum (**Fig. 8.52**) may also occur.

In the female there may be complete absence of the uterus and vagina (**Fig. 8.53**). The hymen may be

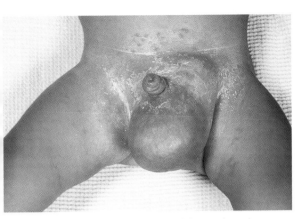

Fig. 8.46 Large inguinal hernia containing testis and Müllerian duct structures.

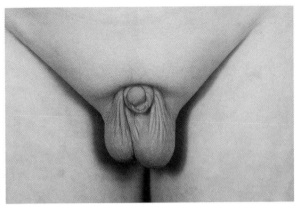

Fig. 8.49 Bifid scrotum.

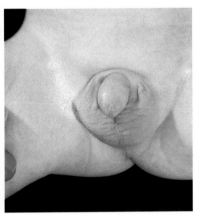

Fig. 8.47 Shawl scrotum (moderate).

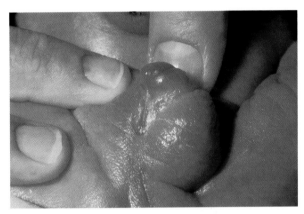

Fig. 8.50 Severe hypospadias and micropenis, 46XY.

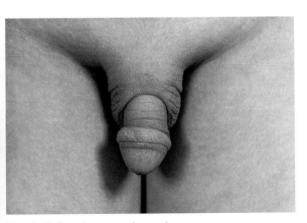

Fig. 8.48 Shawl scrotum (severe).

Fig. 8.51 Reversed male genitalia.

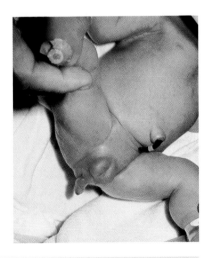

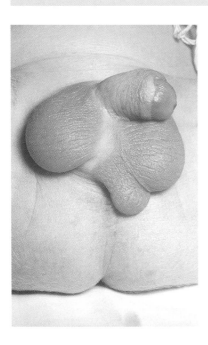

Fig. 8.52 Trifid scrotum, cause unknown.

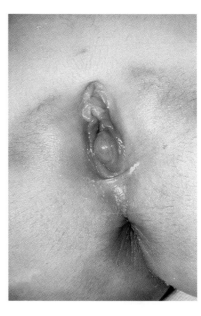

Fig. 8.54 Imperforate hymen in neonate.

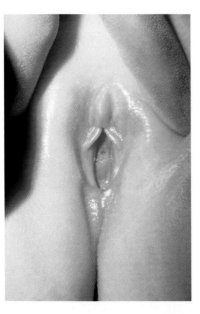

Fig. 8.53 Vaginal atresia, uterus also absent.

side effect. Attempts at parting the adhesions are often painful and result in readhesion.

GONADAL TUMORS

OVARIAN

Large cysts may present with torsion as an abdominal emergency or as a palpable mass (see **Figs 6.34, 6.35 & 10.18**). They may be seen as incidental findings (**Figs 8.62–8.64**). Because hemorrhage into an incompletely ruptured follicle can mimic tumor, it is important to re-scan at a different stage in the cycle (**Fig. 8.65**) before causing concern in the menstruating female.

Only about 1% of childhood malignancies are ovarian in origin, although other tissues in the pelvis can give rise to lesions (neuroblastoma, sarcoma, adenocarcinoma). Patients with ovarian lesions may present with sexual precocity (see Ch. 6), which can be iso- or hetero-sexual. Germ-cell tumors (dysgerminoma, endodermal sinus tumors, embryonal carcinoma, immature teratomas, choriocarcinoma and mixed forms) and juvenile granulosa cell tumors may be unilateral or bilateral, and present with hormonal effects, abdominal pain and masses, and vaginal bleeding. Dysgerminomas may occur in abnormal ovarian tissue, such as that found in Turner syndrome with an unsuspected Y-cell line.

Ultrasonography, computed tomography and magnetic resonance imaging are required along with laparoscopic biopsy. Multidisciplinary management is required depending on the histologic findings and stage of the

imperforate (**Fig. 8.54**) or there may be a transverse vaginal septum, both of which may present early with distension or late with hydrocolpos (**Figs 8.55 & 8.56**) or primary amenorrhea (**Figs 8.57–8.59**). If vaginal abnormalities are associated with renal and/or skeletal abnormalities, this forms the Rokitansky syndrome (**Fig. 8.60**).

Labial adhesions are a common finding and of no pathologic significance (**Fig. 8.61**). They resolve spontaneously and surgical intervention should be discouraged. Topical treatment with estrogen cream will result in resolution but with local pigmentation as a

Fig. 8.55
Hydrocolpos
secondary to
transverse vaginal
septum.

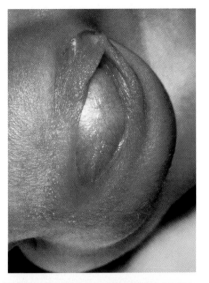

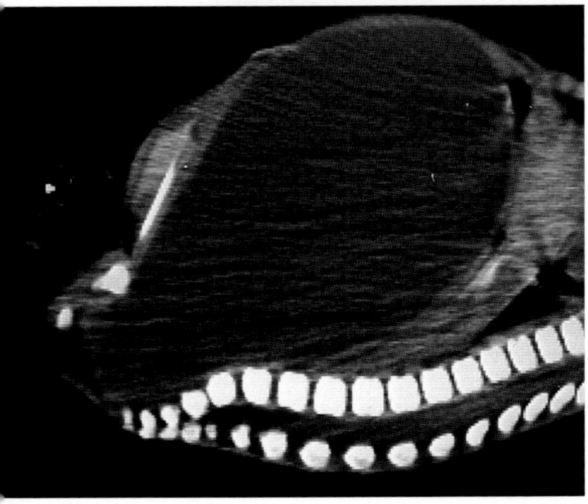

Fig. 8.58 Same
patient as in
Fig. 8.57 at
operation,
showing blueish
discoloration of
imperforate
hymen.

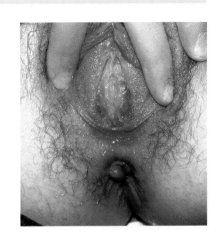

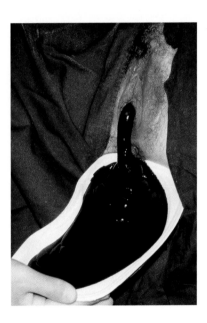

Fig. 8.59
Resulting
discharge of old
blood following
surgical incision
of patient in
Fig. 8.57.

Fig. 8.56 CT scan of same case showing massive
hydrocolpos.

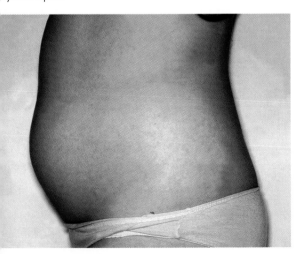

Fig. 8.57 Imperforate hymen presenting as primary
amenorrhea with abdominal distension.

Fig. 8.60
Rokitansky
syndrome.

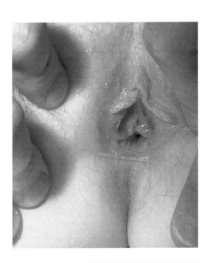

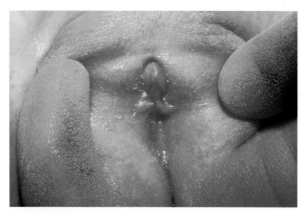

Fig. 8.61 Labial adhesions – spontaneous resolution will always occur.

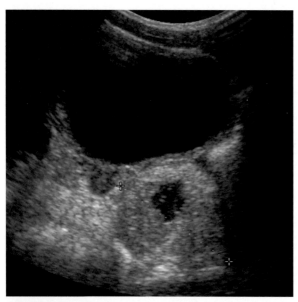

Fig. 8.62 Simple ovarian cyst.

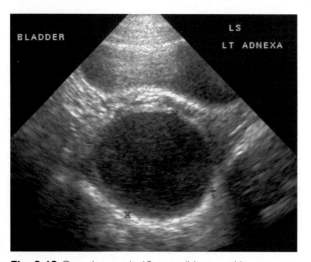

Fig. 8.63 Complex cyst in 12-cm solid mass with some ovarian tissue stretched over superior surface.

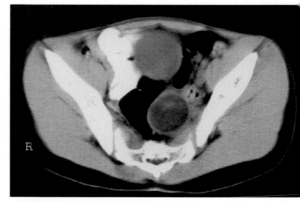

Fig. 8.64 CT scan of patient in Fig. 8.63 showing large cyst containing both lipid-dense and more solid components, typical of a mature teratoma.

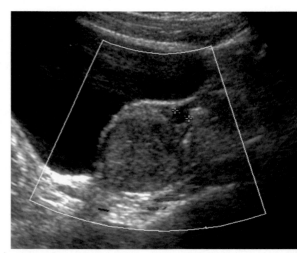

Fig. 8.65 Dense cyst that could represent a tumor or bleeding into an incompletely ruptured follicle. On re-scanning on day 7 of the second subsequent cycle, the cyst had resolved.

lesion. Tumor markers such as α-fetoprotein, hCG, lactate dehydrogenase (LDH) and carcinoembryonic antigen may be helpful in diagnosis and at follow-up.

TESTICULAR

Testicular tumors are rare in childhood. The majority of testicular tumors arise from germ cells. Undescended testes (especially bilateral) are a risk factor. Any dysgenetic internal testis in the undervirilized male may lead to gonadoblastoma. Dysgerminomas and seminomas also occur in childhood, more in primarily abnormal testes than in normal testes. Adrenal rests may hypertrophy in poorly controlled CAH, leading to palpable scrotal masses.

PRENATAL MANAGEMENT OF 21-HYDROXYLASE DEFICIENCY

As 21-hydroxylase deficiency is an autosomal recessive disease, the risk for subsequent siblings of an affected proband is 25%. The most serious consequence of the disorder is the genital ambiguity in females. Therefore it is most important to prevent masculinization of the external genitalia in affected female fetuses. The following strategy has been developed in specialist centers.

Identifying the HLA genotype of the index case and parents along with the restriction fragment length polymorphisms (RFLPs) of the 21-hydroxylase gene or detection of the exact mutation will allow for later identification of affected fetuses in informative kindreds. The mother is instructed to start dexamethasone therapy at a dose of 20 µg per kg body weight per day when she is sure she is pregnant. A chorionic biopsy is performed at 9–10 weeks' gestation, or amniocentesis at 15–18 weeks, which allows the fetus to be sexed and the HLA type and genotype to be assessed. If the fetus is female *and* affected, dexamethasone is continued throughout pregnancy; otherwise treatment is discontinued. After birth the infant is carefully reassessed and treatment with hydrocortisone and 9α-fluorocortisone is commenced if the diagnosis is confirmed.

Chapter 9

Goiter

ASSESSMENT OF THYROID SIZE AND FUNCTION

The thyroid can best be palpated whilst standing behind the sitting patient or with the patient lying with the head falling backwards slightly over the edge of the couch. For accurate documentation of size, one practical method is to draw a line on the skin around the contours of the thyroid gland and to copy this on to a sheet of thin plastic. This plastic can be stored in the case records so that the size can be assessed longitudinally.

Thyromegaly (**Fig. 9.1**) can occur as a result of stimulation, infiltration or inflammation, and may be diffuse or nodular (localized) (**Table 9.1**).

ETIOLOGY

■ **Endemic iodine deficiency** – the main cause of goiter, either euthyroid or with hypothyroidism, in areas of the world with poor natural sources of iodine and in the absence of an iodized salt supplementation program.

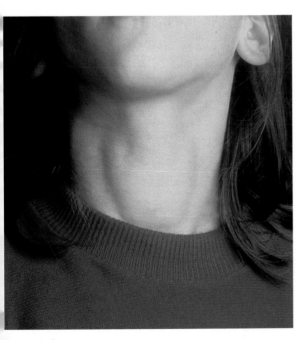

Fig. 9.1 Goiter.

Diffuse thyromegaly
Autoimmune thyroiditis (Hashimoto disease)
Thyrotoxicosis (Graves disease)
Toxic thyroiditis (Hashitoxicosis)
Idiopathic (simple) thyromegaly

Iodine deficiency in endemic areas
Goitrogen ingestion
Antithyroid drugs
Familial dyshormonogenesis
Acute and subacute thyroiditis

TSH-secreting pituitary adenoma (very rare)
Pituitary resistance to thyroid hormone (PRTH) (very rare)

Nodular thyromegaly
Autoimmune thyroiditis
Simple thyroid cyst
Thyroid tumors
   Adenoma – hyperfunctioning (hot)
              non-functioning (cold)
   Carcinoma (medullary thyroid carcinoma or papillary)
   Other tumor
Non-thyroidal masses
Lymphadenopathy
Branchial cleft cyst
Thyroglossal duct cyst

Table 9.1 Causes of thyromegaly

■ **Autoimmune thyroiditis (Hashimoto disease)** – the commonest cause of goiter in areas that are not iodine deficient. The pathogenesis of this disorder is uncertain, but a deficiency in antigen-specific suppressor T lymphocytes may be present. Antithyroid antibodies are usually present in high titers. It may be associated with other autoimmune disorders (**Figs 9.2 & 9.3**) and antibodies against adrenal cortex, parathyroid, gastric parietal cells, etc. (polyglandular syndrome type II or III; **Table 9.2**). Patients with euthyroid

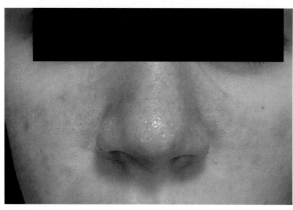

Fig. 9.2 Systemic lupus erythematosus (SLE) coexisting with Hashimoto thyroiditis.

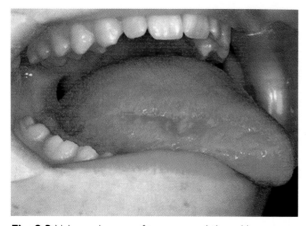

Fig. 9.3 Lichen sclerosus of tongue coexisting with Hashimoto thyroiditis.

Hashimoto disease should be followed for a few years to see whether they develop hypothyroidism or hyperthyroidism (see below).

■ **Idiopathic simple goiter or adolescent goiter (Fig. 9.4)** – enlargement of the gland at the time of puberty to form a visible goiter is not uncommon in euthyroid individuals, often with a positive family history of goiter. Regression is usual but nodular changes may occur three or four decades later.

■ **Acute bacterial thyroiditis** – with fever and tenderness.

■ **Subacute thyroiditis** – with lymphocytic infiltration, tenderness and often evidence of intercurrent upper respiratory tract infection.

■ **Ingestion of goitrogens** – either as antithyroid drugs or as naturally occurring compounds in the diet, such as large amounts of soya and cabbage, or unidentified agents in specific geographic areas.

■ **Dyshormonogenesis** – usually presents as goitrous neonatal hypothyroidism (see Ch. 11) but may occasionally present with goiter in later life.

Hypothyroidism and hyperthyroidism will now be discussed as the most important clinical causes of goiter; congenital hypothyroidism with or without goiter is discussed in Chapter 11.

JUVENILE HYPOTHYROIDISM

Juvenile hypothyroidism most commonly occurs in patients with Hashimoto disease. It is also strongly

Type	Features
1	Two or more of candidiasis, hypoparathyroidism, Addisonism
2	Addisonism plus type 1 diabetes mellitus and/or thyroid antibodies
3	a) Thyroid antibodies plus type 1 diabetes mellitus
	b) Thyroid antibodies plus pernicious anemia
	c) Thyroid antibodies plus vitiligo and alopecia plus other autoimmune disease
Vitiligo may be a component of any of the syndromes	

Table 9.2 The polyglandular syndromes

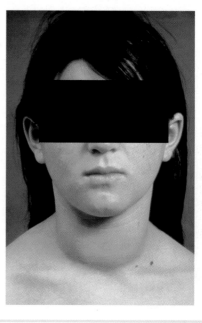

Fig. 9.4 Simple pubertal goiter.

ssociated with several syndromes with abnormal karyotype, such as Ullrich–Turner, Klinefelter and Down syndromes, in which there is also an increased incidence of thyroid dysgenesis (see Ch. 11), with non-chromosomal disorders, for instance the Noonan syndrome, and also metabolic disorders such as cystinosis.

HISTORY AND EXAMINATION

The exploration of the presenting history of suspected hypothyroidism should include:

- Family history of overactive or underactive thyroid glands; any other familial autoimmune disease.
- A history of recent growth failure and any tendency to weight gain.
- Any tiredness or weakness.
- Any change in activity levels, school performance or mental state.
- Constipation.
- Any hair loss or changes in the skin.
- Heat preference and intolerance of cold.
- Deepening of the voice.
- In females post-menarche, any menstrual irregularity or long, heavy periods.

On examination search for:

- Height reduced in relation to weight centile (**Fig. 9.5**).
- Back relatively longer than the legs.
- If old records exist, low height velocity.
- Goiter (not always present if thyroid has involuted).
- Delayed or arrested puberty *or* advanced sexual maturation – in boys manifested by enlarging testicles and penis with little hair growth, and in females by sexual precocity and cystic ovarian changes.
- Myxedema – rare in childhood.
- Dry skin, cutis marmorata (**Fig. 9.6**), vitiligo (**Fig. 9.7**).
- Pale skin – noted most on hands in contrast to yellow knuckles (see **Fig. 1.45**).
- Deep voice.
- Hair loss (often in the temporal area) (**Fig. 9.8**).
- Proximal weakness and delayed relaxation of the tendon reflexes (**Fig. 9.9**).
- Rarely the pituitary may enlarge because of hypertrophy of the thyrotropin-producing cells, and produce visual field loss from optic chiasm compression (**Fig. 9.10**).

DIAGNOSTIC WORK-UP

For the detection of hypothyroidism, serum free thyroxine (FT_4) and thyroid-stimulating hormone (TSH) measurements are most valuable. (If no FT_4 assay is available, total T_4 can be used, but it should be borne in mind that the total T_4 level is determined largely by the thyroxine binding globulin (TBG) concentration. The TBG level can be assayed and is low in congenital deficiency without any clinical consequences. Thus, a low total T_4 concentration does not necessarily indicate

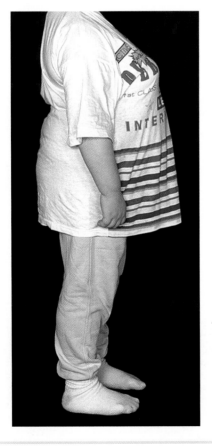

Fig. 9.5 Gross obesity in hypothyroidism. There was a weight loss of 5 kg in the first 2 months of therapy.

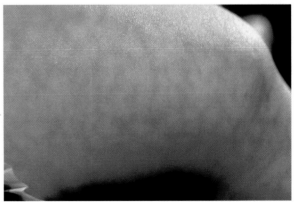

Fig. 9.6 Cutis marmorata in hypothyroidism.

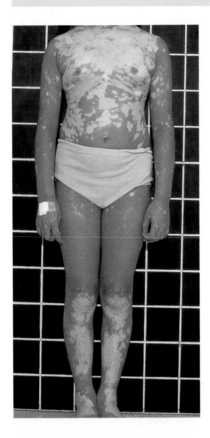

Fig. 9.7 Severe vitiligo.

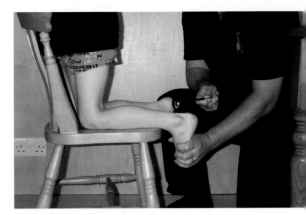

Fig. 9.9 Simple method of demonstrating delayed relaxation of tendon reflexes.

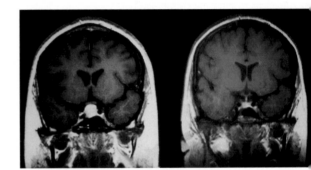

Fig. 9.10 Pituitary enlargement producing compression of the optic chiasm in prolonged hypothyroidism, before and after thyroxine therapy.

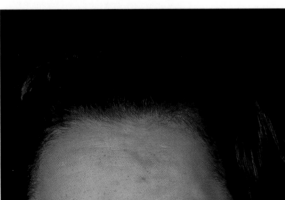

Fig. 9.8 Temporal hair loss in hypothyroidism.

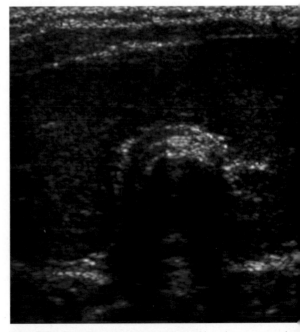

Fig. 9.11 Smooth goiter demonstrated by ultrasonography

hypothyroidism; see Ch. 11.) The combination of a low $(F)T_4$ with an increased TSH concentration is proof of primary hypothyroidism. Antithyroid antibodies indicate an autoimmune process in the thyroid and are usually present in Hashimoto thyroiditis, as may be antibodies to other glands in the polyendocrinopathy syndromes.

Ultrasonography will help to distinguish smooth from nodular goiter and allow serial measurement of volume (**Fig. 9.11**).

The bone age is often markedly delayed and the epiphyses are wider than normal, dysgenetic or eroded. In the presence of early sexual maturation the luteinizing hormone (LH) : follicle stimulating hormone (FSH) ratio may be less than 1, which is abnormal (see Ch. 6).

Although with modern TSH assays this is rarely required, a thyrotropin releasing hormone (TRH) test can sometimes be helpful (see Appendix). If compensated hypothyroidism is suspected with euthyroidism at the expense of mildly raised TSH levels, there will be an exuberant rise of TSH. The test can also be used to differentiate the non-goitrous or artefactual causes of hypothyroidism. An extremely low TSH level during the whole test indicates a pituitary (secondary) deficiency. A pattern in which TSH continues to rise after 20 minutes is indicative for a hypothalamic (tertiary) defect. A normal TRH test result is seen in TBG deficiency. It should be noted that patients with secondary or tertiary hypothyroidism may show few symptoms or signs and that serum $(F)T_4$ is usually not far below the normal range. Urinary iodine excretion can be measured to document iodine deficiency.

THERAPY

Treatment consists of L-thyroxine in sufficient dosage, to normalize serum TSH levels (which will keep the serum $(F)T_4$ in the upper normal range, or even somewhat higher). The child is checked initially at frequent intervals (1–3 months) and then yearly, when a correct dose is determined. The dosage should be individually titrated but is usually in the order of 2–3 µg/kg daily depending on age (or around 100 µg/m²). After the onset of therapy weight often reduces markedly (**Figs 9.12 & 9.13**). Catch-up growth in height is usually seen, but final height is often not as tall as may be expected from the very delayed bone age.

THYROTOXICOSIS

This condition is almost always caused by Graves disease and the presence of thyroid-stimulating antibodies. There is a strong association with infiltration of the orbit by mucopolysaccharide material, which produces the characteristic eye signs. Eye disease is usually less pronounced in children than in adults, and the infiltrative dermopathy seen in adults is very rare indeed in children. Thyrotoxicosis is much more common in females and is strongly familial.

'Hot' secreting adenomas may occur, and in the rare syndrome of pituitary resistance to thyroid hormones (PRTH) there is hyperthyroidism because

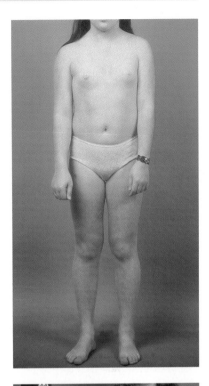

Fig. 9.12 Hypothyroidism before therapy.

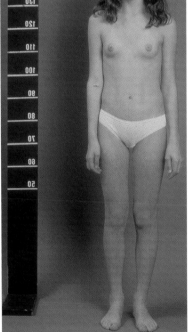

Fig. 9.13 Same patient as in Fig. 9.12, 6 months after starting treatment. There has been weight loss, progression of puberty and improvement of the lank, greasy hair.

of a lack of feedback inhibition of the pituitary. TSH-secreting pituitary adenomas have been described but are exceedingly rare in childhood.

HISTORY AND EXAMINATION

The exploration of the presenting history of suspected hyperthyroidism should include:

- Family history of overactive or underactive thyroid glands; any other familial autoimmune disease (**Fig. 9.14**).
- A history of recent growth acceleration and any tendency to lose weight, *often in the presence of increased appetite* (**Fig. 9.15**).
- Any tiredness or weakness.
- Any increase in activity levels or change in mental state (decreased ability to concentrate on mental tasks).
- Anxiety (and sometimes frank psychosis).
- Poor school performance.
- Fidgety foot and hand movements, generally increased activity.
- Frequent stools.
- Palpitations.
- Any diplopia, eye pain or redness.
- Cold preference and intolerance of heat.
- In females post-menarche, any menstrual irregularity, scanty periods or amenorrhea.
- Any thinning of the hair.

On examination search for:

- Weight reduced in relation to height centile.
- If old records exist, increased height velocity (see Fig. 3.32).
- Goiter (**Fig. 9.16**).
- Chemosis, exophthalmos, lid lag, ophthalmoplegia, especially in inability to converge the eyes (**Figs 9.17 & 9.18**).
- Tachycardia.
- Increased systolic and decreased diastolic blood pressure, leading to a wide pulse pressure.
- Sweatiness.
- Anxiety or abnormal behavior.
- Tremor – this is best appreciated as a buzz transmitted from the outstretched, spread fingers of the patient to the palm of the examiner's hand, it is of high frequency and may not be visible to the eye.
- Proximal weakness and brisk tendon reflexes.
- Thinning of the hair.

DIAGNOSTIC WORK-UP

Thyroid stimulating immunoglobulins (TSIs), also called thyrotropin receptor antibodies (TRabs), are almost always present, but require specialized laboratories for their measurement. In clinical practice these assays are rarely necessary as the signs and symptoms are so typical. The diagnosis is confirmed by high $(F)T_4$ levels in the presence of suppressed TSH levels. New, ultra-sensitive TSH assays can distinguish a low TSH level from one in the normal range.

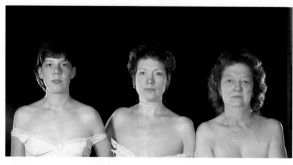

Fig. 9.14 Three generations of patients with autoimmune thyroid disease. Mother and daughter hypothyroid, grandmother thyrotoxic.

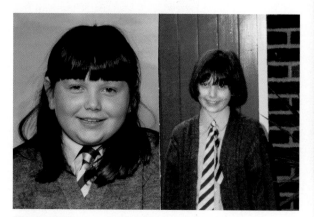

Fig. 9.15 Thyrotoxicosis before and after presentation.

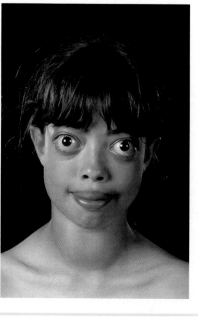

Fig. 9.16 Goiter in Graves disease.

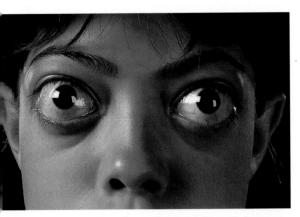

Fig. 9.17 Exophthalmos in a patient with Graves disease.

Fig. 9.18
Chemosis in the
same patient as in
Fig. 9.17.

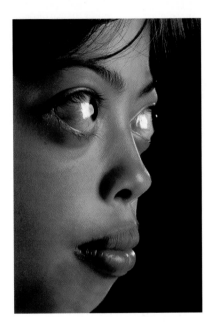

If used, total T_4 levels may again cause confusion in rare congenital situations of TBG excess, or more commonly secondary to pregnancy or various drug therapies such as the contraceptive pill, where T_4 levels will appear high whilst FT_4 levels will be normal (see Ch. 11).

In rare cases of doubt, a TRH test can be done, which will show a suppressed TSH response in the earliest stages of the disease (see Appendix).

Serum total or free triiodothyronine (FT_3) levels may occasionally be valuable in the rare diagnosis of 'T_3 toxicosis' in which FT_3 levels are raised inappropriately for the levels of FT_4 detected on standard assays.

THERAPY

There are four forms of therapy. All have their advantages and disadvantages, and require the supervision of an experienced endocrinologist, especially in the early stages of treatment.

Symptomatic relief

In addition to therapies directed against the thyroid itself, it may be necessary in the early stages of treatment, before lowered FT_4 levels are achieved, to administer a beta-blocker – usually propranolol in a daily dosage of 1–2 mg/kg three times daily – to alleviate the symptoms of hyperthyroidism. This strategy cannot be used in the presence of a history of asthma.

Antithyroid drugs

Propylthiouracil (PTU), methimazole and carbimazole may be used. PTU may have the theoretic advantage of blocking peripheral $T_4 \rightarrow T_3$ conversion and may reduce the titers of thyrotropin receptor antibodies. It is also less likely to exacerbate hair loss if this is a presenting feature of the condition.

PTU is given in a daily dosage of 5–10 mg/kg in three divided doses. The equivalent dosages for methimazole and carbimazole are approximately one-tenth of the PTU dosage, but have the advantage that they can be administered once daily.

There is some evidence that the chances of later relapse are reduced if the antithyroid drugs are given in a dosage sufficient to suppress FT_4 and in combination with L-thyroxine at a replacement dose. This 'blocking' regimen also has the advantage that it is not necessary constantly to increase and decrease drug dosage to try to titrate antithyroid therapy to maintain euthyroid FT_4 levels.

Therapy is usually continued for 2–3 years, after which remission is achieved in about 50% of cases. The dosage can then be slowly tapered. If relapse occurs, antithyroid therapy may be resumed or the patient may be offered the choice of surgical or radio-iodine therapy (see below). The major disadvantages of drug therapy are its long duration, compliance and the risk of toxic side effects (**Table 9.3**); these require the estimation of full blood count in the first 4 weeks of therapy when myelotoxicity is most likely to occur. If any serious side effects are suspected, therapy must be stopped immediately.

Subtotal thyroidectomy

This can occasionally be a first-line therapy, but is more commonly used in cases of relapse after initial drug treatment. The surgeon must have experience of this procedure in children. Permanent hypoparathyroidism and damage to the recurrent laryngeal nerve are possible hazards of surgical intervention.

Side effects of antithyroid drugs (PTU and carbimazole/methimazole)

Rashes: *common* – exchange drugs or, if no substitution possible, treat with antihistamines and continue therapy

Nausea

Headache

Pruritus

Arthralgia

Alopecia (less with PTU)

Jaundice

Lupus (with PTU)

Agranulocytosis: *Patient told to report ANY symptoms of infection, especially sore throat, as soon as they occur. White cell count should be checked immediately and therapy discontinued if there is any clinical or laboratory evidence suggestive of neutropenia*

Table 9.3 Side effects of antithyroid drugs (PTU and carbimazole/methimazole)

Iodine-131 treatment

This has the advantage that it is effective in around 85% of patients and, once administered, requires merely surveillance for the development of later hypothyroidism (20% within 1 year increasing to around 60% after a decade). There are few short-term risks, and 40 years of experience in some centers indicates that there is little risk of later malignant change. It should, however, be considered only in experienced centers.

Treatment of the eye disease is rarely required in childhood. Occasionally intraorbital steroid injections or surgical decompression may be necessary to preserve vision.

In some cases of Graves disease there are detectable levels of antithyroid antibodies of the same kind as found in Hashimoto thyroiditis. In these cases spontaneous hypothyroidism may ensue after initial toxicosis, so-called 'Hashitoxicosis'.

NEONATAL THYROTOXICOSIS

If mothers with Graves disease become pregnant, the circulating thyrotropin receptor antibodies can cross the placenta in the last trimester and cause fetal thyrotoxicosis. This is *not* dependent on the current thyroid status of the mother (the antibodies persist after spontaneous or therapeutically induced hypothyroidism)

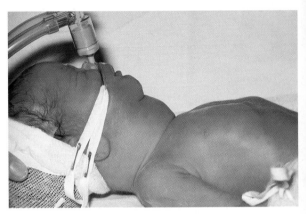

Fig. 9.19 Neonatal goiter secondary to maternal PTU treatment for thyrotoxicosis. The goiter has compressed the trachea, requiring endotracheal intubation to maintain the airway.

and so obstetric staff should be alert to the possibility in any mother with a past history suggestive of thyrotoxicosis.

The incidence is approximately 1 in 25 000 pregnancies. During pregnancy, fetal size and heart rate have to be monitored closely. In case of fetal tachycardia, low-dose PTU (25–50 mg) may be given to the mother to treat the fetus *in utero*. If the mother is being treated with antithyroid drugs, these can also cross the placenta and cause fetal hypothyroidism and goiter (**Fig. 9.19**).

Whether or not fetal thyrotoxicosis has been detected and treated *in utero*, after birth the infant may develop the symptoms of thyrotoxicosis with tachycardia, hyperkinesis, restlessness, diarrhea, poor weight gain, premature craniostenosis and advanced bone age (**Fig. 9.20**). The diagnosis is confirmed by high $(F)T_4$ and suppressed TSH levels. As the maternally administered antithyroid drugs will be metabolized by the fifth day, but the TSIs will persist for 3–5 months, the neonate requires frequent reassessment in the first 10 days of life.

Therapy is with PTU 5–10 mg/kg and propranolol 2 mg/kg to achieve symptomatic control, or alternatively saturated potassium iodide (Lugol's solution), one drop every 8 h.

THYROGLOSSAL CYST

These cysts form in remnants of the embryonic thyroglossal duct and are rarely associated with thyroid disease. They lie in, or just to one side of, the midline and may transilluminate brightly (see **Fig. 1.86**). They move upwards on protruding the tongue. They are separate from underlying thyroid tissue on

Fig. 9.20
Neonatal
thyrotoxicosis.

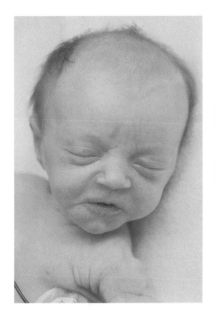

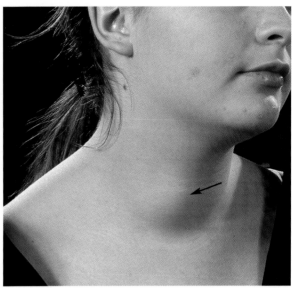

Fig. 9.22 'Cold' thyroid nodule.

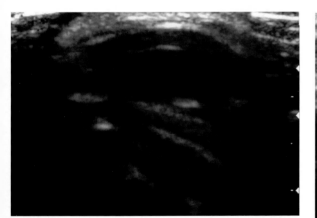

Fig. 9.21 Thyroglossal cyst, separate from underlying thyroid tissue.

ultrasonography (**Fig. 9.21**). They require surgical excision to prevent infection.

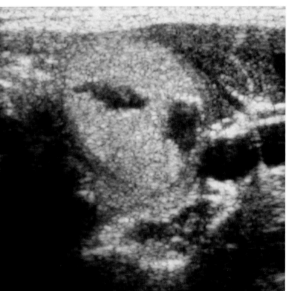

Fig. 9.23 Non-secreting thyroid adenoma on ultrasonography.

AUTONOMOUS THYROID NODULE

Thyroid nodules in childhood are rare (**Figs 9.22 & 9.23**). They are often not associated with hormone excess but may occasionally produce thyrotoxicosis and require surgical removal. It is wise to consider ultrasonography and Doppler studies (**Fig. 9.24**) in all cases as well as a needle biopsy to exclude carcinoma of the thyroid.

Multiple nodules are extremely uncommon and may arise from chronically TSH-stimulated goitrous tissue in areas of iodine deficiency or untreated hypothyroidism,

and in the McCune–Albright syndrome. Ultrasonography and needle biopsy are advisable (**Fig. 9.25**).

THYROID CARCINOMA

Thyroid carcinoma usually presents as an asymmetric thyroid mass in teenage life. Females are three times more likely than males to be affected. These tumors are seen after thyroid irradiation (i.e. in Eastern Europe after the Chernobyl disaster) and occasionally

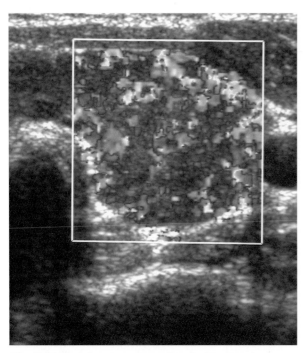

Fig. 9.24 Doppler ultrasonography of goiter showing diffuse vascularity and no regional flow, which may indicate a neoplastic lesion.

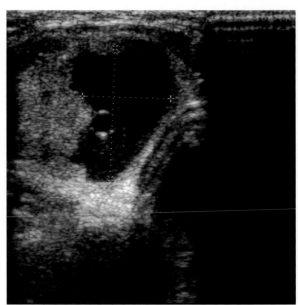

Fig. 9.26 Papillary carcinoma of the thyroid on ultrasonography.

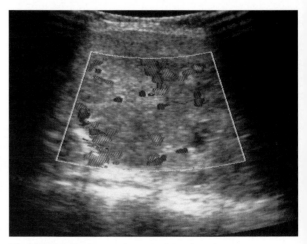

Fig. 9.27 Follicular carcinoma of the thyroid on ultrasonography.

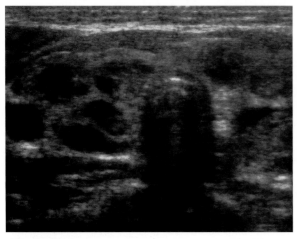

Fig. 9.25 Multinodular goiter on ultrasonography.

in thyroid hormone dyshormonogenesis (see Ch. 11).

Ultrasonography, Doppler studies (which show increased flow around the edge of malignant nodules in comparison to benign adenomas), followed by needle aspiration are mandatory (**Figs 9.26–9.28**). Antithyroid antibodies may be present.

The carcinoma arises from the follicular epithelium and at histologic examination may show papillary (commonest in children) or follicular changes, or a mixture of the two. Anaplastic cancers are extremely unusual in children. They are often micrometastatic at presentation, but the prognosis is excellent in childhood as they are extremely slow-growing. Treatment involves thyroidectomy followed by iodine-131 treatment and then complete suppression of TSH levels by L-thyroxine. The cells are well differentiated and produce thyroglobulin, which can be used as a marker of the disease process. The outlook with adequate treatment and monitoring is excellent.

Medullary cell carcinoma arising from the calcitonin-producing parafollicular C cells is almost

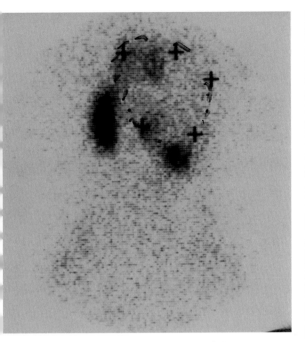

Fig. 9.28 Follicular carcinoma of the thyroid shown on technetium scan.

Syndrome	Description
MEA-I	Parathyroid (97%), pituitary (30% – prolactin, non-functioning, growth hormone, adrenocorticotropic hormone), pancreatic adenomas (50% – gastrin, insulin, glucagon), carcinoid and lipomata. There is a degree of familial uniformity
MEA-IIa (i)	Medullary cell carcinoma of the thyroid, pheochromocytoma, parathyroid adenomas
MEA-IIa (ii)	Medullary cell carcinoma of the thyroid and pheochromocytoma
MEA-IIa (iii)	Medullary cell carcinoma of the thyroid and parathyroid adenomas
Familial isolated medullary cell carcinoma of the thyroid	
MEA-IIb (III)	Medullary cell carcinoma of the thyroid, pheochromocytoma, mucosal neuromas, intestinal neuronal dysplasia, marfanoid habitus

Table 9.4 Multiple endocrine adenomatosis (MEA) (or multiple endocrine neoplasia; MEN) syndromes

always a component of multiple endocrine adenomatosis (MEA) II or IIb (see **Figs 1.72, 1.73 & 3.33**). Diagnosis of this condition on clinical presentation of other components of the syndrome (**Table 9.4**) should prompt immediate removal of the thyroid gland because the risk of malignant change is so great and treatment of distant disease is currently ineffective. Octreotide scanning may help locate malignant metastases. It is now possible to screen relatives of affected individuals by DNA analysis for abnormalities of the *ret* oncogene on chromosome 10q, in informative families, to allow presymptomatic thyroid resection.

Chapter 10

The Child with Diabetes Mellitus

CLASSIFICATION AND PHYSIOLOGY

Diabetes mellitus is present when the blood sugar level is greater than 11 mmol/L on a random blood sample (or at 2 h in a glucose tolerance test; see Appendix) or greater than 7 mmol/L on a fasting sample. Random values between these figures suggest 'impaired' glucose tolerance. Children may show occasional values of more than 11 mmol/L after severe stress, such as a convulsion, but in the absence of a suggestive history and with prompt return to normoglycemia the diagnosis of diabetes should not be made in these cases. There is some evidence that a proportion of these children with stress-induced hyperglycemia are at risk of later diabetes, but it is not usual to institute further investigations and follow-up outside research programs.

Diabetes mellitus results from a relative deficiency of insulin, which is required for normal glucose homeostasis. Insulin is secreted as a single-chain polypeptide called pro-insulin from the beta cells of the pancreas. This is cleaved to yield insulin and C peptide, both of which enter the circulation. Plasma C-peptide levels indicate the residual insulin production by the pancreas, as there is no C peptide in commercially manufactured insulin. The release of insulin is controlled largely by glucose entry into the beta cell via an active transport mechanism (Glut2). This leads to a rise in intracellular adenosine triphosphate (ATP) levels and the closure of a two-component potassium channel (Kir6.2 and Sur1). In turn this leads to membrane depolarization and influx of calcium through a voltage-dependent calcium channel. Exocytosis of insulin is stimulated from storage granules, and insulin is released into the portal circulation.

The rate of insulin production and release is determined mainly by the level of blood glucose, a rise in the blood glucose concentration causing a rise in insulin production. Amino acid levels rise after eating and also stimulate insulin secretion, controlled by a number of different gut hormones such as gastric inhibitory polypeptide (GIP).

Insulin is removed rapidly from the plasma, with a half-life of about 4 min. Insulin normally causes synthesis of glycogen, protein, triglycerides and glucose oxidation. Thus a relative deficiency causes a rise in blood glucose levels and ketones along with reduced glucose oxidation. This in turn leads to a rise in blood glucose concentration, glycosuria when the renal threshold is exceeded, an osmotic diuresis and dehydration, wasting of fat and muscle, and ketosis.

Several other hormones have an effect on blood glucose levels. Amylin is a small 37-amino-acid peptide co-secreted with insulin that controls gastric emptying and hepatic glucose release. Resistin is a 750-amino-acid peptide hormone (coded by a gene on chromosome 19) secreted from white fat that modifies insulin sensitivity in the periphery. In humans it is more highly expressed by fat from central rather than peripheral sites. Tumor necrosis factor (TNF) α is a cytokine secreted by adipocytes that may also modify insulin sensitivity. Glucagon, growth hormone, cortisol and epinephrine (adrenaline) all produce a rise in blood glucose concentration by inhibiting glucose uptake by muscle and by stimulating the production of glucose from amino acids, glycerol and glycogen stored in the liver. Epinephrine also inhibits insulin release from the pancreas. During fasting, the blood sugar and amino acid levels fall, and this results in a fall in insulin levels. However, there is a rise in glucagon, growth hormone and cortisol levels, producing an increase in the breakdown of glycogen and in blood glucose production from lactate, amino acids and glycerol. These counterregulatory hormones continue to operate even in a child with diabetes (certainly during the early phases of the illness) and will be produced in response to hypoglycemia.

Diabetes mellitus can be produced in a number of different ways. Type 1 diabetes is caused by immune-mediated or idiopathic islet cell destruction, resulting in insulin deficiency. In type 2 diabetes there is a relative insulin resistance or a combination of insulin resistance with a secretory failure. Type 3 diabetes includes several different mechanisms for abnormal glucose homeostasis: genetic defects of beta-cell function and insulin action, diseases and infections of, and toxicity to, the exocrine pancreas, defects in counterregulation caused by other endocrine disorders, immune-modulated conditions, and associations with genetic syndromes. Type 4 diabetes (gestational diabetes) is not considered in this chapter.

TYPE I DIABETES

EPIDEMIOLOGY OF CHILDHOOD DIABETES

The incidence of type 1 diabetes varies considerably across the world, being highest in the Scandinavian countries (>20 per 100 000 population per year), intermediate in countries such as the UK, USA and New Zealand (7–19 per 100 000 per year), and lowest in Asian and South American countries (<7 per 100 000 per year). Finland has the highest incidence in the world (43 per 100 000 per year) where the risk is 60 times greater than in China, which has the lowest incidence (0.7 per 100 000 per year). In temperate latitudes about 2–3 per 1000 children aged under 16 years are affected by childhood diabetes, so it is a relatively uncommon disorder in primary care. The incidence is slowly rising in the Western world. When families migrate from an area of low incidence to one where the disease is common, they acquire the risk of their new homeland, suggesting an environmental trigger.

Type 1 diabetes is very rare in the first few months of life, the incidence rising from 9 months of age until puberty, with a fall in adult life. There are peaks occurring at around 5 years of age and again at around the time of puberty, and these patterns are seen around the world. A seasonal variation has been observed worldwide, with a reduction in the warm summer months. The northern and southern hemispheres are 6 months out of phase. These patterns indicate that triggers such as virus infections may be important. However, there is also evidence of an important genetic contribution in the development of diabetes as a first-degree relative with insulin-dependent diabetes mellitus (IDDM) increases the risk to 3–10%, and in monozygotic twins the concordance rate is 36%. Although the risk of developing diabetes is roughly equal for males and females, the inheritance of risk is less from a mother with IDDM (2%) compared with a father with IDDM (6%).

Chromosome 6 carries genes encoding for human leukocyte antigens (HLAs) expressed on the surface of most nucleated cells and they present processed antigens to cytotoxic T lymphocytes. A strong relationship has been demonstrated between type 1 diabetes and the HLA-DR locus, with approximately 95% of IDDM cases having either DR3 and/or DR4 antigens. Some HLA types are 'protective' (i.e. 2 and 5). There is some variation in phenotype with different HLA type; for instance, DR3 has more of an association with other autoimmune disease and a longer honeymoon period in comparison with that in patients with DR4, who are also younger. If individuals are positive for both DR3 and DR4, their risk of diabetes is 25%.

Antibodies against pancreatic islet cells (islet cell autoantibodies; ICAs) and insulin have been detected in 65–100% of newly diagnosed patients with IDDM. As yet it is not known whether these antibodies play a direct role in the disease process or whether they serve simply as a marker for damage by other etiologic agents. However, fewer than 50% of ICA-positive individuals develop IDDM, so it is likely that other genetic and environmental factors influence the development of the disease. Anti-glutamic acid decarboxylase (anti-GAD) antibodies are even more sensitive markers for the development of type 1 diabetes than ICAs. They may be detected up to 10 years before the onset of the disease and persist for longer than ICAs, which may disappear after several years of the disease.

A number of different environmental triggers has been proposed. Viral infections such as retroviruses and coxsackie B4 have been implicated, but are not identified in the majority of IDDM cases. There does appear to be some evidence for nutritional triggers. An increased incidence of IDDM has been demonstrated in rats with early exposure to cow's milk protein, and in Scandinavia the incidence is significantly higher in children who were fed on formula from an early age. It is suggested that a whey protein, bovine serum albumin, is conformationally similar to a surface protein of beta cells of genetically susceptible children, thus sensitizing the immune system. At times of stress or viral infection, the pancreas is exposed to the sensitized immune system and anti-islet cell antibodies are produced, leading to beta-cell destruction.

After presentation there is commonly a phase of relatively preserved post-meal insulin secretion, the 'honeymoon phase', which may persist for months to 1–2 years before insulin production ceases totally.

PRESENTATION OF TYPE I DIABETES

The so-called 'classical triad' of diabetes is:

- polyuria.
- polydipsia.
- weight loss.

Less commonly (5% in a recent series) in the developed world the child may present with diabetic ketoacidosis (DKA), usually at a time of intercurrent illness or hot weather. DKA may present classically with acidotic, ketone-laden respiration and dehydration, but can sometimes present as shock, acute abdominal pain or an apparent respiratory illness (**Figs 10.1 & 10.2**).

In retrospect the child will have been lethargic, miserable and may have suffered from candidiasis or recurrent staphylococcal skin infections. There may be

Fig. 10.1 Severe diabetic ketoacidosis and dehydration.

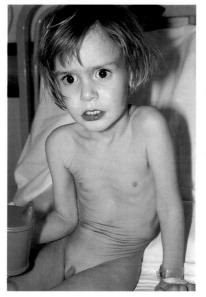

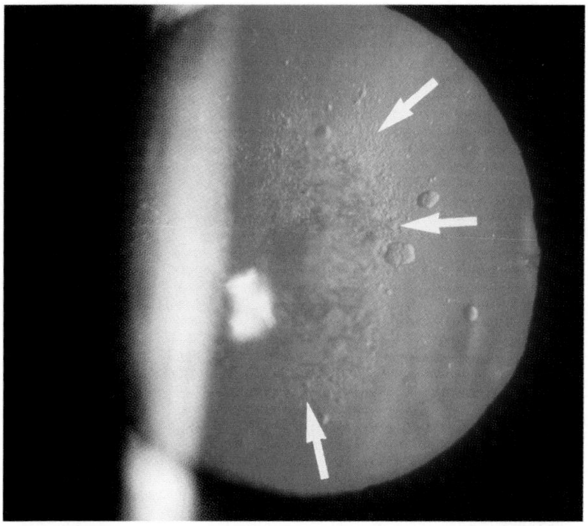

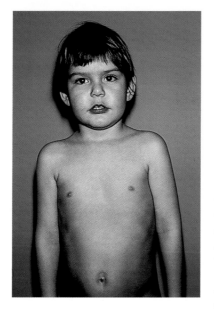

Fig. 10.3 Posterior subcapsular cataract at presentation of diabetes.

Fig. 10.2 The same child as in Fig. 10.1, 4 months later.

and education are undertaken at home. This increases the family's confidence to manage their child's diabetes and reduces the 'medicalization' of the disease. Other centers feel that a prolonged admission for initial education results in later improved control. Local circumstances will dictate the appropriate approach.

Subsequent outpatient care should include frequent multidisciplinary follow-up from physicians, specialist nurses, dieticians and psychologists. Ideally an age-banded clinic allows for the differing educational, physiologic and psychologic needs of the child to be provided in a planned and logical manner. This is particularly true of adolescence, when there is often particular resistance to external control and resentment of perceived differences from peers.

Educational 'camps' and holidays are organized in many countries and allow for peer-led education and direct experience of coping with vigorous exercise (**Fig. 10.4**).

secondary nocturnal enuresis. If there is a long prodromal phase, there may be cataracts at presentation (**Fig. 10.3**).

Type 1 diabetes is not infrequently diagnosed by the serendipitous demonstration of glycosuria during attendance at primary care or by 'screening' of children with previously affected relatives.

MANAGEMENT OF THE CHILD WITH NEWLY DIAGNOSED TYPE I DIABETES

Some studies have demonstrated there is a lower readmission rate in families where the early management

Education

The most important component of management is education, to empower the family and child to care for their own diabetes and make adjustments to diet and insulin in response to changes in daily activity, growth and health. The most predictive factors about long-term control relate to the abilities and stability of the family and child, and the degree of support they receive from a multidisciplinary medical team. The education should be age and language appropriate and delivered frequently at a rate that can be assimilated by the family. It needs to include other carers, the school and leisure

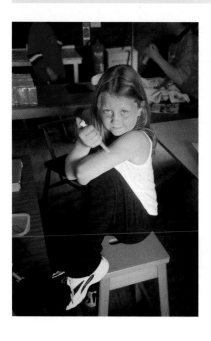

Fig. 10.4
Participant in diabetes education camp learning self-injection.

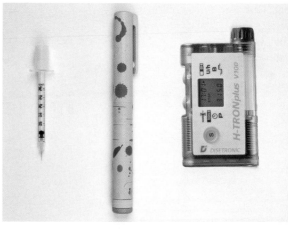

Fig. 10.5 Three methods of insulin administration: conventional low-volume syringe with high-gauge needle; insulin 'pen' with cartridge; pump for continuous subcutaneous insulin infusion (CSII).

organizations. Ideally patients should be able to inject insulin as needed for their diet and activity, and make appropriate adjustments to maintain as near-normal sugar levels as is possible without severe hypoglycemia.

Insulin

In most developed countries biosynthetic human insulin is used. Of the unmodified types there are basically two forms: 'short acting' or 'medium–long acting'. Short-acting insulin is, in reality, a misnomer because it forms a hexameric crystal that must dissociate to a monomer to be active, and has a peak of action at around 2–4 hours if given subcutaneously, lasting for 8 h post-injection. These insulins are used as 'bolus' injections with food (although now being replaced by genetically modified insulins; see below) or mixed with the longer-acting varieties and given two or three times a day.

Increased absorption time is created by binding insulin to a simple peptide, protamine, to form the isophane insulins or to crystallize the insulin in the presence of zinc to form the lente insulins (the bigger the particles formed, the longer the half-life). Isophane insulin, being bound 1 : 1 to protamine, can be mixed in various ratios with soluble insulin to derive pre-mixed preparations. The excess of zinc in the lente insulins combines with soluble insulin to delay its action, and so must be mixed by the patient shortly before administration. These insulins have peaks of action after 4 h and may persist for 18–24 h after injection. Mostly they are designed to be given twice a day.

Modern genetically modified insulins are becoming widely available in both truly short- and long-acting

forms. In the short-acting modified insulins there are amino acid substitutions that result in conformational changes that inhibit crystal formation and hence remain monomeric. The speed of action is around 1 h to peak, with an action to 4–6 h depending on the preparation used. They are very suitable for bolus injection, as required to normalize sugar levels, and for use in pumps (see below). The long-acting modified insulins are altered to change their solubility at physiologic pH levels and precipitate in tissue after injection to form a reservoir, which effectively provides a constant background level.

Insulin (**Fig. 10.5**) can be administered parenterally, usually by subcutaneous injection, or intravenously in DKA. High-gauge needles and low-volume syringes make the injection relatively painless, and the injection may be packaged as a pen device for patient convenience. Pressurized sprays are sometimes used as an alternative to needles. Increasingly, continuous subcutaneous infusions of (modified short-acting) insulin (CSII) are used with a programmable external pump which can be set at different rates for day and night, and also used to deliver boluses of insulin with food. Inhaled insulin is being currently investigated for safety and efficacy, delivered at around 10 times the subcutaneous dose by a special inhaler device for bolus use.

The exact insulin regimen chosen needs to be modified to be appropriate for the age and capabilities of the child and family. In young children with a persistent honeymoon period, twice-daily medium-acting insulin may be all that is required for the first few years. After the honeymoon, short-acting insulin will be required to cover the post-meal peaks of glucose and can be delivered pre-mixed with medium-acting insulin in various combinations or as individual boluses tailored to the carbohydrate content of the meal or snack (in which case twice-daily medium–long-acting insulin will be required for 'basal' cover).

Islet cell transplants, either from cadaveric donors or from modified animal tissue, are being investigated as a curative treatment for type 1 diabetes, but are not yet available for use in children.

A usual starting dose of insulin is around 0.5 units per kg per day. In puberty, requirements may climb to 2 units per kg per day, before settling by 50% at sexual maturity.

Diet

A high-fiber, high-carbohydrate (50–55% of calories), low-fat (35% of calories) diet is recommended. This may be prescribed as 'portions' appropriate for the age and growth of a child, or given more liberally as a 'healthy' diet. There is some evidence that the ability to match specific input to bolus levels of insulin results in better control, but this requires considerable training to achieve. If twice-daily insulin regimens are used, carbohydrate must be eaten at three main meals and at three snacks – mid-morning, afternoon and bedtime – to prevent the unopposed action of insulin and therefore hypoglycemia between main meals.

Monitoring control

To vary insulin dosage sensibly, the patient must be able to test blood (or sometimes urine) glucose levels. Modern lancets and finger-pricking devices, coupled with rapid-reading meters, make this easier than in previous times, but monitoring remains one of the main barriers to achieving good control in childhood. Sensible, achievable goals for control need to be set (particularly in adolescence) and there is evidence to suggest that the best control is possible only with frequent testing (and then subsequent alteration of insulin dose or diet).

In the longer term, measurement of glycosylated hemoglobin levels (HbA1c) is required to assess the risk of complications (see below). All proteins are glycosylated at the time of synthesis in proportion to the ambient glucose level. Other proteins have been used (e.g. serum albumin-'fructosamine'), but most information regarding risk is related to HbA1c and this is becoming the standard test. The red cell extrudes its nucleus as it leaves the bone marrow, halting hemoglobin synthesis. A sample of blood will therefore include a population of cells from 0 to 120 days of 'age,' and the HbA1c level (the percentage of the hemoglobin A1c fraction on chromatography that is glycosylated)

will represent the average control over this period (with a bias to the first 40 days). The normal range is usually less than 6%, but caution should be used in interpreting levels in populations or patients that may have abnormal hemoglobin (e.g. HbF) due to hemoglobinopathies. The Diabetes Control and Complications Trial (DCCT) showed that the risk of complications is related to HbA1c level in a curvilinear fashion, with rapidly increasing risk of retinopathy and nephropathy after 8% and an approximate doubling of risk for every percentage point thereafter.

Hypoglycemia

A relative excess of insulin for the dietary intake of the child or energy expenditure may result in rapid hypoglycemia. Early warning symptoms vary from child to child but include pallor, tremor, hunger, change in mood and sweating. The blood sugar level needed to produce these symptoms is very variable. Some children with poor long-term control may feel 'hypo' at levels of 7 to 8 mmol/L. In patients with excellent long-term control and frequent hypoglycemic episodes, this early warning may be lost and occur only at the same time as CNS symptoms. CNS signs with a reduced level of consciousness leading to coma and convulsions reliably occur as the blood sugar level drops below 2.6 mmol/L.

Nocturnal hypoglycemia is extremely common in childhood, although often unrecognized (**Fig. 10.6**). It may produce nightmares, bed-wetting or morning headaches secondary to unrecognized convulsions.

The DCCT showed that the risk of hypoglycemia was inversely related to HbA1c level, although patients do get better at predicting hypoglycemia with experience. Young children with a growing brain are particularly at risk of CNS damage from severe hypoglycemia in the first 5 years of life. This may result in later learning difficulties and epilepsy.

Treatment of hypoglycemia is by a staged approach (**Fig. 10.7**). Initially a short-acting sugary drink or snack should be eaten, followed by a complex carbohydrate meal or snack. If the child is uncooperative because of the hypoglycemia, then sugary gel can be placed in the mouth or, if consciousness is being lost, glucagon can be administered to raise sugar levels (although this often results in vomiting and so parenteral dextrose may be subsequently required).

Sick-day rules

During illness counterregulatory hormone levels rise and lead to an increase in blood glucose concentration. The child is at high risk of ketoacidosis during illness. Insulin must always be given during illness, even if the child is eating little, although the dose may need to be

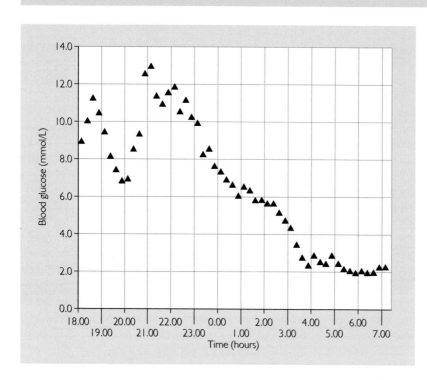

Fig. 10.6 Overnight blood glucose profile showing unrecognized asymptomatic hypoglycemia from 0400 to 0600 hours. Such profiles are found commonly in childhood. (Data courtesy of Professor David Dunger.)

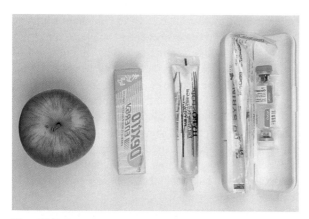

Fig. 10.7 Staged approach to hypoglycemia (food; dextrose tablets or sugary drink; dextrose polymer gel; glucagon).

reduced in gastroenteritis. Glucose-containing food and drink should be offered frequently and the blood glucose levels checked regularly, along with urinary ketones. Rising levels of sugar and ketosis should prompt seeking medical advice.

Psychological support

Many parents go through a period of 'bereavement' following the diagnosis of diabetes in their child, including the classic feelings of guilt, denial, anger and disbelief. Young children and adolescents in particular may find it very difficult to come to terms with their illness. Diabetes affects not just the child but the whole family, and other siblings must also be considered. Access to expert psychological support is hence vital.

Complications

Clinically significant complications of diabetes are rare in childhood, although joint stiffness (see **Fig. 1.22**) may be seen after only a few years of diabetes due to glycosylation of collagen. Lipohypertrophy is common if the injection sites are not 'rotated' frequently (**Figs 10.8 & 10.9**). As the hypertrophied site becomes relatively anesthetized, there is a vicious circle of continuing use and subsequent poor absorption of insulin. More rarely, lipoatrophy can occur, even with sole use of human insulin (**Fig. 10.10**).

Diabetic nephropathy is predicted by the appearance of macroalbuminuria (>300 mg albumin per 24 h); 50% of patients will develop renal failure within the next 10 years. Some 40% of patients may develop renal complications that can occur any time after 5 years of diabetes, but usually after 15 years of age. Microalbuminuria is the presence of >30 mg and <300 mg albumin per 24 h in the urine, which may also be detected on screening early morning urine and measuring an albumin : creatinine ratio. A ratio greater than 4 requires further investigation. However, in children, unlike adults, the presence of microalbuminuria may be variable and not as predictive of later progression of renal involvement, and so should be

"""

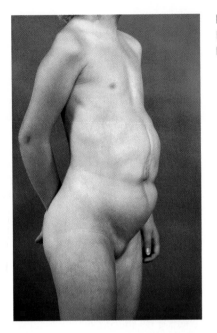

Fig. 10.8
Lipohypertrophy
of abdomen.

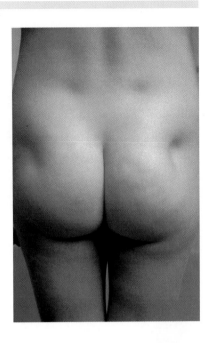

Fig. 10.10
Lipoatrophy of
buttocks.

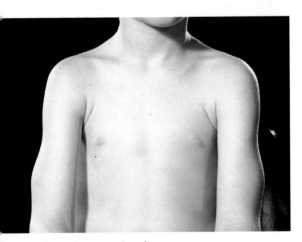

Fig. 10.9 Lipohypertrophy of arms.

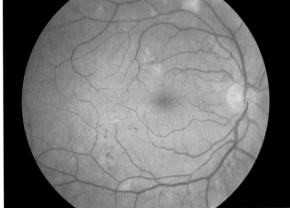

Fig. 10.11 Mild diabetic retinopathy found at presentation of childhood type I diabetes.

treated only if persistent or accompanied by hypertension. The evidence that angiotensin converting enzyme (ACE) inhibitors prevent or slow the progression of nephropathy in children is not available.

Diabetic retinopathy (**Fig. 10.11**) may rarely be present at, or soon after, presentation in some individuals, presumably representing an inherent genetic susceptibility to this complication. Usually it occurs after 5 years of diabetes and in the teenage and young adult years when detectable changes become almost universal. Only the minority of these changes will require laser photocoagulation, however. All patients should have their dilated fundi examined yearly after 5 years of diabetes, and teenagers. Diabetic posterior subcapsular cataract may be seen at presentation in children who had

a long prodromal phase, and this should be looked for at diagnosis (**Fig. 10.3**).

Skin manifestations of diabetes tend to be nonspecific as they can occur alone or in combination with other systemic disorders, but include necrobiosis lipoidica (**Fig. 10.12**) and granuloma annulare (**Fig. 10.13**), which are seen more frequently in type 1 diabetes.

Other autoimmune conditions occur with increased frequency, such as Hashimoto disease (in >5%), vitiligo and systemic lupus erythematosus (SLE) (see **Figs 9.2, 9.3 & 9.7**) as well as rheumatoid arthritis (**Fig. 10.14**). Regular (4–5 yearly) measurement of antithyroid antibody status and further yearly checking of thyroid stimulating hormone (TSH) levels in antibody-positive

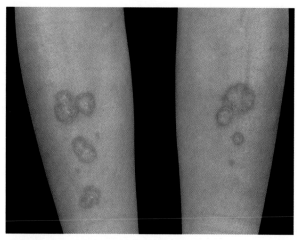

Fig. 10.12 Necrobiosis lipoidica.

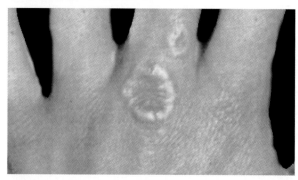

Fig. 10.13 Granuloma annulare.

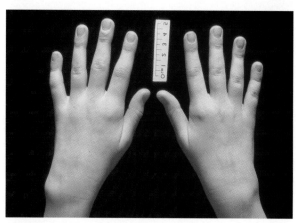

Fig. 10.14 Rheumatoid arthritis in association with type 1 diabetes.

individuals is routine in many clinics. Adrenal antibody-positive Addison's disease developing in a child with type 1 diabetes is rare, but serious, and may present with unexplained hypoglycemia and weight loss. Celiac disease is sufficiently common (2–4%) for some clinics to recommend screening by regular measurement of endomysial antibodies. It is commonly asymptomatic when detected this way and there is little evidence for the long-term benefit of an extra dietary therapy in these cases. Certainly all children with type 1 diabetes and gastrointestinal symptoms or unexplained weight loss should have their serology checked.

Mauriac syndrome secondary to long-term poor control is now rarely seen in the developed world, although it still occurs in those areas where insulin supply is limited for economic reasons (see **Figs 4.17 & 4.18**).

Diabetic ketoacidosis

The treatment of DKA is outlined in the notes and algorithm shown in **Fig. 10.15**.

TYPE 2 DIABETES

There is no specific diagnostic test for type 2 diabetes and its diagnosis in childhood is often confirmed only in retrospect. Some patients with type 1 diabetes have a slow evolution and may manage without insulin for months after diagnosis. In some children with one of the type 3 maturity-onset diabetes of youth (MODY) syndromes (see below) it may be impossible initially to delineate a mutation or exact phenotype because of the heterogeneity of the condition. Classically a child with type 2 diabetes will be overweight (**Fig. 10.16**), have signs of insulin resistance (acanthosis) (**Fig. 10.17**) and a positive family history of type 2 diabetes in one or more first-degree relatives. Type 2 diabetes is much commoner in some ethnic groups (from the Indian subcontinent and Mexico, in particular). On testing they will not be DR3/4 positive, will be islet cell and GAD antibody negative and may have a raised fasting insulin: glucose ratio. They remain C-peptide positive for many years. The associated features of dyslipidemia and hypertension may already be present in childhood.

The role of the recently discovered hormone, resistin, in type 2 diabetes remains to be elucidated, but this secretion from white fat, along with free fatty acids and TNF-α release, appears to modulate peripheral insulin resistance and may explain partly the link between type 2 diabetes and obesity. A failure of insulin secretion may follow a period of insulin resistance, making retrospective diagnosis of type 2 diabetes very difficult. The inheritance is polygenic with some gene polymorphisms appearing important in particular populations, but not others.

Type 2 diabetes used to be extremely uncommon in children but its incidence is rising along with the incidence of obesity and inactivity.

TREATMENT OF TYPE 2 DIABETES

Lifestyle modification, with increased exercise in particular, is important. Muscle can clear glucose more efficiently in the active child and this contributes as much as oral drug therapy to control. A diet should be introduced that comprises a high unrefined carbohydrate, low fat intake and is coupled with weight stabilization or reduction as appropriate. If glycosylated hemoglobin levels can be maintained at a satisfactory level, initially exercise and dietary therapy may be all that is required. If control is poor, then monotherapy should be initiated with an oral hypoglycemic agent. Metformin is probably the drug of choice as it has anorectic properties, no hypoglycemia risk and is usually well tolerated (although gastrointestinal side effects may limit the dose used). Metformin acts by reducing hepatic glucose production and increasing peripheral insulin sensitivity. It also has a role in restoring ovulation in those obese girls with a polycystic ovarian phenotype in addition to their diabetes. Sulfonylureas have the advantage of once-daily dosing, but may lead to weight gain and hypoglycemia. They act by increasing insulin release from the pancreas. Dual therapy with metformin and sulfonylureas may subsequently be required, and the place of newer agents such as the glitazones (insulin 'sensitizers'), repaglinide (postprandial insulin secretagogues) or acarbose (an α-glucosidase inhibitor that slows down glucose absorption from food), alone or in addition to one of the older agents, has yet to be established in children, although their effect on control is likely to be small. If HbA1c is consistently high, insulin may be required as for type 1 diabetes.

TYPE 3 DIABETES

The commonest genetic defects of beta-cell function are often called the maturity-onset diabetes of youth (MODY) syndromes. There are currently at least six subtypes caused by different mutations, usually transmitted in a dominant fashion. They are characterized by a primary defect in insulin secretion and the onset of often mild non-ketotic diabetes at age less than 25 years in the context of a familial history. The onset may be at younger ages in successive generations. The patients are DR3/4 negative and antibody negative, and remain C-peptide positive. Treatment is usually dietary, but some forms may require metformin or insulin therapy. Sulfonylureas may produce severe hypoglycemia, especially in type 3 MODY. **Table 10.1** shows the various currently recognized subtypes of MODY, although new mutations are being described.

Mitochondrial DNA abnormalities can also result in defects of beta-cell function and should be suspected if diabetes, neuromuscular and retinal abnormalities such as retinitis pigmentosa (see **Fig. 1.117**) coexist in a child.

Genetic defects of insulin action can result from defects in the insulin receptor, or post-receptor signaling (and, extremely rarely, from structural abnormalities of insulin itself, although most described cases are euglycemic). In type A insulin resistance there is an

	Genes	Severity	Other
MODY 1 and 3	*HNF4* and *HNF1α*	Similar; worsen with age and may become severe	May progress from oral agents to insulin. Complications occur
MODY 2	Glucokinase	Mild	Dietary treatment. Homozygous state results in permanent neonatal diabetes
MODY 4	*IPF1*	Very rare, mild. Beta-cell development altered	Homozygous state causes pancreatic agenesis
MODY 5	*HNF1β*	Moderately severe	Diabetes and renal cysts. Female Müllerian abnormalities
MODY 6/others	Various transcription factors	Moderately severe	May account for more than 50% of cases of MODY in some populations

Table 10.1 Type 3a diabetes – maturity-onset diabetes of youth (MODY) subtypes

Algorithm for treatment of diabetic

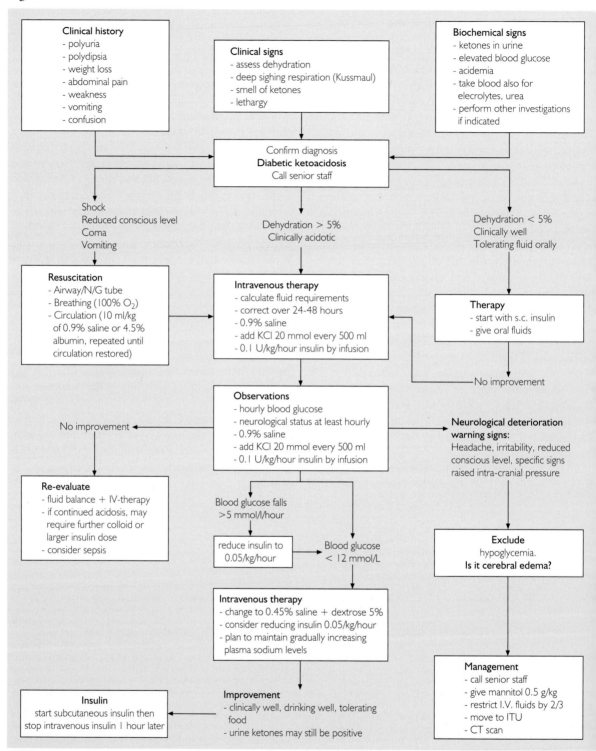

Fig. 10.15 Algorithm for the management of diabetic ketoacidosis. Notes and algorithm designed for Diabetes UK © by Dr Julie Edge and a working party of the British Society for Paediatric Endocrinology and Diabetes including the author (J.W.). This information is reproduced with the kind permission of Diabetes UK, the charity for people with diabetes (**www.diabetes.org.uk**). Initially adapted by Diabetes UK and reproduced here from *Practical Algorithms in Pediatric Endocrinology*, ed. Z. Hochberg, Karger, Basel, 1999, with permission.

NOTES

These guidelines are recommended to be used for children who are

■ more than 5% dehydrated and acidotic

■ and/or vomiting.

No guidelines have been shown to eliminate the risk of cerebral edema, but the principles outlined in these guidelines are believed to be as safe as possible in the light of current research and clinical practice. Guidelines should not replace intelligent thought and should be tailored to meet the needs of each individual patient; junior medical staff should always be encouraged to contact a more senior member of the medical team as soon as DKA is suspected.

The algorithm should not be used in isolation, and the following notes are an essential adjunct.

Diagnosis

■ This is usually not difficult, but the combination of hyperglycemia, acidosis and ketones must be found.

■ Severe metabolic acidosis in the absence of hyperglycemia (or other obvious causes of acidosis such as renal failure) raises the possibility of lactic acidosis (including glycogen storage disease type I), alcoholic ketoacidosis, salicylate overdose, other inborn error of metabolism (propionic acidemia, methylmalonic acidemia) and sepsis (Gram negative).

Resuscitation

■ There are theoretical reasons why colloid (such as 4.5% human albumin solution) may be preferable to saline in restoring circulating volume. However, in the light of recent concerns 0.9% saline is used more frequently. The choice should be left to individual units.

Dehydration

■ To evaluate the degree of dehydration the usual clinical signs should be used, but over-estimation may occur; first signs appear at 3% and a capillary refill time of more than 3 seconds indicates 10% dehydration. Use a maximum of 10% dehydration for the initial calculations.

Coma on admission

■ Always document conscious level in the notes, Glasgow Coma Score if depressed.

■ True coma at admission is rare (less than 10%), but conscious level may be impaired at presentation.

■ If the child presents with coma, other possible causes must be considered (DKA may have been precipitated secondarily).

■ Very rarely cerebral edema may occur early in the disease, before any intravenous treatment has been given.

Nursing and Observations

■ Consider early on whether the child should be nursed on the intensive treatment unit (ITU) (if shocked, very acidotic or very young, or ward staff stretched or inexperienced).

■ Regular observations should be carried out from the start, and doctors informed of significant changes; neurologic observations may be required every half hour initially, and doctors should be informed of headache or behavior change promptly, even during the night, as these may indicate cerebral edema.

Fluid requirements

■ The volume of fluid to be replaced is based on the deficit (degree of dehydration) plus the maintenance (basal 24-h requirement), given at a constant steady rate over the first 24 h; ongoing losses should be replaced if excessive and balance remains negative.

■ The debate over the duration of fluid replacement (24, 36 or even 48 h) is still ongoing; rapid infusion of large volumes of fluids has been suggested but not proven as a risk factor for the development of cerebral edema. In general, 24 h is suggested as the rehydration period, but if the child is very young or the blood glucose level very high, a longer duration may be appropriate.

■ 0.9% saline is used at the start of intravenous therapy until the blood glucose level falls to around 12 mmol/L.

■ Once the blood glucose level falls to 12 mmol/L, 0.45% saline is preferable to 0.18% saline, because there is some evidence that falling plasma sodium concentrations may be associated with cerebral edema.

Insulin dose

■ 0.1 units/kg/h have been chosen as the standard insulin infusion rate. Some suggest using a lower dose (0.05 units/kg/h), particularly in younger children. There is no good evidence to support either regimen, but lower doses may be insufficient to switch off ketogenesis.

■ If blood glucose concentration falls by more than 5 mmol/L/h, then the insulin dose may be reduced to 0.05 units/kg/h.

■ **Do not** switch off the insulin infusion rate if the blood glucose falls: add more dextrose to the infusate – insulin is needed to reverse the ketosis.

continued on next page

Fig. 10.15 *continued*

Bicarbonate

- There is no experimental evidence to support the use of bicarbonate in the treatment of the metabolic acidosis in DKA.
- If acidosis persists, consider giving further colloid, increasing the dose of insulin (more glucose may need to be added to the fluids), or the possibility that the child is septic.

Cerebral edema

- This complication of DKA is almost exclusively a condition of childhood.
- The pathophysiology is still not completely understood.
- Usually occurs between 4 and 12 h from the start of treatment, but may be present at onset of DKA and can occur up to 24 h later.
- The clinical signs are variable: gradual deterioration and worsening of conscious level from admission, or more commonly a gradual general improvement followed by sudden neurologic deterioration.
- Requires urgent recognition and intervention; the treatment of choice is mannitol (0.5–1.0 g/kg; 2.5–5 mL/kg mannitol 20%), which should be given immediately there is neurologic deterioration.
- Headache may be a symptom; severe headache should also be treated with mannitol.
- Admit to ITU. Intubation and hyperventilation may be required. Computed tomography to rule out other diagnoses.

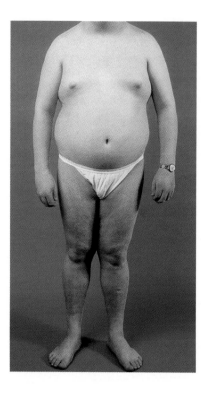

Fig. 10.16 Insulin resistance and obesity.

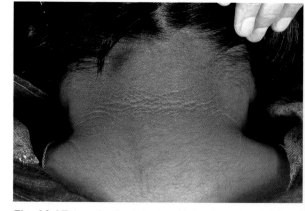

Fig. 10.17 Acanthosis nigricans with insulin resistance.

abnormal receptor or post-receptor signaling mechanism and greatly increased insulin levels in the presence of usually moderate hyperglycemia. There is acanthosis, and females present more often than males with virilization, hirsutism, skin tags and oligomenorrhea (the HAIR-AN syndrome of hyperandrogenization, acrochordons, insulin resistance and acanthosis nigricans; **Fig. 10.18**). There is an increase in free insulin-like growth factor (IGF) 1 concentration, which may result in rapid late childhood growth with acromegaloid

features and very low sex hormone binding globulin (SHBG) levels, worsening the free testosterone index. In a specific phenotype of abnormal dentition, precocious puberty, abnormal skin and nails, hirsutism and pineal hyperplasia, there are also insulin receptor abnormalities (the Rabson–Mendenhall syndrome).

Insulin resistance is also seen in association with the Leprechaun syndrome (see **Figs 4.19 & 4.20**) and other congenital generalized lipoatrophies.

The possibility now exists of treating these forms of resistance due to abnormal insulin receptors with recombinant IGF-1, although availability is limited, and work is being performed to bypass the receptor by stimulating post-receptor signaling.

Diseases of the pancreas, such as pancreatitis, neoplasia, trauma (including surgery for hyperinsulinism; see Ch. 11) and stones may result in endocrine pancreatic insufficiency and diabetes. In cystic fibrosis the

Fig. 10.18
Acanthosis
nigricans in
severe insulin
resistance (type
A) leading to
HAIR-AN
syndrome (see
also Figs 6.34 &
6.35).

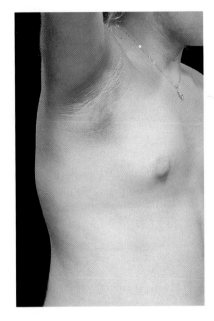

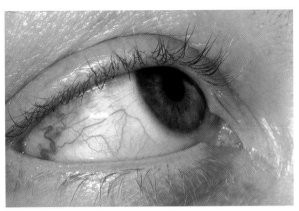

Fig. 10.20 Ataxia telangiectasia.

Fig. 10.19
Congenital
rubella may lead
to later diabetes.

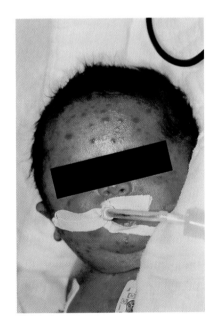

pancreatic fibrosis results in cystic fibrosis-related diabetes (CFRD) in about 10% of adolescents with the condition, although the incidence increases with increasing survival. Glucagon secretion is also affected, resulting in a tendency to hypoglycemia on treatment but also a lessening of the risk of ketosis. If undetected, the catabolism produced by incipient diabetes will cause a reduction in respiratory function and so CFRD should be prospectively screened for in all teenagers with cystic fibrosis. Sulfonylurea therapy or insulin should be instituted early to prevent catabolism and coupled with a high-calorie diet (with no restriction on intake of fat), designed to reverse any weight loss.

Hemochromatosis causes diabetes through iron overload, as does thalassemia in about 10% of cases. Cystinosis damages the pancreas (and thyroid) as a result of the intracellular accumulation of free cystine.

Endocrine abnormalities covered elsewhere in this book can result in glucose intolerance or frank diabetes. Gigantism, Cushing syndrome and thyrotoxicosis can all affect glucose metabolism. Iatrogenic Cushing syndrome, especially in the early phases of treatment of brain tumors and following bone marrow transplantation, can result in intermittent frank diabetes requiring insulin during each 'pulse' of therapy. Asparaginase has an additive toxic effect on the pancreas. Very rare tumors such as glucagon- and somatostatin-producing tumors of the pancreas, and occasionally pheochromocytomas, can all result in diabetes.

Drug- or chemical-induced diabetes and glucose intolerance may be seen with thiazide diuretics and diazoxide (which are used in the treatment of hyperinsulinism; see Ch. 11). Specific drugs such as pentamidine, dilantin, α-interferon, β-adrenergic agents and toxins in some foods can damage the pancreas.

Congenital infections such as rubella (**Fig. 10.19**) and cytomegalovirus may result in diabetes from an early age, and rare systemic infections such as with Nocardia can destroy the pancreas.

Immune-modulated diabetes is due to antibodies against the insulin receptor. Type B insulin resistance and 'stiff man syndrome' usually occur late in life, but in 60% of patients with ataxia telangiectasia (**Fig. 10.20**) there is glucose intolerance associated with anti-insulin receptor antibodies.

Syndromic associations of diabetes include the Klinefelter (Ch. 3), Ullrich–Turner and Down syndromes (Ch. 2), and a number of non-chromosomal disorders. Insulin resistance may be a feature of several dysmorphic conditions associated with obesity, including the Bardet–Biedl, Alstrom and Prader–Labhart–Willi syndromes (Ch. 5). Glucose intolerance is seen in many cases of dystrophia myotonica, and occasionally in Huntington's disease. The DIDMOAD (or Wolfram) syndrome of diabetes insipidus, diabetes mellitus, optic atrophy (see **Fig. 1.111**) and deafness is a severe autosomal recessive disorder characterized by diabetes mellitus and optic atrophy in the first decade. Diabetes insipidus and deafness occur in the second decade, psychiatric and renal abnormalities in the third decade, and finally CNS degeneration with myoclonus and ataxia. About 25% have gastrointestinal dysmotility and 25% of males are hypogonadal. Death occurs between 25 and 50 years of age. It is a heterogeneous syndrome caused by mutations at two different sites on chromosome 4, and a mitochondrial form has also been described. Roger syndrome has a superficially similar presentation with early visual and eighth nerve abnormalities and diabetes, but no other CNS involvement. There may be an accompanying sideroblastic anemia. It is due to an autosomal recessive thiamine transporter defect; the diabetes and anemia respond to high doses of thiamine. Most kindreds have originated from Kashmir.

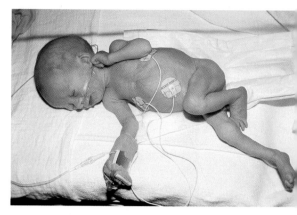

Fig. 10.21 Neonatal diabetes, whole body view.

NEONATAL DIABETES

Transient neonatal diabetes is characterized by the early onset (<6 weeks) of glycosuria and wasting. The children are often small for gestational age and look alert and anxious (**Figs 10.21 & 10.22**). The blood sugar level is often markedly raised and ketosis is mild or absent. Thrombotic events may occur secondarily to the dehydration. The illness is of unknown etiology, and patients are antibody negative, although familial occurrence is described. Insulin and C-peptide levels are low and it is postulated that there may be 'delayed maturation' of the pancreas. Treatment is with insulin (although the infant may be very sensitive to this). The condition remits spontaneously after a few weeks or months, and rising C-peptide levels can be used as a clue to the timing of discontinuation of treatment. Later, permanent diabetes occurs in the second decade in many infants, suggesting the mechanism may be related to permanent abnormalities of beta-cell mass or function. Permanent diabetes may occur from the neonatal period, and can be differentiated from the transient form only in retrospect, unless there is complete pancreatic agenesis in which case exocrine pancreatic function is also abnormal. Isolated beta-cell aplasia may rarely occur. In DR3/4 and antibody-positive individuals, type 1 diabetes has been rarely described dating from the

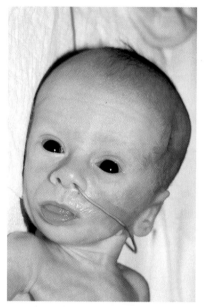

Fig. 10.22 Face of baby shown in Fig. 10.21.

neonatal period. The Wolcott–Rallison syndrome consists of neonatal diabetes mellitus and epiphyseal dysplasia due to a mutation of a translational factor.

TYPE 4 DIABETES

Type 4, gestational, diabetes occurring in 3–5% of pregnancies may represent the unmasking of glucose intolerance during prenatal care. Glucose homeostasis returns to normal post-partum, although the risk of subsequent type 2 diabetes is high.

TYPE 5 DIABETES

Type 5 diabetes (malnutrition related or tropical diabetes) is seen in adolescents and young adults who are thin and have a history of previous malnutrition (see Ch. 4). They often require large amounts of insulin but are surprisingly ketosis free. They may be difficult to distinguish from patients with type 1 diabetes. Fibrocalculous pancreatic disease again often results in diabetes in young adult males with a history of past malnutrition and abdominal pain. It may be related to cyanide ingestion from foodstuffs such as cassava on a genetically susceptible background.

HISTORY AND EXAMINATION

- Family history of type 1 diabetes or autoimmune disease, of type 2 diabetes in a first-degree relative or of MODY.
- Polyuria, polydipsia = glycosuria, diabetes insipidus in DIDMOAD syndrome.
- Weight loss = type 1 diabetes, or autoimmune process in syndrome.
- Drug history, chemotherapy.
- Known cystic fibrosis, thalassemia, Down or Turner syndrome, etc.
- History of past malnutrition = possible tropical diabetes.
- Ethnic subgroup = predisposition to type 2 diabetes in Asians, Polynesians, etc. Roger syndrome in Kashmiris.
- Dehydration and ketosis = type 1 with DKA.
- Acanthosis = insulin resistance.
- Candidiasis, staphylococcal skin infection = poorly controlled diabetes.
- Retinal pigmentary changes, neurologic signs = mitochondrial abnormality.
- Deafness, optic atrophy = DIDMOAD or Roger syndrome.
- Diabetes insipidus, psychiatric features = DIDMOAD.
- Hirsutism, skin tags, acanthosis = HAIR-AN syndrome.
- Cushingoid appearance = Cushing syndrome.

WORK-UP

Most childhood diabetes will be type 1, and little diagnostic testing is required. If resources allow, it is useful to measure anti-islet cell, anti-GAD antibodies; other autoantibodies (including antithyroid and anti-gliadin antibodies) should be measured at diagnosis (then 4 yearly), in addition to true blood sugar and glycosylated hemoglobin levels (which gives an indication of length of prodromal phase). At follow-up glycosylated hemoglobin should be measured regularly and thyroid function checked 3–4 yearly if antibody positive.

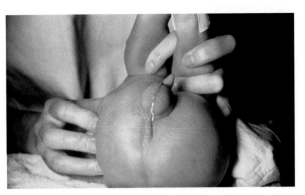

Fig. 10.23 Imperforate anus in infant of a diabetic mother.

To differentiate between type 2 diabetes and the various forms of MODY, it is usual to genotype the individual, looking for the known MODY mutations or confirm the same genotype as in an affected relative (see Appendix). Insulin levels (or the insulin : glucose ratio) will be moderately raised in type 2 diabetes, but massively so in insulin receptor defects.

The two common mutations for DIDMOAD (4p and 4q) are known (although a mitochondrial form has also been described), and Roger syndrome (1q) may be analyzed.

THE INFANT OF A DIABETIC MOTHER

It is important to educate potential mothers with any form of diabetes about the need for planned conception at a time of assiduous control. Periconceptional diabetes clinic attendance can improve fetal malformation rates from 10% to 2%. The teratogenic effects of maternal diabetes have their effects in the first 8 weeks of pregnancy and are related to the glycosylated hemoglobin levels in the first trimester. The mechanisms for the effects on the developing fetus are ill understood. The congenital abnormalities seen include:

- Caudal regression and recto-anal atresia (**Fig. 10.23**).
- Spina bifida, hydrocephalus and anencephaly.
- Situs inversus, transposition of the great arteries, ventricular septal defects.
- Renal abnormalities.

Later control influences birth size (see Ch. 3) and hence complications of macrosomia such as shoulder dystocia, birth asphyxia and birth injury. The incidence of respiratory distress syndrome, neonatal hypoglycemia, jaundice and hypocalcemia is also related to fetal hyperinsulinism in the last trimester.

Chapter 11

Abnormal Laboratory Values

CONGENITAL HYPOTHYROIDISM

The majority of infants with congenital hypothyroidism present as a result of routine neonatal screening and hence are discussed in this chapter.

PHYSIOLOGY

The thyroid forms as a midline outpouching from between the first and second pharyngeal pouches and descends into the neck just above the developing lung bud between 4 and 7 weeks gestation. The parathyroid glands condense from the third and fourth pharyngeal pouches and move into the migrated thyroid tissue. C cells are derived from separate neuroectodermal tissue in the ultimobranchial body. These events are under the control of a series of transcription factors and 'patterning' genes that can be mutated to produce maldevelopment at any stage of descent. However, it is rare for there to be associated hypoparathyroidism as the derivation of the tissue is separate. The gland may fail to develop or may be an abnormal midline structure anywhere from the base of the tongue (see **Fig. 1.85**) to the upper thorax.

During fetal life the thyroid starts to produce thyroid hormone from 20 weeks onwards, stimulated by pituitary thyroid stimulating hormone (TSH) secretion. Thyroxine (T_4) is first primarily metabolized to inactive reverse triiodothyronine (rT_3) by the placenta, and only after 30 weeks does the active T_3 level starts to rise. It was thought for many years that maternal T_4 does not cross the placenta, but there is now good evidence that some bioactive and necessary T_4 can pass to the fetal circulation as mothers with borderline hypothyroidism have infants with slightly, but significantly, lower developmental quotients. The majority of release of thyroid hormones from the thyroid gland is in the form of T_4 that is de-iodinated to T_3 in the peripheral tissues or deactivated by the formation of rT_3 and then further de-iodinated. Most of the activity of the hormones is mediated by the action of T_3 on intranuclear receptors.

Most T_4 circulates bound to a specific protein, thyroxine binding globulin (TBG), and albumin. Assays of total T_4 are strongly influenced by states that affect this binding such as drugs, liver disease, and pregnancy. Modern assays of free T_4 (FT_4) and T_3 (FT_3) are largely free of interference from other conditions, although some antiepileptic drugs do speed up the conversion of FT_4 to FT_3 and can alter circulating levels in the assay. Normal levels of thyroid hormones in infancy and childhood are given in the Appendix; there is an immediate postnatal surge in TSH, and FT_4 levels are higher in the neonatal period than later in life.

Congenital hypothyroidism can be divided into primary and secondary–tertiary forms. Primary hypothyroidism is caused either by embryonic defects (agenesis, dysgenesis, ectopia), accounting for 90% of cases, or by dyshormonogenesis – this category comprises several enzyme deficiencies, which are usually transmitted as an autosomal recessive trait and are commoner in some ethnic subpopulations and with consanguinity. Secondary or tertiary hypothyroidism is usually associated with other pituitary hormone deficiencies and accounts for only 1–2% of cases.

Down syndrome is associated with an increased incidence of thyroid agenesis.

CLINICAL FINDINGS

In most developed nations all neonates are screened for hypothyroidism. The cost : benefit ratio is high because the incidence is around 1 in 4000, and early detection and treatment prevent later cretinism – many affected children are asymptomatic in the first months of life. Thyrotropin (TSH) screening is the simplest and least expensive strategy with a low number of false-positive results. With such screening, secondary and tertiary hypothyroidism is not detected, but these account for only a small proportion of cases and are often suspected on the basis of other clinical features of pituitary dysfunction (such as prolonged jaundice, micropenis, hypoglycemia). In some countries T_4 levels are measured along with TSH, and all forms of congenital hypothyroidism may be detected.

Because of screening, the majority of infants are asymptomatic at diagnosis. The signs that may be evident soon after birth and those that can further develop if the diagnosis is not made early are shown in **Table 11.1**. These physical features will regress on

Early symptoms[a]	Late symptoms[b]
Umbilical hernia	persists
Pallor and hypothermia	persists
Enlarged tongue	increases to 100%
Hypotonia	worsens
Prolonged jaundice	decreases
Rough, dry skin	persists
Open posterior fontanelle	closes
Relative constipation	persists
Mild post-maturity	
Birth weight > 3.5 kg	
	Facial puffiness
	Hoarse cry
	Growth retardation
	Poor development
	Myxedema

[a] All or none of these may be present in the first month of life).
[b] At 1 month or more.

Table 11.1 Signs and symptoms in congenital hypothyroidism

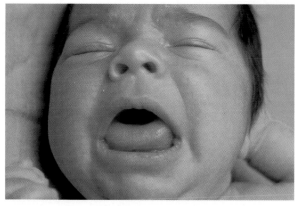

Fig. 11.2 Congenital hypothyroidism presenting at 5 months of age.

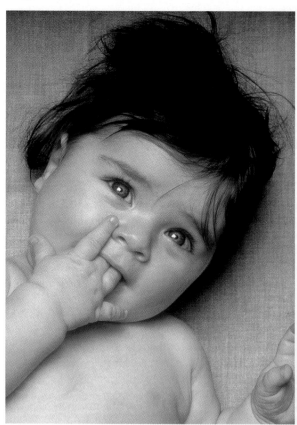

Fig. 11.3 Patient in Fig. 11.2 at 2 years of age.

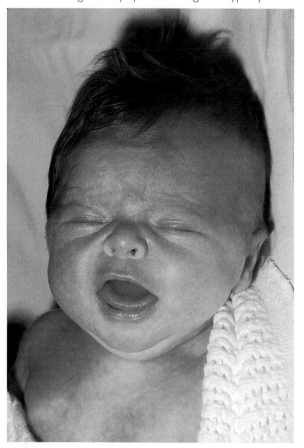

Fig. 11.1 Congenital hypothyroidism at presentation (1 month).

treatment (**Figs 11.1–11.3**), but the later therapy is commenced the worse is the outlook for normal mental development. Full-blown cretinism with severe intellectual impairment, dwarfing and the characteristic facial features (**Figs 11.4–11.6**) is now rarely seen in the developed world (**Fig. 11.7**).

Neonatal goiter (**Figs 11.8 & 11.9**) will be present in dyshormonogenesis but not in thyroid dysplasia or secondary–tertiary hypothyroidism.

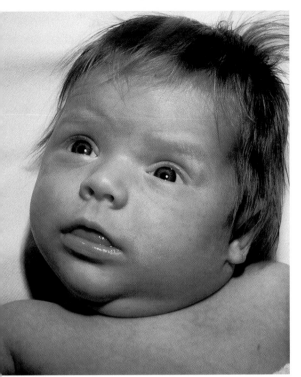

Fig. 11.4 Cretinism in an infant aged 6 months.

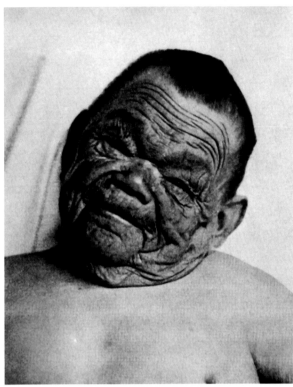

Fig. 11.6 Cretinism in an adult.

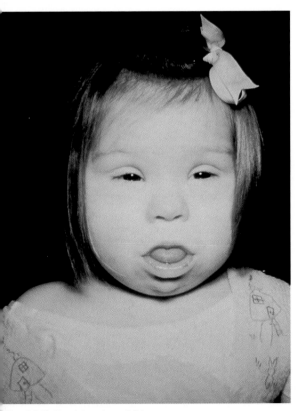

Fig. 11.5 Cretinism in a child.

Occasionally dyshormonogenesis can present in later childhood, especially in the Pendred syndrome (see below) where the onset of hypothyroidism can be very variable.

DIAGNOSTIC WORK-UP

From a radiograph of the knee and foot, the skeletal age can be assessed; it is usually delayed. A radio-iodine scan or a technetium scan (which delivers a lower radiation dose) can visualize the thyroid, so that agenesis or ectopia can be demonstrated (**Fig. 11.10**). This is not necessary in most straightforward cases of congenital hypothyroidism. Serum thyroglobulin levels can be measured to differentiate between aplasia and partial presence of the gland, but this is rarely necessary.

Radiography and ultrasonography of an enlarged thyroid by an experienced radiologist can assist in the detection of the thyroid gland and in assessing its size (**Figs 11.11 & 11.12**).

If dyshormonogenesis is suspected, the radio-iodine scan (but not technetium) will provide information about causality. If there is failure of uptake of iodine into salivary or thyroid tissue then there is a defect in the concentration of iodine. This rare disorder carries a poor prognosis even with therapy. To assess whether organification is defective because of an enzyme defi-

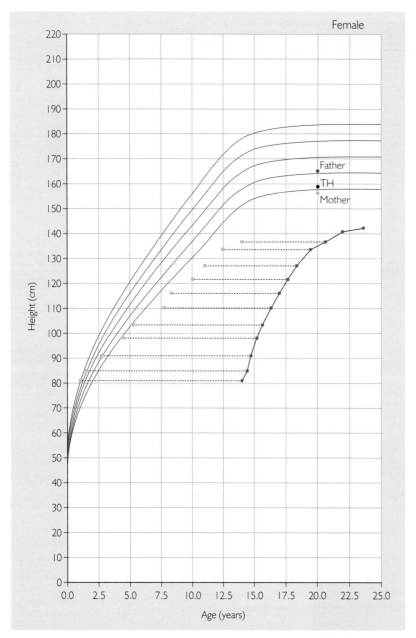

Fig. 11.7 Female with congenital hypothyroidism diagnosed in the neonatal period and treated for first 4 months. Treatment was discontinued until age 14 years, when the patient was unable to walk or speak. Re-presenting height SDS −12.5 and bone age 1.0. Pubertal signs evident 8 months after recommencing treatment. Height catch-up to −4.4 adult height.

ciency, a perchlorate discharge test may be performed (**Figs 11.13 & 11.14**). The perchlorate ion will compete with iodide for trapping by the thyroid follicular cell plasma membrane, and discharge of iodine will occur that can be monitored by release of radiation from the gland. If discharge occurs, the child and family should be screened for asymptomatic goiter or hypothyroidism and high tone deafness (Pendred syndrome), which can have very variable expression in different members of a kindred. It is rare for Pendred syndrome to present with a rasied TSH level and/or goiter in the neonatal period. If uptake

occurs and there is no discharge, one of the other enzyme defects causing failure of de-iodination, storage or transport of thyroid hormones is present. There is no practical reason to differentiate between these conditions, as they have no associated features.

TREATMENT

The first task of the physician is to treat the hypothyroid infant as soon as possible. Treatment should be started immediately. A diagnosis made on neonatal screening should be confirmed by low (F)T$_4$ and increased TSH

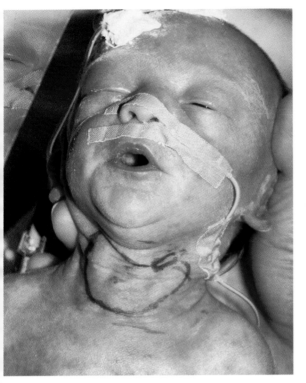

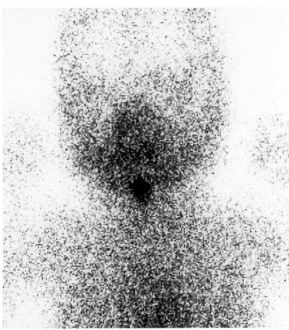

Fig. 11.10 Technetium scan showing small midline gland in child presenting with raised TSH level on screening and evidence of compensated hypothyroidism at 2 years of age.

Fig. 11.8 Small neonatal goiter.

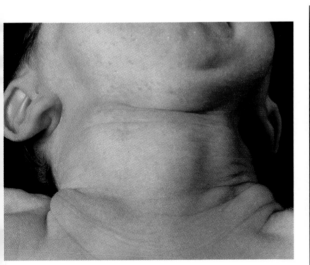

Fig. 11.9 Larger neonatal goiter.

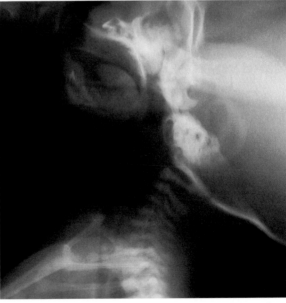

Fig. 11.11 Lateral neck radiograph showing neonatal goiter enveloping trachea.

levels. Whilst awaiting these results L-thyroxine is started in a dosage of 10–15 µg/kg body weight, and then tapered to 7–5 µg/kg to maintain the $(F)T_4$ at the higher end of the age-specific normal range and maintain a normal TSH concentration. Overtreatment can lead to craniostenosis. In some cases the TSH levels may remain high for many months, despite adequate treatment, because of acquired hypothalamic feedback insensitivity. In rare cases of mistaken screening-based diagnosis, therapy can be discontinued with no ill effect. Therapy is continued life-long, although there is an argument for reinvestigating the occasional case where early control is achieved and then no high levels of TSH

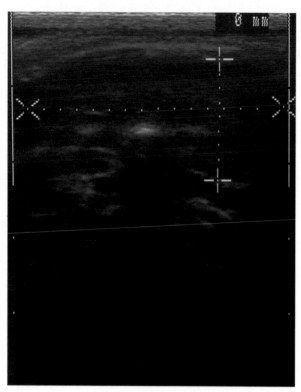

Fig. 11.12 Ultrasonographic scan of same case as in Fig. 11.11. Trachea in center of film; goiter measures 35 mm by at least 16 mm.

are detected during the first 2 years of follow-up (for instance because of non-compliance or inadequate dosage with growth). In this situation gradual reduction of dose and the demonstration of a rising TSH concentration will demonstrate that the hypothyroidism persists. If this TSH rise does not occur, then occasionally the early defect will prove to have been transient and due to maternal goitrogens or placental transfer of TSH blocking antibodies, and treatment can be discontinued.

If the TSH level rises to the upper end of the normal range with a FT_4 at the lower end of the range (evidence of compensated hypothyroidism), a technetium scan or computed tomography (CT) may demonstrate a small midline (**Fig. 11.10**) or lingual gland (**Figs 1.85, 11.15–11.17**). L-Thyroxine should then be recommenced to remove the theoretical risk of later malignant change from chronic TSH hyperstimulation.

HYPONATREMIA AND HYPERNATREMIA

WATER REGULATION

Anatomic and physiologic considerations

The osmoregulatory system is controlled by the hypothalamic–neurohypophyseal axis, which includes osmoreceptors (near the supraoptic nuclei) and the neurones for the synthesis, storage and secretion of arginine vasopressin (AVP) (mainly in supraoptic nuclei, some in paraventricular nuclei). It also includes osmoreceptors of thirst, which control drinking behavior. The second component involves the kidney, where the renal collecting duct is sensitive to the action of AVP.

AVP secretion is controlled by changes in water balance, particularly through changes in plasma osmolality, to which the osmoreceptor is extremely sensitive. The 'osmotic threshold' for the release of AVP is 280 mOsm/kg water. Between 280 and 295 mOsm/kg, the AVP level rises steeply. Beyond 295 mOsm/kg, AVP concentration cannot rise further and thirst is perceived, leading to increased water intake.

The baroregulatory system is the secondary mechanism for controlling AVP secretion. The baroreceptor system (carotid sinus, aortic arch, left

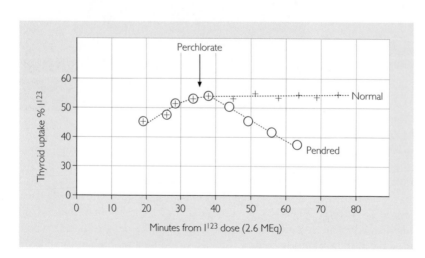

Fig. 11.13 Perchlorate discharge test. Graphical representation between normal or non-organification defect and organification defect such as the Pendred syndrome.

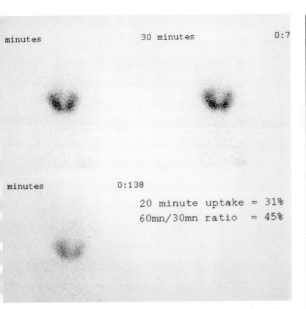

Fig. 11.14 Perchlorate discharge test showing uptake of radio-iodine into goitrous gland and discharge between 30 and 60 minute image in organification defect.

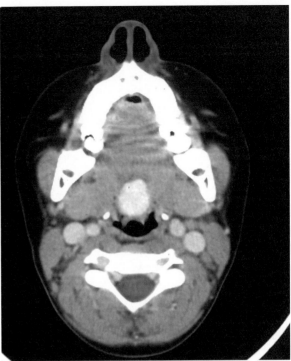

Fig. 11.16 Cross-sectional CT of neck showing extent of goitrous lingual thyroid tissue, see Fig. 1.85.

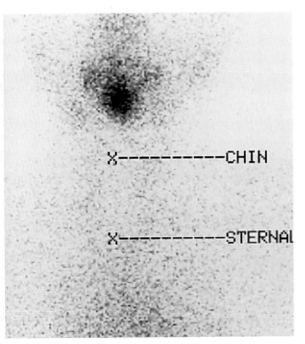

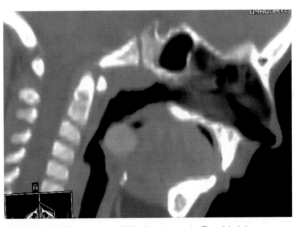

Fig. 11.17 Transverse CT of neck, as in Fig. 11.16.

Fig. 11.15 Lingual CT, technetium scan confirming no thyroid tissue in neck. (Parathyroid glands present in neck as derived from separate embryonic structures.)

atrium) is much less sensitive than the osmoreceptor, as a change in blood volume of 5–10% is necessary before AVP is released. Once this threshold is exceeded, release of AVP may reach levels 10 times higher than those reached after osmotic stimulation.

Atrial and brain natriuretic peptides act as secondary regulators of blood volume, but may become important in some pathologic states.

1-Deamino-8-D-arginine vasopressin (DDAVP) is a synthetic analog of AVP with more antidiuretic activity and no pressor activity; it is used for diagnosis and treatment of central diabetes insipidus (DI).

Hypernatremia due to diabetes insipidus

Definition and etiology

Diabetes Insipidus (DI) describes different disorders of water regulation due to vasopressin deficiency or lack of action and manifested by polyuria and polydipsia with varying degrees of plasma hypertonicity. Clinical features include:

■ constipation.
■ vomiting.
■ fever.
■ loss of weight or failure to thrive.
■ dehydration.

When caused by insufficient AVP secretion, this state is called central DI. A lack of peripheral response to AVP results in nephrogenic DI.

Central DI is rare in childhood and is most commonly due to intracranial tumors, or as a result of neurosurgery for these tumors. Craniopharyngioma may rarely present with polyuria and polydipsia, but this is common after operation. Other tumors such as Langerhans cell histiocytosis (**Figs 11.18–11.20**) and germinoma (see **Fig. 2.76**) along with non-neoplastic infiltration (such as sarcoid) are also causes of DI. Midline anatomic defects, such as septo-optic dysplasia (see **Fig. 2.81**) cause DI in around 30% of cases that may precede or follow other pituitary hormone deficiencies. Posterior pituitary damage can occur post-traumatically with disruption of the vulnerable pituitary stalk by trauma or after meningitis. After trauma there is a characteristic triphasic initial antidiuretic hormone (ADH) deficiency followed after 7 days by inappropriate ADH secretion then either recovery or permanent DI in the third week. The neurosecretory granules of AVP show up brightly on magnetic resonance imaging (MRI), and following stalk transection the lesion can be demonstrated by a 'hold-up' of this material in the

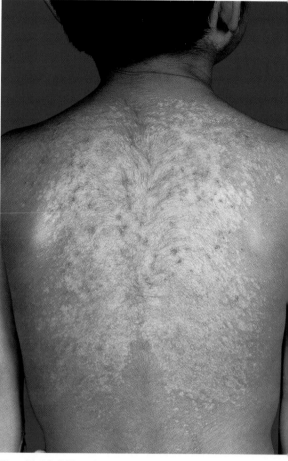

Fig. 11.19 Diffuse Langerhans cell histiocytosis with skin infiltration.

proximal part of the stalk (see **Fig. 2.78**). Idiopathic, autoimmune and familial cases also occur. Adipsic DI is a rare but serious entity, where the condition exists in a patient with impaired thirst mechanisms.

Nephrogenic DI can be inherited as an X-linked abnormality or be secondary to renal damage from metabolic disease (cystinosis, hypophosphatemia), sickle cell disease, drug therapy and chronic renal failure from any cause.

Primary polydipsia is due to a specific disorder of thirst regulation or psychogenic causes and will not result in hypernatremia.

Diagnostic work-up

Many cases of primary polydipsia can de differentiated from DI by a simple morning paired plasma and serum osmolarity. In primary polydipsia there will often be hyponatremia and a low serum osmolarity, in contrast to DI where the opposite is found.

The surest way to differentiate the forms of DI (which can occur in varying degrees of severity) is a

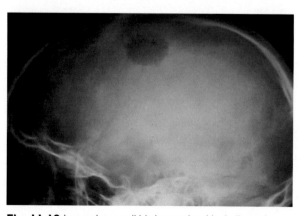

Fig. 11.18 Langerhans cell histiocytosis with skull erosions.

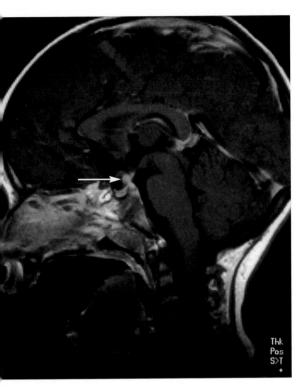

Fig. 11.20 Langerhans cell histiocytosis with involvement of pituitary stalk and diabetes insipidus (followed later by hypopituitarism).

dehydration test with measurements of plasma osmolality, urine osmolality and plasma AVP level (see Appendix). If there is no AVP assay available, an acceptable alternative is a dehydration test with measurements of plasma and urine osmolality, followed by a short desmopressin (DDAVP) test.

If, after dehydration, a high plasma osmolality is found (>295 mOsm/L) with a low urine osmolality (<400 mOsm/L), there is complete central DI. Following desmopressin administration the urine osmolality increases steeply. In cases of nephrogenic DI, there is only a partial rise of urine osmolality after dehydration (<800 mOsm/L) and a subnormal response to DDAVP. AVP levels will be high in nephrogenic DI.

During the dehydration test patients with primary polydipsia usually show an increase in urine osmolality that is close to normal values, and administration of desmopressin causes an increase in urine osmolality of less than 10%. In some cases the test result can be abnormal after a prolonged polyuric state (due to a 'wash-out effect' in the renal medulla), and can be difficult to distinguish from partial central DI. The water deprivation test can be repeated after several days of DDAVP treatment, or a hypertonic saline infusion test can be performed. Here slight hypertonicity is induced by strong saline infusion and AVP levels measured; in primary polydipsia there will be an appropriate rise, which will be absent in central DI.

Treatment

Central DI Central DI is treated with DDAVP intramuscularly or intravenously (usually only in the postoperative phase of management), intranasally or orally. The intranasal solution contains 100 μg in 1 mL, but can be diluted for use in neonates. The usual daily dosage is 0.25–10 μg/kg, given in two or three doses. Given orally, the dosage is around 10 to 20 times higher, but very variable, and tablets of 0.1 or 0.2 mg are used. Because there is no clear relationship between the previously needed intranasal dose and the oral dose, start at the lowest dose and increase under hospital supervision. The dosage should be adjusted according to response and should permit normal drinking behavior and sleep. Overdosage or continued habit polydipsia during treatment will lead to severe water intoxication and hyponatremia.

In adipsic DI, strict weight, fluid input and output records must be kept and an obligate intake maintained.

Indomethacin, chlorpropamide and the anticonvulsants carbamazepine and lamotrigine interfere with water excretion, and co-treatment may lead to dangerous hyponatremia.

During intercurrent illness in children with hypopituitarism there is relative hypocortisolemia. Cortisol is needed to excrete salt-free water and so there is often dilutional hyponatremia. It is safest to stop DDAVP treatment until the hypocortisolemia has been corrected.

Nephrogenic DI Nephrogenic DI is treated with a low-solute diet, restricted protein and salt intake, and water at frequent intervals. In severe cases chlorothiazide (100 mg/m² body surface per day) can be given in three divided doses.

Hyponatremia due to inappropriate secretion of ADH

The syndrome of inappropriate secretion of ADH (SIADH) can be caused by many systemic illnesses, burns, drugs or trauma to the CNS. It is characterized by hyponatremia and water retention in the presence of non-dilute urine.

Treatment relies on removing the cause, if possible, combined with fluid restriction. If severe, phenytoin (in young children) or demeclocycline (in older children) can be used; these drugs antagonize the actions of ADH. In life-threatening situations hypertonic saline and even combinations of furosemide (frusemide) and fludrocortisone may be used to reverse the hyponatremia.

Hyponatremia due to cerebral salt wasting

After severe brain injury there may be natriuresis and extracellular volume depletion secondary to the release of several natriuretic peptides and other unknown factors. The differentiation from SIADH (which often occurs in similar situations) is usually straightforward, as there is a diuresis and concentrated blood, but formal measurement of blood volume may be needed (by central venous pressure, echocardiography or isotope dilution).

SALT REGULATION

Physiological considerations and laboratory test

The renin–angiotensin–aldosterone system (RAAS) is the most important mediator in the endocrine regulation of sodium and water balance. Another component is atrial natriuretic factor (ANF), which inhibits aldosteronogenesis physiologically.

The determination of plasma renin activity is thus an important investigation in hyponatremic or hypernatremic states. Levels are strongly dependent on age, with the highest values in the first year of life, and they also vary according to the time of day, posture and sodium intake.

Aldosterone can be measured in plasma and in a 24-h urine collection. Plasma levels are also highest in the first year of life. Diagnostic accuracy can be enhanced by relating aldosterone excretion in the urine to sodium excretion.

Cortisol is the only hormone that produces feedback inhibition of adrenocorticotropic hormone (ACTH) secretion, and hence an increase in ACTH concentration is useful in distinguishing salt-losing states with primary adrenal failure.

Hyponatremia secondary to salt-losing syndromes

Loss of salt occurs in gastrointestinal, renal and adrenal disorders. Gastrointestinal diseases may be easy to diagnose, whereas the differential diagnosis of renal and adrenal diseases can be difficult.

Clinical symptoms of salt loss comprise:

- wasting.
- dehydration.
- intermittent fever.
- salt craving.
- shock.

Renal disease

Many chronic renal disorders can lead to salt-losing states. The clinical symptoms of renal salt-losing syndromes may be accompanied by the biochemical changes of proteinuria, aminoaciduria and glycosuria. Hypokalemia due to renal loss of potassium is common. In infants, salt loss can occur in cases of urethral obstruction with or without secondary infection, and the clinical and laboratory presentation may be very similar to that of CAH. Sonography of the kidney and bladder is thus an important investigation in infancy, accompanied by determination of plasma renin activity and aldosterone measurements in uncertain cases.

Adrenal disorders

These comprise various defects in the synthesis of mineralocorticoid and glucocorticoid hormones (see also Ch. 8 for a discussion of CAH causing intersex conditions).

In functional terms the adrenal consists of two parts: the cortex, which produces steroid hormones, and the medulla, which secretes catecholamines. Although interactions between both parts appear to exist, the physiologic functions can be considered as separate. In fetal life the adrenal cortex plays an important role in producing hormones that appear to be vital for placental function. After birth the adrenal cortex diminishes quickly in relative size, with atrophy of the hyperplastic fetal cortex. The remaining definitive cortex consists of three layers: the outer zona glomerulosa, the zona fasciculata and the zona reticularis. There are five groups of hormones produced in the adrenal cortex: corticosteroids, mineralocorticoids, androgens, estrogens and progestagens (see **Fig. 8.5**). The three groups of hormones are regulated differently. Glucocorticoid secretion is stimulated by ACTH from the pituitary in a classic negative feedback pattern. Mineralocorticoid secretion is mainly stimulated by the renin–angiotensin system. Androgen production is stimulated physiologically during early adolescence, probably under the control of ACTH or another central stimulating hormone, producing 'adrenarche' (see Ch. 6). ACTH, and hence cortisol, is produced in a circadian rhythm, with the highest levels in the early morning. ACTH can also be quickly secreted in times of stress.

Failure of aldosterone secretion

Congenital isolated defects of aldosterone biosynthesis with a normal glucocorticoid production are caused by abnormalities in methyloxidases I and II, which transform corticosterone into aldosterone. Investigations will reveal hyperkalemia, low-normal or diminished serum sodium levels, metabolic alkalosis and progressive reduction of kidney function, resulting finally in central shock and acidosis. Plasma renin activity is high and aldosterone low. Measurement of plasma corticosterone, 18-hydroxycorticosterone and aldosterone levels along with a urinary steroid profile can demonstrate the precise enzymatic defect. Fludrocortisone acetate is used as replacement therapy (see Ch. 8).

Pseudohypoaldosteronism is caused by a defect of type I aldosterone receptors. The symptoms are the same as those of hypoaldosteronism, but aldosterone levels are very high. Administration of fludrocortisone acetate has no effect and high doses of oral sodium chloride are necessary for treatment.

Mineralocorticoid deficiency as part of salt-wasting CAH is discussed in Chapter 8.

Hypoadrenalism

Although hypoadrenalism *per se* does not invariably cause hyponatremia, this is often a major component of the presentation of the causes of hypoadrenocorticism that are listed in **Table 11.2**. Primary hypoadreno-corticism is caused by a disorder in the adrenal itself, and manifests biochemically by a low serum cortisol level and a high serum ACTH concentration. The secondary forms are associated with low ACTH levels.

Adrenal hypoplasia is usually an X-linked condition associated with deletion of the same *DAX1* gene that produces XY sex reversal when duplicated (see Ch. 8).

Primary hypoadrenocorticism
Aplasia or hypoplasia of the adrenals
Adrenal hemorrhage of the newborn
Congenital adrenal hyperplasia caused by
   21-Hydroxylase deficiency
   17-Hydroxylase deficiency
   3β-Hydroxysteroid dehydrogenase deficiency
   Lipoid hyperplasia
Adrenal crisis of acute infection
Congenital adrenocortical unresponsiveness to ACTH
Chronic hypoadrenocorticism (Addison's disease)
The 3A syndrome
Primary familial xanthomatosis
Adrenoleukodystrophy
Secondary to insufficient ACTH secretion
Suppression by glucocorticoid therapy
Removal of unilateral secreting adrenal tumors
Starvation, anorexia nervosa
Infants born to mothers treated with steroids
Anencephaly
Secondary to drug therapy (ketoconazole, cyproterone)

Table 11.2 Syndromes of hypoadrenocorticism

Clinical presentation Infants with *aplasia or hypoplasia of the adrenal glands* present with:

- shock, tachycardia, cold and clammy skin, rapid respiration, vascular collapse.
- hyperpyrexia.
- cyanosis.
- skin pigmentation in the later presenting cases.

Depending on the involvement of the zona glomerulosa, salt loss can occur with hyponatremia and hyperkalemia. The differential diagnosis lies between septicemia, intracranial hemorrhage and pulmonary infections.

This disorder can be sex-linked recessive or sporadic.

Adrenal hemorrhage

This occurs mainly after prolonged labor and/or traumatic deliveries of large infants, and occurs more in boys than in girls. Severe clinical signs, similar to those described above, are seen only if hemorrhages have occurred bilaterally. On physical examination there may be a mass in the flank. On ultrasonography the kidney can be seen to be displaced downward by a hyperechoic adrenal. Usually calcification is seen after 3–6 weeks. During fulminating infections (particularly meningococcemia, but also during pneumococcal, streptococcal, Hemophilus and diphtheric infections), acute adrenal failure may occur. The clinical presentation is with shock and purpura, and if the child dies bilateral adrenal hemorrhage can be seen at autopsy.

Chronic hypoadrenocorticism (Addison's disease)

The symptoms of this chronic progressive debilitating illness consist of:

- weight loss and gastrointestinal complaints (anorexia, nausea, vomiting, diarrhea).
- cardiovascular problems (hypotension, decrease in heart size).
- skin hyperpigmentation due to ACTH oversecretion (particularly on pressure areas and scars, buccal mucosa, axilla, nipples, groin and the borders of the lips) (see **Figs 1.138 & 1.139**).

Because of the slow progression of the disease, diagnosis may be delayed. It is often not suspected until an acute adrenal crisis with dehydration and shock is precipitated by surgery, trauma or infection. Addison's disease can be a result of tuberculosis; AIDS; other rare infections such as coccidiomycosis, blastomycosis and histoplasmosis; amyloidosis and malignant infiltration. It can result from autoimmune disease, which may be due to isolated antiadrenal antibodies but is more often as part of the polyglandular syndrome type 1 (or HAM syndrome, with *H*ypoparathyroidism, *A*ddisonism and *M*oniliasis; see Ch. 9).

Hypoadrenocorticism secondary to insufficient ACTH secretion

This is usually part of multiple pituitary endocrinopathy, but can rarely occur as an isolated event. It may follow cranial irradiation.

Congenital unresponsiveness to ACTH has also been described.

3A syndrome

The Algrove syndrome, or 3A syndrome of alacrima, achalasia and adrenal hypofunction (see **Figs 1.150 & 1.151**), is a rare multisystem disorder affecting the autonomic nervous system and is associated with later neurodevelopmental abnormalities. It is caused by a mutation in a regulatory gene that is expressed ubiquitously in neuroendocrine and cerebral tissue.

Adrenal calcification

Adrenal calcification is not an uncommon finding, especially after neonatal sepsis. It is almost always discovered coincidentally and hardly ever results in adrenal insufficiency (**Fig. 11.21**).

Diagnostic work-up

Measurements of serum sodium and potassium concentrations are obviously necessary, sometimes in association with an estimation of urinary salt excretion. An early morning (0800–0900 hours) serum cortisol measurement allows for simple exclusion of cortical insufficiency (preferably paired with a simultaneous measurement of ACTH concentration; see below).

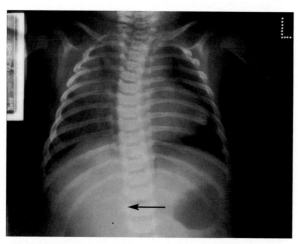

Fig. 11.21 Adrenal calcification seen coincidentally on radiograph of ex-premature neonate.

Note that infants up to 3 months of age do not show a circadian rhythm; consequently, below this age the timing of the sample is not critical and repeated measurements during the day or an ACTH (Synacthen) test will give useful information.

A paired serum ACTH determination will discriminate the primary and secondary forms of hypoadrenalism.

In response to Synacthen (see Appendix), primary defects will show an absent or low serum cortisol response. A suboptimal rise is also seen in long-standing central defects although, if Synacthen is continued for 48 h, a response will be seen. To discriminate between pituitary or hypothalamic problems, a stimulation test with corticotropin releasing factor (CRF) may be performed (see Appendix).

A urinary steroid profile and measurements of plasma adrenal steroids will help to discriminate between the various biosynthetic disorders. An autoantibody screen should be performed along with at least ultrasonic imaging of the adrenals, although abdominal CT may give more detail. Very long-chain fatty acid (VLCFA) levels are abnormal in adrenoleukodystrophy.

Treatment

Acute adrenal insufficiency is treated with fluid and electrolyte replacement, for example 20 mL normal (0.9%) saline per kg body weight in the first hour followed by a regimen tailored to the circulating volume and serum electrolytes. If there is continuing salt loss, oral sodium chloride supplements are required (1 g per 10 kg body weight), both for the initial therapy and until stabilized on mineralocorticoid replacement. For this, use deoxycorticosterone acetate (DOCA) at an approximate dose of 2 mg per day intramuscularly, then changing to twice-daily 9α-fludrocortisone acetate (0.15–0.25 mg/m^2 in 24 h) when the patient is able to take oral fluids. This dose should then be tailored to maintain normal plasma renin activity and blood pressure.

Hydrocortisone sodium hemisuccinate is given intravenously in a daily dose of 120 mg/m^2 or prednisolone 25 mg/m^2. This dosage is approximately 10 times the physiologic secretion rate. Maintenance therapy consists of hydrocortisone, 12–15 mg/m^2 daily, orally every 8 h, commonly divided 2 : 1 : 1 to try to mimic the natural circadian secretion. The first dose should be given on waking, the second in the early afternoon and the last dose after supper. Infants and small toddlers may require a four times a day dose or the use of a pre-bedtime equivalent dose of prednisolone (with a longer half-life) to allow safe levels during sleep. At times of stress the body responds with an increased ACTH and cortisol production; therefore, children with hypoadrenocorticism should be treated at times of fever, minor infections and trauma, and even psychologic upset, with a double dose of hydrocortisone. For elective surgery, with serious infections or trauma, and if a vomiting illness occurs, parenteral therapy is required, at 10 times the physiologic rate (as at diagnosis). The parents of all hypoadrenocortical children should be instructed on how to seek immediate medical help and advice, and how to give an initial intramuscular injection of 50–100 mg hydrocortisone, which may be life-saving in some situations. It is advisable to wear some form of Medicalert identification.

Hypernatremia due to mineralocorticoid excess

In 11β-hydroxysteroid dehydrogenase (and to a lesser extent in 17α-hydroxylase deficiency), there is sufficient accumulation of deoxycorticosterone (DOC) to produce salt retention, hypokalemia and hypertension, as well as cortisol deficiency and pseudo-hermaphroditism (see Ch. 8).

Overtreatment of 21-hydroxylase deficiency with fludrocortisone will produce salt retention and hypertension.

Other endocrine causes of hypertension

Primary hyperaldosteronism is very rare in childhood, but when it occurs is most likely due to bilateral nodular adrenal hyperplasia or tumor. Plasma expansion, hypernatremia and renin suppression occur.

Cushing syndrome in childhood is often accompanied by hypertension.

Tumors of neural crest origin (pheochromocytoma, neuroblastoma or ganglioneuroma) may produce hypertension secondary to catecholamine excess. They may occur sporadically or in association with neurofibromatosis, von Hippel–Lindau syndrome and multiple endocrine adenomatosis (MEA) II and IIb. The hypertension may be intermittent or sustained and accompanied by:

- headaches.
- pallor and sweating.
- nausea.
- abdominal pain.
- visual loss or diplopia.
- fits.

Diagnosis is by determination of plasma catecholamine levels or their urinary metabolites vanillylmandelic acid (VMA) and homovanillic acid (HVA). The radio-isotope MIBG (^{131}I-*m*-iodobenzylguanidine) and CT can be used to localize the tumor. Treatment is by surgical resection after combined α- and β-blockade in a specialist unit.

CALCIUM AND PHOSPHATE

PHYSIOLOGY

The main regulator of calcium and phosphate levels is parathyroid hormone (PTH), which is secreted in response to reduced serum calcium concentrations. It increases bone mobilization of calcium and renal calcium reabsorption, and (less immediately) increases calcium absorption in the intestine (through its action on vitamin D metabolism). It also decreases the reabsorption of phosphate from the proximal tubules of the kidney. The effect of PTH on vitamin D metabolism is mediated through an increase of the renal 1-hydroxylase enzyme activity, which transforms 25-(OH) vitamin D into 1,25-(OH)$_2$ vitamin D.

Vitamin D (calciferol) is synthesized from cholesterol in the skin and taken in food, and is then transformed to 25-(OH) vitamin D in the liver. In the kidney it is transformed either to the 1,25-(OH)$_2$D (active) or 24,25-(OH)$_2$D (inactive) forms. The activity of 1-hydroxylase is upregulated by PTH, and downregulated by both raised 1,25-(OH)$_2$D and serum phosphate concentrations. It acts on the intestine to increase calcium absorption, mobilizes calcium from bone and reabsorbs calcium in the kidney. Hepatic and renal disease will lead to secondary hypocalcemia by disrupting the synthesis of active vitamin D metabolites and tubular reabsorption of calcium.

The skeleton serves as a store of calcium and phosphate. PTH and 1,25-(OH)$_2$D act synergistically to promote bone resorption.

Calcitonin decreases calcium mobilization and increases calcium excretion by the kidney. It is secreted in response to hypercalcemia. It has only a minor role in calcium homeostasis.

Phosphate levels are maintained in a complex manner. Mutations in the gene for a fibroblast growth factor (FGF-23) lead to autosomal dominant hypophosphatemic rickets by causing relative over-expression of this phosphaturic compound. FGF-23 is also produced in some tumors, leading to phosphate loss and tumor-induced osteomalacia. FGF-23 is itself metabolized by an endopeptidase and *PHEX* mutations (which code for this protein) cause X-linked hypophosphatemia.

The calcium-sensing receptor (CASR) is a membrane G protein-coupled receptor expressed in the parathyroid gland and kidney tubule. It detects changes in calcium concentration and modifies PTH secretion or renal cation handling.

INVESTIGATION OF HYPOCALCEMIA OR HYPERCALCEMIA

Serum calcium and phosphate measurements should be determined. After the neonatal period, serum calcium levels remain constant throughout childhood (2.1–2.85 mmol/L, 8.4–10.6 mg/dL), whereas serum phosphate concentration is age dependent, with high levels in early childhood (1.3–2.3 mmol/L, 4–7 mg/dL), decreasing to adult levels (0.6–1.5 mmol/L, 2.0–4.6 mg/dL) only after adolescence. Total serum calcium levels should be interpreted in relation to serum albumin, and corrected in states of hypoalbuminemia or hyperalbuminemia by the formula:

$$\text{Corrected Ca} = \text{total Ca in mmol/l} - (0.25 \times \text{Albumin g/L}) + 1$$

If abnormalities are detected, further investigations are warranted. Intact PTH, 25(OH)D, 1,25(OH)$_2$D and urine cyclic adenosine monophosphate (cAMP) levels should be measured. An indirect measure of PTH secretion is an estimation of renal phosphate reabsorption. Renal phosphate excretion occurs mainly by means of failure of reabsorption in the proximal tubule of the kidney. This process is saturable, and the ratio of the maximal rate of tubular phosphate reabsorption to the glomerular filtration rate (Tmp/GFR) can easily be determined by simultaneous measurement of fasting urine and serum phosphate and creatinine concentrations. Normal levels of the Tmp/GFR ratio are age dependent, with high values during childhood (1.3–2.6 mmol/L, 4–8 mg/dL), declining to adult levels (0.8–1.4 mmol/L, 2.5–4.2 mg/dL) after the age of 18 years. PTH is one of the many factors influencing renal handling of phosphate (in that it resets the Tmp/GFR ratio at a lower level, resulting in increased urinary phosphate excretion and decreased serum phosphate concentrations); accordingly the Tmp/GFR ratio is high in hypoparathyroidism and low in hyperparathyroidism.

Hypocalcemia

The clinical symptoms and signs of hypocalcemia occur earlier when the calcium level falls rapidly, when serum magnesium concentration is low, when there is an alkalosis, or when the serum potassium level is high, and comprise:

- tetany (increased neurologic excitability), which can express itself in atypical forms, such as paresthesia, cramps.
- stridor, from laryngospasm.
- Chvostek's sign (spasm around the mouth and eyes from percussion of the temporomandibular branch of the facial nerve; this sign may be present in normal individuals, but is exaggerated in hypocalcemia).
- Trousseau's sign (spasm of the hand and thumb in response to relative ischemia from a tourniquet).
- smooth muscle spasm.
- persistent diarrhea.
- seizures.
- extrapyramidal signs due to basal ganglion calcification.
- papilledema.
- raised intracranial pressure.
- psychiatric disorders.
- dermal and dental changes (dry skin, brittle nails, coarse hair).
- cataracts.

Differential diagnosis

A list of causes of hypocalcemia in the neonate and later childhood is given in **Table 11.3**.

Deficient PTH secretion results in hypocalcemia (due to decreased bone mobilization, renal reabsorption and intestinal absorption). Hyperphosphatemia results from increased renal reabsorption due to inadequate inhibition by PTH. The causes of hypoparathyroidism are given in **Table 11.4**. A plain radiograph in early infancy may demonstrate thymic aplasia (**Fig. 11.22**), which may be confirmed by ultrasonography. (Further investigations should be undertaken to evaluate the immune system and to look for cardiac defects if DiGeorge syndrome is a possibility. The hypocalcemia is usually mild and requires treatment for only the first 2 years of life.)

Age	Etiological factors
Early neonatal	Prematurity; asphyxia; infants of diabetic mothers; maternal vitamin D deficiency
Late neonatal	Hypoparathyroidism (transient or permanent); high milk phosphate load; hypomagnesemia; parenteral nutrition; exchange transfusions; chronic alkalosis or bicarbonate treatment; maternal hyperparathyroidism
Childhood	Vitamin D deficiency (in early or latest stages); vitamin D-dependent rickets (types I and II); hypoparathyroidism; pseudo-hypoparathyroidism; AIDS

Table 11.3 Causes of hypocalcemia, by age

Aplasia and hypoplasia

Isolated (sporadic, X-linked, autosomal recessive, maternal ¹³¹I therapy)

Dysbranchiogenesis – the DiGeorge syndrome (in association with hypoplastic thymus, cardiac defects and abnormalities on chromosome 22q)

Kenny syndrome (in association with hypermetropia, short stature and tubular bone stenosis)

Transient hypoparathyroidism

Transient congenital parathyroid gland dysplasia

Maternal hyperparathyroidism

Hypomagnesemia

Polyglandular syndrome type I (or HAM syndrome)

Isolated idiopathic hypoparathyroidism

Acquired hypoparathyroidism

Surgical

Irradiation

Infiltration (iron storage in the hemoglobinopathies)

AIDS

Pseudohypoparathyroidism

(Albright hereditary osteodystrophy)

Table 11.4 Causes of hypoparathyroidism

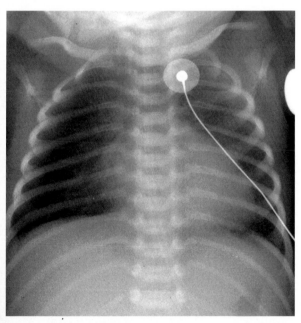

Fig. 11.22 Thymic aplasia in DiGeorge syndrome (confirmed on ultrasonography).

Various PTH receptor defects will result in PTH-resistant hypocalcemia, pseudo-hypoparathyroidism (see Ch. 2). Many cases are associated with learning difficulties, short stature, a round face with a short neck, a short fourth metacarpal (see **Figs 1.28 & 1.29**) and nodular subcutaneous calcification (osteoma cutis).

Autosomal dominant familial hypocalcemia is caused by a mild activating mutation of the CASR.

Maternal hyperparathyroidism will cause transient hypocalcemia in the infant due to exposure to a hypercalcemic environment *in utero* and PTH suppression.

Treatment

Acute The treatment of tetany consists of a 10% calcium gluconate infusion at a dosage of 0.20 mL/kg body weight, followed by 1.6 mL/kg (15 mg/kg) over 6–12 h. Extravasation leads to tissue necrosis (**Fig. 11.23**), so the solution should preferably be diluted (1 : 10). If there are no neurologic symptoms, oral calcium (50 mg/kg over 24 h in four divided doses) should be used.

Long-term The aim of therapy is to maintain serum calcium levels at the lower limit of normal. Vitamin D is given as dihydrotachysterol, 1α-hydroxycholecalciferol or 1,25-dihydroxycholecalciferol, usually in combination with calcium supplements (20 mg/kg daily). Overtreatment will result in nephrocalcinosis, so regular checks are needed of serum calcium, phosphate and creatinine levels, as well as urinary calcium excretion over 24 h. The calcium excretion should not exceed 0.1 mmol/kg (4 mg/kg), and the fasting urinary calcium : creatinine ratio (both in mmol/L) should be less than 0.7. Annual renal ultrasonography is also recommended.

Rickets

Rickets is a state of faulty mineralization of bone matrix in a growing child. It may result in hypocalcemia, but the biochemical manifestations are variable. The various causes of rickets are shown in **Table 11.5**.

Clinical signs

- Hard expansion of the bone ends (see **Figs 4.5 & 4.6**).

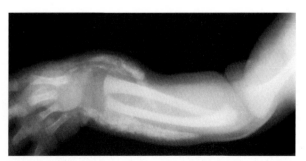

Fig. 11.23 Radiograph showing extravasated calcium; this required later forearm amputation.

- Skull deformities with frontal bossing and brachycephaly.
- Rachitic rosary (**Fig. 11.24**).
- Leg deformities, often with bowing (**Figs 11.25 & 11.26**), although there may be a wind-swept deformity and knock knees.
- Leg pain and refusal to walk (not seen in hypophosphatemic rickets).
- Growth retardation (see **Fig. 2.52**).
- Myopathy.

Radiography

Radiographs of any of the large joints show widening of the growth plate with 'cupping' and irregular concavity at the metaphysis (**Fig. 11.27**). There may be reduced bone mineralization.

Therapy and prevention

Simple vitamin D-deficient rickets is treated by either 20 μg vitamin D (800 IU), given daily for 3–4 months, or by a single intramuscular dose of 15 000 IU vitamin D (375 μg) (ergocalciferol).

Vitamin D-dependent rickets type I (secondary to a deficiency or absence of 1α-hydroxylating enzyme) is treated with calcitriol or 1α-calcidol, 0.25–2 μg per 24 h in two divided doses. Vitamin D-dependent rickets type II due to defects in the vitamin D receptor can be treated with large doses of calcitriol. If ineffective, extra calcium must be given via a central line, overnight, 1–2 mmol/kg daily.

Hypophosphatemic rickets is treated with oral phosphate supplements coupled with calcitriol. It is essential to monitor PTH levels and urinary calcium

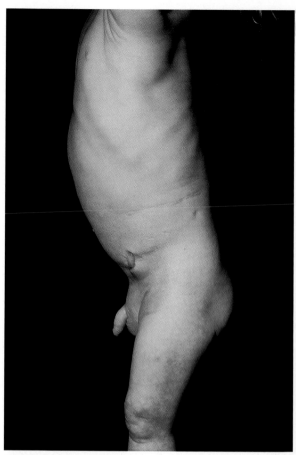

Fig. 11.24 'Rickety rosary' visible in child with malnutrition secondary to bowel resection.

	Calcium	Phosphate	PTH
Vitamin D deficiency			
Stage 1, early	Low	Normal	Normal
Stage 2	Normal	Low	High
Stage 3, late	Low	Low	Low
X-linked hypophosphatemia	Normal	Very low	Normal (may be raised initially. Monitor during treatment)
Type 1, vitamin D dependent	Low	Low	High
Type 2, as above plus alopecia	Low	Low	High
Calcium deficiency	Low	Normal	

Table 11.5 Causes of rickets

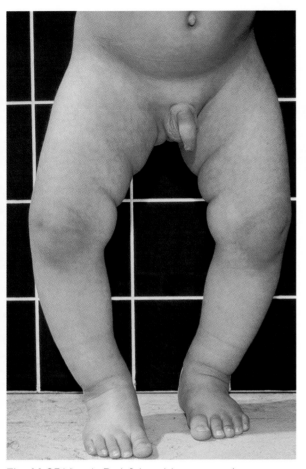

Fig. 11.25 Vitamin D-deficient rickets, external appearance.

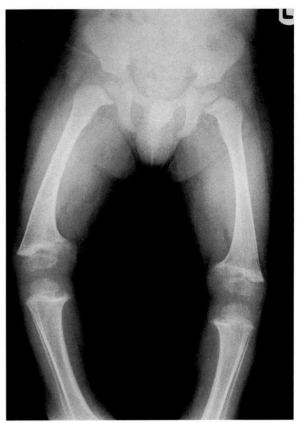

Fig. 11.26 Radiograph of patient in Fig. 11.25.

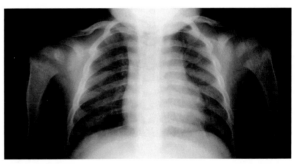

Fig. 11.27 Chest radiograph showing widened epiphyses, cupping of the metaphyses and abnormal bone formation in hypophosphatemic rickets.

excretion, and to perform a yearly renal ultra-sonographic scan. The evidence that growth hormone will improve the tubular phosphate loss or improve the rate of growth is poor outside the youngest child, and data on long-term follow-up are not available.

Osteoporosis

Juvenile idiopathic osteoporosis (**Fig. 11.28**) is a condition of unknown cause that produces bone pain and fractures in the prepubertal child, but seems distinct from osteogenesis imperfecta. It remits after several years but can leave residual deformity and short stature. The serum calcium levels are usually normal, but may be slightly low whilst the disease is most active.

Osteogenesis imperfecta (see **Figs 2.53, 2.61 & 2.62**) produces severe osteoporosis.

Any causes of pubertal delay (see Ch. 7) can produce undermineralization of the skeleton, detectable on estimation of bone mineral density, which tends to be more severe with later presentation. Whether this produces clinically important later effects is unknown, but spontaneous fractures have been reported in adults with the Ullrich–Turner syndrome.

Cushing syndrome can produce vertebral collapse and permanent stunting due to low mineral density.

Treatment of all causes of osteoporosis is with a normal, but monitored, calcium and vitamin D intake, with the bone-strengthening bisphosphonates under specialist supervision.

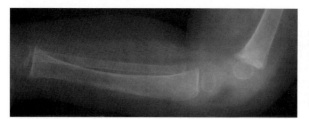

Fig. 11.28 Juvenile idiopathic osteoporosis; very low bone mineral content.

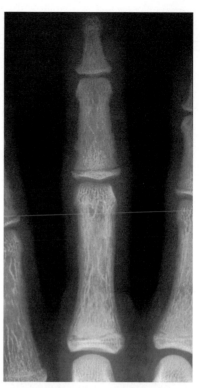

Fig. 11.29 Hyperpara-thyroidism with bony erosions of phalanges.

Hypercalcemia

The clinical symptoms and signs of hypercalcemia are:

- weakness.
- vomiting and constipation.
- polyuria and polydipsia.

Nephrocalcinosis may occur, leading to renal failure and secondary hypertension.

Hyperparathyroidism may be caused by an adenoma or general hyperplasia of the glands and is rare in childhood (**Fig. 11.29**). Adenomas are sporadic, but hyperplasia may be familial and associated with MEA I or II (see **Table 9.4**). Sestamibi imaging may help to locate non-thyroidal parathyroid tissue (i.e. thoracic). The genes associated with MEA I and II are located on 11q and 10q respectively, and may be analyzed to confirm the diagnosis or exclude siblings and children from unnecessary screening. Further screening tests in genetically identified teenage individuals with MEA I include yearly PTH and calcium estimation, gut peptides (vasoactive intestinal peptide (VIP), pancreatic poly-peptide, glucagon, gastrin and somatostatin), prolactin and insulin-like growth factor (IGF) 1 with 5-yearly MRI of the pituitary and pancreas, and the neuroendocine tumor markers chromogranin A and neurone-specific enolase.

Vitamin D intoxication and malignancy may also cause hypercalcemia.

In infancy, transient idiopathic hypercalcemia is associated with characteristic facial features (**Fig. 11.30**) and neurologic (**Fig. 11.31**) and cardiovascular defects (Williams syndrome).

An infantile form of severe primary hyperpara-thyroidism due to hyperplasia of the glands may occur. It presents with marked hypotonia, feeding problems, chest deformity and respiratory distress. It may be familial or sporadic; usually the cause is unknown, although some cases may be due to mutations of the calcium-sensing receptor. It is severe enough to warrant emergency total parathyroidectomy. Milder reduction in

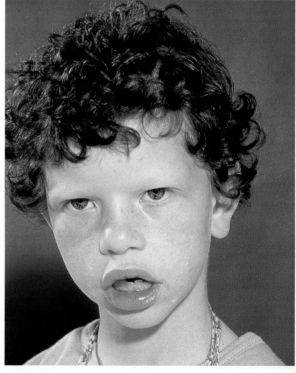

Fig. 11.30 The Williams syndrome – note abnormal mid-face and wide, open, mouth. The iris has a stellate appearance. The voice is hoarse and there may be hyperacusis.

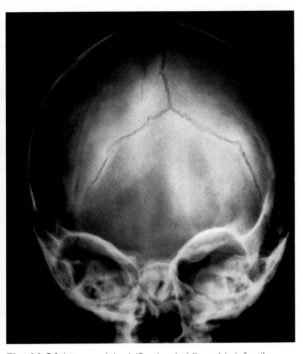

Fig. 11.31 Intracranial calcification in idiopathic infantile hypercalcemia.

the activity of the calcium-sensing receptor produces familial hypocalciuric hypercalcemia.

Maternal hypocalcemia due to hypoparathyroidism or other causes will result in transient reactive hypercalcemia after birth. Phosphate depletion in the preterm infant may also cause infantile hypercalcemia.

GLUCOSE

Glucose input from the diet and tissue stores is balanced against utilization by the tissues. Pancreatic endocrine secretion of insulin, as well as glucagon, somatostatin and pancreatic polypeptide, is modulated by nutrient levels (glucose and amino acids), autonomic neural input and paracrine influences. The secretion of insulin is secondary to rising intracellular adenosine triphosphate (ATP) levels. This in turn closes membrane potassium channels and leads to cell depolarization. In response to the voltage change there is calcium influx and exocytosis of insulin from storage granules.

In the circulation, insulin acts to move glucose into fat and muscle, to promote liver glycogen synthesis, and has an anabolic action on muscle protein synthesis. These actions result in a lowering of glucose, ketone body, free fatty acid and branched-chain amino acid levels. Resistin, secreted from white fat, antagonizes these peripheral insulin actions.

Glucagon concentration rises at the expense of insulin during periods of starvation, possibly in part

modulated by the effects of pancreatic somatostatin. As glucose concentrations fall there is a reciprocal rise in the extrapancreatic counterregulatory hormones cortisol, growth hormone and epinephrine (adrenaline), which act in various ways to stabilize blood glucose levels. Growth is adaptively inhibited, despite the rise in growth hormone levels, by an increase in levels of IGF binding protein 1 and thus reduced growth factor availability. It follows that any relative excess of insulin or lack of counterregulatory hormones will tend to produce hypoglycemia. Insulin deficiency (usually seen in type 1 insulin-dependent diabetes mellitus) or insulin resistance (seen much more rarely in childhood as maturity-onset diabetes of youth (MODY), or with other syndromic associations) will produce hyperglycemia (see Ch. 10). Cortisol excess, either iatrogenic or as part of the Cushing syndrome, will also produce hyperglycemia (as can iatrogenic overdosage with growth hormone in rare clinical situations).

HYPOGLYCEMIA

Hypoglycemia triggers a set of counterregulatory and neurobehavioral responses. The blood glucose level that achieves these effects is to an extent dependent on age, disease and situation, but may be taken approximately as <2.2 mmol/L (40 mg/dL) in the older child or adult and as <2.8 mmol/L (50 mg/dL) in the neonate, although levels lower than 3.5 mmol/L (62 mg/dL) may be of concern in the sick, premature infant.

Hypoglycemia itself modifies especially the metabolic responses to subsequent episodes of low blood sugar levels, in both the long and short term, and there may also be changes in disease duration and activity. Some metabolic disorders that cause hypoglycemia also affect normal counterregulation, further complicating the predictability of symptoms.

Clinical presentation

The presenting features of hypoglycemia in childhood are:

- pallor and sweating.
- confusion and irritability, proceeding to loss of consciousness.
- hunger, abdominal pain or nausea.
- convulsions.

In the neonate, additionally:

- jitteriness.
- hypotonia.
- hypothermia.
- apnea and oxygen desaturation.
- tachypnea.

A drug history should be taken as steroid withdrawal, even inhaled steroids, can occasionally precipitate symptomatic hypoglycemia. Ingestion or administration of sulfonylureas and insulin can cause factitious hypoglycemia.

Severe hypoglycemia can be devastating to a developing brain and result in severe damage. There is a tendency for this to be most severe in the occipital region of the brain, resulting in a syndrome of cortical blindness along with spastic quadriplegia, severe delay and fits (**Fig. 11.32**).

Differential diagnosis

In the neonate, hyperinsulinism caused by diabetes in the mother or by persistent hyperinsulinemic hypoglycemia of infancy (PHHI) should be associated with macrosomia (see **Figs 3.26 & 3.28**). PHHI can be caused by a number of genetic mechanisms affecting the membrane potassium channels and the abnormal coupling of release of insulin to glucose levels. These defects may be inherited in both an autosomal dominant and recessive manner. The recessive form is particularly common in the Arabian peninsula. One form associated with an abnormality of glutamate dehydrogenase presents with mild hyperinsulinism and hyperammonemia. The histologic changes of diffuse beta-cell hyperplasia (**Fig. 11.33**) are no longer thought to be a primary anatomic abnormality ('nesidioblastosis'), but secondary to the assorted gene defects described above.

Neonatal hyperinsulinism can also be secondary to hydrops fetalis. Premature babies and small-for-dates infants (see **Fig. 2.22**) have decreased energy stores in the presence of increased utilization. The Beckwith–Wiedemann or EMG syndrome (exomphalos, macroglossia, gigantism) (see **Figs 3.17–3.19**) may be associated with an abnormality of chromosome 11 in a proportion of patients, and there is a risk of Wilms tumor and other malignancies (see Ch. 3).

Panhypopituitarism producing hypoglycaemia in the male neonate may be evident from micropenis or cryptorchidism (see **Fig. 8.12**).

Although the importance of growth hormone as a counterregulatory hormone wanes after the first year of life, there is genetic variability in mechanisms of glucose homeostasis, and hypoglycemia may be a presenting feature of isolated growth hormone deficiency or hypopituitarism even in the older child (who will also manifest a poor rate of growth, short stature or hypogonadism).

There may be hepatomegaly associated with the glycogen storage disorders both in the neonatal period and at later presentation (see **Fig. 2.49**). Fatty acid oxidation disorders, galactosemia and some other metabolic disorders will produce hypoglycemia as a consequence of decreased production of glucose, as will severe liver disease. Alcohol ingestion in childhood may be associated with severe hypoglycemia.

Pancreatic adenomas may occur in later childhood *de novo* or as part of MEA I.

Diagnostic work-up

At the time of hypoglycemia (which may need to be induced by starvation in some carefully supervised

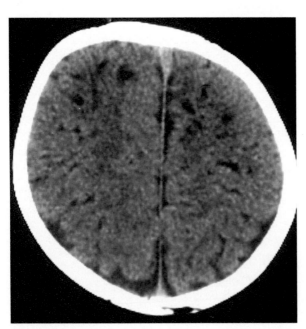

Fig. 11.32 Brain CT showing cortical defects and loss of gray matter, predominantly in the occipital region, following a single event of severe hypoglycemia.

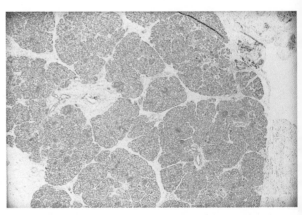

Fig. 11.33 Diffuse beta-cell hyperplasia, showing insulin-secreting tissue as brown – a condition formerly called nesidioblastosis.

situations in specialized centers), blood should be obtained to allow comparison of the low blood glucose levels to insulin, cortisol and growth hormone. Also estimate levels of ammonia, branched-chain amino acids, hydroxybutarate, lactate and free fatty acids. The first urine passed after the episode should be analyzed for dicarboxylic acids, glycine conjugates, organic acids and acylcarnitine. If there is any possibility of factitious hypoglycemia, assay C-peptide levels (which will be low at the same time as a raised insulin concentration if this is being administered by a carer), and for alcohol, salicylate or oral hypoglycemic agents such as sulfonylurea.

Hypoglycemia can be broadly classified as ketotic or non-ketotic, and a summary of the interpretation of these investigations is given in **Table 11.6**.

Treatment

Treatment of PHHI involves immediate restoration of normoglycemia. Intravenous dextrose utilization may exceed 10 mg/kg/min and may need central line placement. Glucagon up to 200 µg/kg will raise the blood sugar level for up to 12 h whilst more definitive therapy is instituted. Diazoxide opens the pancreatic potassium channels and should be started at a low dose (5 mg/kg daily) to avoid the heart failure that occurs with doses up to 20 mg/kg daily. With chronic use, hypertrichosis occurs (**Fig. 11.34**). Diazoxide is often combined with chlorthiazide, 7–10 mg/kg daily, which ameliorates the heart failure and has independent membrane polarization effects. Nifedipine is a calcium channel antagonist that may be useful in isolated cases. Octreotide (a synthetic analog of somatostatin) inhibits insulin release but needs to be given by injection and causes suppression of other peptide hormone release and gallstones. If medical treatment fails to suppress symptoms, then pancreatectomy of 95% or more may be required. There is evidence that the pathology is focal in at least 40% of cases, and preoperative venous sampling for insulin may remove the need for total pancreatectomy and subsequent diabetes with exocrine pancreatic failure. Many children with PHHI have gastric dysmotility and require prokinetic agents.

SCREENING SURVIVORS OF PEDIATRIC MALIGNANCY

The success of treatment for various childhood malignancies means that increasing numbers of long-

Finding at the time of hypoglycemia	Interpretation
Ketosis with low fatty acids	Ketone body utilization defects
Ketosis plus fatty acid increase, normal lactate level	Growth hormone deficiency (In the neonate the growth hormone response to hypoglycemia is variable and may require later provocation testing to confirm. Treatment with growth hormone and restoration of normoglycemia is an initial pragmatic approach) Cortisol deficiency, confirmed by low cortisol level Glycogen storage disease types 3, 6 and 9 'Ketotic hypoglycemia'
Ketosis plus fatty acid increase, raised lactate level	Organic acidemias Gluconeogenesis defects
No ketosis plus low fatty acid level	Hyperinsulinism – confirm with detectable (not necessarily absolutely raised) insulin level Sometimes panhypopituitarism in the neonate
No ketosis plus raised fatty acids, normal lactate levels	Fatty acid oxidation defects
No ketosis plus raised fatty acids, lactate level raised	Glycogen storage disease type 1 Respiratory chain defects
C-peptide level low whilst insulin level high	Factitious administration of insulin

Table 11.6 Investigation of hypoglycemia.

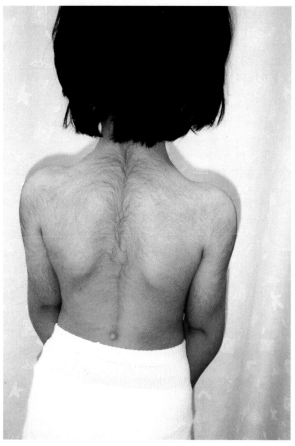

Fig. 11.34 Hypertrichosis following diazoxide treatment for PHHI.

term survivors require follow-up. It is estimated that by the year 2010 almost 1 in 800 of the young adult population will fall into this category.

The cost of the cure is related to the chemotherapy and radiotherapy received during initial treatment. Many survivors will have short stature and endocrine dysfunction (see Ch. 2). The exact nature of the later endocrine and growth-inhibiting effects will depend on the nature, dosage, age of administration and sex of the patient. The relative contributions of drug- and radiation-induced effects is still far from clear. Only active surveillance for the development of these problems at an early stage will allow for early detection and treatment before avoidable morbidity occurs.

An outline of the endocrine and other problems that will require prospective surveillance in these survivors is given in **Table 11.7**.

ARTEFACTUAL ENDOCRINOPATHIES

Any laboratory assay has an inbuilt error of estimation. If the results obtained on testing do not agree with the clinical picture, it is always wise to raise the possibility of laboratory error or repeat the estimation. Many diagnostic 'kits' come with inappropriate reference ranges for children and it is wise to establish local experience and 'normal' values with an assay before routine use. It should be remembered that 'normality' is usually defined as a value ± 2 standard deviations from the mean, and some outliers will, by definition, be healthy individuals.

'Adequate' responses to stimulation tests (especially with respect to growth hormone) are often defined in an arbitrary way and change with availability of treatment and medical practice. Apparent lack of response may reflect poor investigative methodology more than pathology. Failure to appreciate changes in hormone levels with time of day, age, stage of pubertal development, weight or surface area will also lead to confusion.

Some international hormone standards measured in units referable to a biologic standard also change from time to time and require revision of normal values.

There are some apparent endocrine abnormalities that are due to more predictable laboratory artefacts or to biological/induced variation in binding protein levels or hormone metabolism. These are briefly discussed below.

DRUGS AND DIET

Many drugs will induce liver enzymes and hence increase hormone clearance or binding protein levels and thus interfere with free hormone estimations. Alkaline phosphatase levels may also be altered. The H_2 histamine blockers such as cimetidine interfere with the measurement of serum calcium. *It is thus essential that a drug history is provided for the laboratory.* Food with a high vanilla content and a number of drugs will interfere with urinary estimation of VMA and HVA.

HYPERLIPIDEMIA

Hyperlipidemia (**Fig. 11.35**) may be seen in diabetic ketoacidosis and interferes with some laboratory electrochemical methods of sodium analysis to produce apparent hyponatremia.

BINDING PROTEIN ABNORMALITIES

Cortisol, testosterone and thyroxine are bound to specific circulating binding proteins as well as serum albumin. Measurement of total levels of these hormones will therefore overestimate biologic activity in states of binding protein excess, and underestimate activity with low binding protein levels. General states of protein loss

Growth impairment	
Proportionate loss (GHD)	Cranial irradiation – onset of GHD in proportion to the dose and young age of treatment
± Short spine (GHD + spinal damage) (?epiphyseal toxicity)	Spinal irradiation; abdominal or thoracic irradiation; TBI ?Chemotherapy including 6-mercaptopurine
Gonadal dysfunction	
Females	
Primary ovarian failure	
Premature ovarian failure	TBI, abdominal irradiation, cyclophosphamide
Central precocious puberty (contributes to height loss)	Low-dose cranial irradiation (18–24 Gy)
Males	
Testicular failure (Leydig cells + germinal epithelium)	Direct irradiation (as in some ALL treatment regimens and testicular tumors; TBI) Scatter irradiation from abdominal tumor
Infertility (germinal epithelium)	Chemotherapy, especially cyclophosphamide, vinblastine and procarbazine Direct irradiation
Thyroid dysfunction	
Thyroid failure	Direct irradiation (Hodgkin's disease), or as part of craniospinal irradiation and TBI. TSH lack secondary to cranial irradiation
Thyroid malignancy	In proportion to dose received by gland; special risk if TSH level is raised
Adrenal insufficiency	
Hypocortisolemia	Rare, but can occur after high-dose irradiation for cranial tumors
Posterior pituitary	
Diabetes insipidus	Rare, usually after neurosurgery for cranial tumors
Other	
Renal damage and hypertension	Chemotherapy, direct irradiation
Cardiac toxicity	Anthracycline chemotherapy ± radiation damage
CNS damage	Irradiation, in proportion to dose received, more with early age of therapy. Direct trauma from surgery
Vision	Cataracts from irradiation. Damage to optic tracts from irradiation and surgery
Second malignancy	Skin and soft tissue in irradiation field. Second tumors with alkylating agents or genetic predisposition
Dental caries and enamel hypoplasia (see Fig. 1.78)	Most chemotherapy

GHD, growth hormone deficiency; TBI, total body irradiation; ALL, acute lymphoblastic leukemia.

Table 11.7 Surveillance in survivors of childhood malignancy

such as nephrotic syndrome, or decreased production as in cirrhosis of the liver will affect all the levels of binding proteins.

Corticosteroid binding globulin (CBG) levels are increased by estrogen, producing high levels of measured cortisol in pregnancy and with estrogen therapy. Low levels are seen in hypothyroidism and obesity. Genetic disorders producing high and low CBG levels have been described.

Testosterone–estrogen binding protein (or sex hormone binding globulin; SHBG) levels are increased in androgen deficiency states, with estrogen treatment and in thyrotoxicosis. Levels are low in obesity, hypothyroidism, Cushing syndrome and after androgen

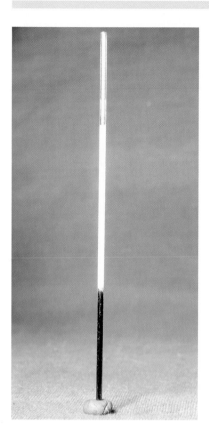

Fig. 11.35
Gross hyperlipidemia in glycogen storage disease type 1.

	T$_4$	FT$_4$	T$_3$	TSH
Renal failure	↓	↓	↓	→
Hepatic failure	↓	↓	↓	→↑
Estrogen therapy	↑	→	→↑	→
Propranolol treatment	↑	→	↑	→
Epilepsy treatment	↓	→	↓	→
High-dose steroids	↓	→	↓	→
Growth hormone therapy	↓	→	↑	↑
hCG treatment or choriocarcinoma	↑	↑	↑	↓

hCG, human chorionic gonadotropin.

Table 11.8 Induced abnormalities of thyroid function tests

HETEROPHILIC ANTIBODIES

As many modern assays are based on anti-hormone antibodies raised in other animals, it is surprisingly common to get interference from anti-mouse, or other animal, antibodies present in the blood of the patient. There may be a history of animal handling, exposure to rat feces, etc, but this is not always the case. If any immunoassay result is surprisingly increased, it is worth rechecking the levels on a second assay based on another animal's antibodies or attempting to dilute or bind the offending antibodies before re-assay.

MATERNAL HORMONE ABNORMALITIES IN PREGNANCY DUE TO FETAL EFFECTS

The fetoplacental axis is 'added on' to the maternal hormone system through pregnancy. The fetal adrenal cortex plays an important role in producing hormones that appear to be vital for placental function. In particular, dehydroepiandrosterone (DHEA) and its sulfate (DHEAS) are produced in large quantities, and further processed to estrogens in the placenta. Maternal urinary excretion of estriol (E$_3$) in particular provides useful information about the fetal pituitary–adrenal axis. Low levels of estriol indicate fetal adrenal insufficiency, either primary or secondary. (Undetectable maternal estriols are found in placental sulfatase deficiency, producing a syndrome of post-maturity and congenital ichthyosis; see **Fig. 1.149**). Maternal virilization has been reported as a consequence of fetal P450 aromatase deficiency (converting testosterone to estradiol), with the later delivery of a female pseudo-hermaphroditic infant.

treatment. Again hereditary abnormalities of production have been described. Estrogen largely circulates bound to albumin and will therefore appear decreased in nephrotic syndrome.

Probably the most clinically important binding protein considerations are in relation to the assessment of thyroid function. It is now common to be able to assay free hormone activity directly, avoiding some of these difficulties. A summary of diseases and drugs that will interfere with the interpretation of thyroid function tests is shown in **Table 11.8**.

Blood calcium levels need to be adjusted for serum albumin:

Total calcium level (mmol/L) – [0.25 × Albumin (g/l)] + 1
= True value

Carbohydrate-deficient glycoprotein syndrome is a rare generalized disorder of serum glycoproteins that is associated with developmental delay, organ failure and adult hypogonadism. There is a deficiency of TBG, CBG and SHBG, and consequently low levels of these hormones on total assay. Associated abnormalities of unbound luteinizing hormone (LH), follicle stimulating hormone (FSH), prolactin and growth hormone have also been described in this complex syndrome.

FETAL/INFANTILE HORMONE ABNORMALITIES DUE TO MATERNAL EFFECTS

Maternal androgen production may virilize the infant in cases of maternal tumor, CAH and even severe polycystic ovary, and also after anabolic steroid abuse – although the associated subfertility makes conception less likely in uncontrolled cases.

Maternal cyproterone therapy can lead to under-virilization of the fetus and so is commonly administered concomitantly with the contraceptive pill.

Neonatal thyrotoxicosis is a consequence of the passage of thyroid receptor stimulating antibodies in late pregnancy (see Ch. 9). Maternal antithyroid medication may suppress the thyroid overactivity either as a deliberate therapeutic maneuver if fetal tachycardia is severe, or lead to potentially adverse late presentation of neonatal thyrotoxicosis if not recognized.

Maternal steroid administration for autoimmune disease, thyrombocytopenia, etc. can produce infantile adrenal suppression severe enough to warrant replacement treatment; it may take up to a year for the infant to show recovery. In familial cases of CAH, dexamethasone is used deliberately to suppress virilization in affected female infants (see Ch. 8).

Maternal hypothyroidism can produce a mild reduction in later developmental quotient, which may be severe if the fetus is also hypothyroid from iodine deficiency or coincidental congenital hypothyroidism (see above).

Maternal phenylketonuria, if not adequately controlled by diet, leads to infantile microcephaly and smallness-for-dates with later short stature.

Suggested Reference Texts

Becker KL, Bilezikian JP, Bremner WJ, Hung W, Kahn CR. *Principles and Practice of Endocrinology and Metabolism*, 2nd edn. Philadelphia, Pennsylvania: Lippincott, 2001.

Beighton P. *Inherited Disorders of the Skeleton*, 2nd edn. Edinburgh: Churchill Livingstone, 1988.

Besser GM, Thorner MO. *Clinical Endocrinology*, 2nd edn. London: Wolfe, 1994.

Brook CDG, Hindmarsh P, eds. *Clinical Paediatric Endocrinology*, 4th edn. Oxford: Blackwell Scientific, 2001.

Hochberg Z, ed. *Practical Algorithms in Pediatric Endocrinology*. Basle: Karger, 1999.

Kappy MS, Blizzard RM, Migeon CJ, eds. *Wilkins: The Diagnosis and Treatment of Endocrine Disorders in Childhood and Adolescence*, 4th edn. Springfield, Illinois: Charles Thomas, 1994 (new edition due 2003).

Kelnar C, ed. *Childhood Diabetes*. London: Chapman and Hall, 1994.

Kelnar CJH, Savage MO, Stirling HF, Saegner P, eds. *Growth Disorders*. London: Chapman and Hall, 1998.

Lifshitz F, ed. *Pediatric Endocrinology*, 3rd edn. New York: Dekker, 1996 (new edition due 2003).

Ranke MB. *Functional Endocrine Diagnostics in Children and Adolescents*. Mannheim: JJ Verlag, 1992.

Sanfillipo JS, Muram D, Dewhurst J, Lee PA. *Pediatric and Adolescent Gynecology*. Philadelphia, Pennsylvania: Saunders, 2001.

Sperling MA, Barlow M, Fletcher J. *Pediatric Endocrinology*. Philadelphia, Pennsylvania: Saunders, 1996.

Wass JAH, Shalet SM, eds. *Oxford Textbook of Endocrinology and Diabetes*. Oxford: Oxford University Press, 2002.

Winter RM, Baraitser M. *Multiple Congenital Abnormalities, A Diagnostic Compendium*. London: Chapman and Hall, 1991 (also available as computerized London Dysmorphology Database).

Appendix

Tests of Endocrine Function and Normal Values

INTRODUCTORY NOTES

These protocols are included for general guidance only. They were designed for use in a specialist children's endocrine unit and may not always be applicable elsewhere. It is the responsibility of clinicians performing the tests to ensure that correct local procedures are followed, particularly in relation to the administration of drugs, patient safety and comfort.

Further information on dynamic testing can be obtained from one of the texts cited in the Foreword.

COMBINED ANTERIOR PITUITARY FUNCTION TEST

PRINCIPLE

A combined provocation test is used to test for adequate excretion of GH, TSH, LH and FSH. Basal levels of GH are of no value because of the pulsatile nature of secretion. Likewise, exercise and sleep are both very poor stimuli for GH secretion and should not be used. IGF-1 and IGFBP-3 levels, if interpreted together, may give some information about GH status, but have an unacceptably high false-positive and false-negative value (especially post-irradiation), and so stimulated secretion, as described below, is required in most cases to confirm or refute GH deficiency and before treatment is commenced. It may be necessary and advisable to perform two tests of GH secretion in cases of isolated GHD.

The 'gold standard' test is still the insulin tolerance test + TRH + GnRH test, which has the advantage of allowing the assessment of ACTH secretion in response to hypoglycemia in a more predictable manner than with clonidine. However, this test has led to death in some circumstances and it should remain confined to experienced units, which will already have an established protocol; it is therefore not described here.

MATERIALS REQUIRED

Pharmaceutical

- Clonidine, TRH and LHRH (separately or combined in a single ampoule).

- Depot testosterone (for boys of TW2 bone age greater than 10 years).

Other

- Lithium heparin containers.

APPROXIMATE LENGTH OF TEST

Three hours, excluding any overnight preparation.

PATIENT PREPARATION

The exact procedure employed in males depends upon the age of the patient. If older than 10 years but with no signs of endogenous sexual development, consideration should be given to prior priming with sex steroids as there is good evidence that false-positive results will result in the relatively hypogonadotropic milieu of delayed puberty. Sex steroid priming is achieved by giving 100-mg depot testosterone esters i.m. 3–5 days before the test. There is no evidence that priming of females is required, but in some countries priming is still performed, for example with 25 µg ethinylestradiol twice a day for 5 days.

The patient is fasted overnight before the test. Venous access is secured and fixed into position along with a three-way stopcock for the duration of the test. The line is kept patent with heparinized saline.

Clonidine may make the subject nauseated, dizzy and hypotensive; young children may become very sleepy. TRH and GnRH can produce flushing and a metallic taste in the mouth. The subject must be fully recovered and have taken a meal before discharge home.

Other tests of GH release

A safe alternative to clonidine is to use arginine mono-hydrochloride, 12.5% solution, 0.5 g/kg infused over 30 min with blood taken at −30 min in addition to the samples described above.

Glucagon, GHRH, L-dopa and metaclopramide have all at some time been used as GH secretagogues.

PROCEDURE

Oral clonidine ($150 \, \mu g/m^2$) is given at time 0.

The standard dose of TRH is 5–7 μg/kg (up to 200 μg) and that of GnRH is 2.5 μg/kg (up to 100 μg) injected over 2 min at time 0, immediately after the clonidine has been taken.

SAMPLES REQUIRED

Blood is collected at each timepoint according to the schedule in **Table A.1**. The volume required will vary according to local laboratory needs. The time of collection of the samples should be carefully recorded.

INTERPRETATION OF RESULTS

Growth hormone

Adequate secretion = more than 7 μg/L (using the 1 mg = 3 IU conversion).

As discussed in Chapter 2, this level is arbitrary and has tended to increase over time. Certainly, levels of 3.5 μg/L or less are indicative of more severe deficiency than intermediate levels.

TSH

Hypopituitary = all levels usually within normal basal range

and an increase to peak level of less than 5 mU/L (when basal level < 2 mU/L)

or an increase to peak level of less than 3-fold basal (when basal level > 2 mU/L).

Hypothalamic = level at 20 min greater than five times the upper limit of the normal basal range

or level at 20 min less than level at 60 min (when both levels are above the normal basal range), with a slow fall from this peak if a 120-min sample is analyzed.

Normal = results that are neither hypopituitary nor hypothalamic.

FSH and LH

Normal pubertal response = peak levels more than 3-fold greater than basal, LH peak > FSH. Must be interpreted in relation to bone age (see below) and physical maturation.

Prolactin

Prolactin is released in response to TRH. A similar rising 'hypothalamic pattern' may be seen. Basal levels should be interpreted in relation to the reference range. Inappropriate increases may be seen secondary to compression of the pituitary stalk or with prolactinomas.

Testosterone, estradiol

Normal = basal levels within the age-appropriate reference ranges (see below).

Cortisol

Cortisol may rise in response to clonidine administration, reflecting an intact hypothalamopituitary axis. If started after an overnight fast, the basal level

Time	GH	TSH	FSH & LH	Cortisol	Prolactin
0	+	+ Give clonidine, TRH & LHRH	+	+	+
20	+	+	+	+	+
60	+	+	+	+	+
90	+	–	–	+	–
120	+	+	–	+	–
150	+	–	–	+	–

Basal samples should be taken at 0900 hours for FT_4, ACTH, IGF-1 and IGFBP-3.

Table A.1 Schedule of sample collection for combined anterior pituitary function test

should be <120 nmol/L and the ACTH detectable, usually <40 pmol/L. However, the combined test described above is not an adequate test of cortisol secretion and if there is a reason to suspect adrenal insufficiency it is the authors' practice to combine it with a short, low-dose Synacthen test.

SHORT, LOW-DOSE SYNACTHEN TEST

PRINCIPLE

A synthetic form of ACTH is given to test the responsiveness of the adrenal cortex by production of cortisol. Older protocols relied on huge doses ($250 \mu g/m^2$) of Synacthen. The high-dose test can still be used in cases where primary adrenal failure is likely and estimation of intermediary adrenal hormones is important. Estimation of intermediary compounds (17α-hydroxyprogesterone) can give information about biosynthetic defects, such as atypical 21-hydroxylase deficiency (see below).

The low-dose test has been shown to generate more physiologic levels of ACTH and can detect subtle adrenal underactivity, for instance secondary to steroid medication. The protocol for the low-dose test is given but differs from the original only in the size of the Synacthen bolus and the need for more frequent, early, timed sampling.

MATERIALS REQUIRED

Pharmaceutical

■ Synacthen – tetracosactrin acetate, 5% dextrose.

Other

■ Lithium heparin tubes for blood.

APPROXIMATE LENGTH OF TEST

Ideally, a midnight sample should be collected at some point prior to the test; otherwise 1 h (or 150 min if combined with pituitary function tests).

PATIENT PREPARATION

In atopic individuals anaphylaxis can occur rarely in response to Synacthen, even at low dose; consequently a supply of emergency drugs should be available and the patient supervised carefully.

SAMPLES REQUIRED

Lithium heparin blood at each timepoint for cortisol, EDTA tube for ACTH (must be spun and frozen within 15 min).

PROCEDURE

Dissolve 125 μg in 500 mL 5% dextrose to give a solution of 250 ng/mL. Mix thoroughly. Give Synacthen i.v. at a dose of $500 \ ng/m^2$. Collect blood 10, 20, 30, 60 and 120 min after dose.

INTERPRETATION OF RESULTS

Primary or secondary hypocortisolemia

The midnight and pre-dose cortisols should show a normal diurnal variation (midnight usually undetectable but up to 280 nmol/L (10 μg/dL); 0800 hours pre-dose 120–660 nmol/L (4.3–23.5 μg/dL) with ACTH detectable but <40 pmol/L; a raised ACTH level at baseline indicates adrenal pathology.

The normal response to Synacthen is a rise of cortisol of at least 280 nmol/L (10 μg/dL) to a peak of at least 550 nmol/L (20 μg/dL). Inadequate response indicates impaired adrenal cortical function.

Suspected adrenal enzyme disorders

Use standard 250-μg dose. A rise in 17α-hydroxyprogesterone to levels >10 nmol/L (5 μg/L) is seen in atypical 21-hydroxylase deficiency. The test can be used to promote secretion of any other adrenal steroid if blocks in the synthesis pathway are suspected, either alone or in combination with a 24-h urinary steroid profile.

CORTICOTROPIN RELEASING FACTOR (CRF) TEST

PRINCIPLE

Human or ovine CRF is given to test the responsiveness of the pituitary in producing ACTH and then cortisol. Ovine CRF has a longer duration of action for the stimulation test. This test is sometimes useful as a means of discriminating pituitary from ectopic ACTH-dependent Cushing's syndrome. It can be used to test pituitary recovery after surgery, irradiation or suppression.

MATERIALS REQUIRED

Pharmaceutical

■ CRF, human or ovine preparations are available.

Other

■ EDTA and lithium–heparin tubes for blood.

APPROXIMATE LENGTH OF TEST

Four hours

PATIENT PREPARATION

The test should commence at 0900 hours.

SAMPLES REQUIRED

Lithium–heparin blood at each timepoint for cortisol, EDTA tube for ACTH (must be spun and frozen within 15 min).

PROCEDURE

Give CRF 100 µg i.v. over 60 s. Collect blood at −15, 5, 15, 30 and 60 min after dose.

INTERPRETATION OF RESULTS

With pituitary adenoma, the mean ACTH and cortisol rise from baseline at 15 and 30 min should be >20% (up to 1000%). There is little response in ectopic ACTH production. In pituitary recovery after operation, etc. the cortisol level should exceed 500 nmol/L at one timepoint.

GROWTH HORMONE SUPPRESSION TEST

PRINCIPLE

Glucose, given as in an oral glucose tolerance test (GTT), will suppress GH production except in situations of pituitary overproduction. With the availability of IGF-1 and IGFBP-3 (which will be raised in pituitary gigantism), this test is rarely necessary.

MATERIALS REQUIRED

Pharmaceutical

- Oral glucose solution.

Other

- Fluoride oxalate and heparinized containers.

APPROXIMATE LENGTH OF TEST

Two hours, excluding overnight fast.

PATIENT PREPARATION

The patient should be admitted after an overnight fast. Venous access should be secured.

PROCEDURE

Samples for glucose and GH are collected at time 0, and then glucose, 1.75 g/kg, is administered orally (maximum dose 75 g). Blood is drawn at 30, 60, 90 and 120 min. Test any urine passed for the presence of glucose.

INTERPRETATION OF RESULTS

Basal GH concentration should be less than 3 µg/L. GH should fall to an undetectable level through the test. Failure to suppress GH levels and an abnormal glucose response (true blood sugar level >10 mmol/L (182 mg/dL) = frank diabetes; >6.7 mmol/L (122 mg/dL) = impaired glucose tolerance) are indicative of a pituitary adenoma.

GH may fail to suppress in chronic severe anemia, hepatic cirrhosis, porphyria and malnutrition.

IGF-1 GENERATION TEST

PRINCIPLE

If GH resistance is suspected, the ability of exogenous GH to stimulate IGF-1 can be measured.

MATERIALS REQUIRED

Pharmaceutical

- Growth hormone.

Other

- Heparinized containers.

APPROXIMATE LENGTH OF TEST

Four days.

PATIENT PREPARATION

Administer GH 0.03 mg/kg daily, for 4 days.

PROCEDURE

Samples for GH, IGF-1 and IGFBP-3 estimation are collected on day 0, and those for IGF-1 and IGFBP-3 on day 5.

INTERPRETATION OF RESULTS

In GH resistant states the basal GH concentration should be more than 3 µg/L. IGF-1 level should be low and not show a rise after 4 days of GH treatment. IGFBP-1 concentration will be low throughout.

ORAL GLUCOSE TOLERANCE TEST

Glucose tolerance tests are required much less commonly in children than in adults. The diagnosis of diabetes can almost always be made by a random fasting plasma glucose level. A 2-h level is all that is required to confirm the diagnosis in rare borderline cases of diabetes. However, delineation of some of the rarer forms of diabetes can be made by simultaneous measurements of insulin and glucose. The procedure is the same as outlined above for a GH suppression test above (omitting the measurement of GH, but including the simultaneous assay of insulin at time 0 and intermediate timepoints to 2 h). Other basal or stimulated testing of C peptide and lactate may be useful in some circumstances.

INTRAVENOUS GLUCOSE TOLERANCE TEST

PRINCIPLE

An intravenous glucose tolerance test eliminates gastrointestinal factors that can affect the oral test. It allows calculation of a disappearance rate for circulating glucose that is related to insulin status. The test is performed only rarely.

MATERIALS REQUIRED

Pharmaceutical

■ D-Glucose as a 50% solution w/v in water.

Other

■ Fluoride oxalate bottles for blood.

APPROXIMATE LENGTH OF TEST

1.5 h plus overnight fast.

PATIENT PREPARATION

Fast patient overnight.

SAMPLES REQUIRED

Blood in fluoride oxalate tubes at each timepoint.

PROCEDURE

Glucose is given i.v. as a 25% solution at a dose of 0.5 g/kg body weight over 5 min. A stopwatch is started when half the dose has been given. Blood samples are collected at exactly 5, 10, 20, 30 and 60 min. All urine passed over 2 h is tested for glucose.

INTERPRETATION OF RESULTS

Blood glucose results versus time are plotted on semi-logarithmic graph paper to calculate the half-life. The

disappearance constant, k, is calculated:

$$k\ (\%\ per\ min) = \frac{(0.693 \times 100)}{half\text{-}life}$$

Disappearance rates are normally 1–3%. They are reduced in diabetes and increased in hyperinsulinism.

WATER DEPRIVATION (URINE CONCENTRATION) AND DDAVP STIMULATION TESTS

PRINCIPLE

Fluid intake is restricted and urine osmolality measured to assess renal concentrating ability. DDAVP may be administered to distinguish renal tubular from posterior pituitary dysfunction. ADH measurement is useful to distinguish nephrogenic (usually raised) from central (low) diabetes insipidus.

MATERIALS REQUIRED

Pharmaceutical

■ DDAVP (1-deamino-8-D-arginine vasopressin).

Other

■ Universal containers for urine.
■ Lithium–heparin tubes for blood.

APPROXIMATE LENGTH OF TEST

1–2 days.

PATIENT PREPARATION

The patient is weighed before and periodically during the test. The frequency of weighing depends on the age of the child and suspected disorder. It should not be less frequent than every 4 h and may have to be hourly or even half-hourly in suspected nephrogenic DI. Calculate 5% of the body weight, subtract it from the starting weight, and discontinue the test if the patient's weight falls below this level. Terminate the test at any time if there are clinical signs of serious dehydration.

SAMPLES REQUIRED

Lithium–heparin blood samples for sodium and serum osmolality. Urine container for osmolality. Note time of collection on tubes. Direct measurement of basal ADH level may be useful in some circumstances.

PROCEDURES

Fluid deprivation

Day 1

Normal diet and fluid intake. Send each specimen of urine passed for measurement of volume and osmolality – at least every 4 h. Note the collection time on the container. If the osmolality of any urine is greater than 700 mmol/L (mOsmol/L), no further testing is required.

Day 2

At 0830 hours give a normal feed. Weigh the patient. Allow no more food or fluid. Collect blood samples for osmolality and sodium. Collect all urine passed and send immediately to the laboratory for the measurement of volume and osmolality as before.

Collect blood for osmolality and sodium at least 4 hourly. Terminate the test as soon as any urine osmolality is greater than 700 mmol/L or if there are clinical signs of significant dehydration.

The length of the test depends on the age of the child and clinical response to dehydration. Careful observation of the child is required throughout the test.

INTERPRETATION OF RESULTS

If any urine sample has an osmolality greater than 700 mmol/L (mOsmol/L), concentrating ability is adequate and the test should be terminated.

If there has been inadequate urinary concentration, proceed to a DDAVP test.

DDAVP test

The patient is allowed to eat normally, but restrict infants to half-normal fluid intake and limit older children to 0.5 L fluids to prevent excessive drinking in the 8 h after DDAVP has been administered to prevent overhydration and hyponatremia. DDAVP is given i.m. at a dose of 0.125 μg for children and one-tenth of this for infants (who may be extremely sensitive to DDAVP in the presence of congenital DI).

INTERPRETATION OF RESULTS

If adequate concentration is achieved after DDAVP, this suggests satisfactory renal concentrating ability but an inadequate secretion of posterior pituitary AVP (central DI). If there is inadequate concentrating ability after DDAVP, renal unresponsiveness to AVP (nephrogenic DI) is demonstrated and the basal ADH level may be raised. In habit polydipsia, if prolonged, there may be dilute urine passed even after a prolonged period of water deprivation, making differentiation from partial central DI difficult. In these cases a hypertonic saline test performed on a specialist unit may help the diagnosis by creating a mild hyperosmolar state and promoting ADH release in the habit drinker.

DEXAMETHASONE SUPPRESSION TESTS

PRINCIPLE

Dexamethasone is a potent steroid that will suppress ACTH secretion, and hence cortisol, in the normal situation but not in Cushing's syndrome.

MATERIALS REQUIRED

Pharmaceutical

- Dexamethasone.

Other

- Lithium–heparin tubes for blood.

APPROXIMATE LENGTH OF TEST

One day for overnight test, 5 days for the high-dose test.

SAMPLES REQUIRED

Lithium–heparin blood at each timepoint for cortisol and ACTH; urine containers for free cortisol estimation and urinary steroid profile.

PROCEDURE AND INTERPRETATION OF RESULTS

Measure basal cortisol and ACTH levels:

- If both are raised, administer oral dexamethasone, 1.0 mg per 1.7 m^2 at 2300 hours. Determine serum cortisol concentration at 0800–0900 hours the following morning. The morning cortisol level should be less than 50 nmol/L (1.8 μg/dL) or at least 50% of the pre-test morning cortisol concentration.
- If ACTH is undetectable and there is hypercortisolemia, an adrenal cause is proven and no further tests are required.
- If ACTH is detectable or raised, and there is failure of suppression of cortisol in response to the overnight test, dexamethasone should be administered in a dosage of 0.5 mg/m^2 four times a day for 2 days, and blood estimations repeated. Then continue with dexamethasone 2.0 mg/m^2 four times daily for a further 2 days.

Collect 24-h urine samples each day for free urinary cortisol and steroid profile.

If cortisol excretion is not suppressed by the low dose of dexamethasone, some form of Cushing syndrome is virtually certain. If there is some suppression on the higher dosage, pituitary Cushing disease is most likely, while a lack of any suppression indicates an adrenal tumor.

INVESTIGATION OF HYPOGLYCEMIA IN CHILDREN

PRINCIPLE

Hypoglycemia has a wide variety of causes in children (see Ch. 11). These include various metabolic problems in which hypoglycemic episodes occur intermittently. To overcome this difficulty in investigation, a suitable approach is the measurement of the intermediary metabolites directly involved in glucose homeostasis after a prolonged, supervised fast (6, 12 or 24 h depending on age) or during an actual hypoglycemic attack.

MATERIALS REQUIRED

Lithium–heparin and fluoride oxalate containers for blood; urine containers.

APPROXIMATE LENGTH OF TEST
Up to 24 h.

PATIENT PREPARATION

For a prolonged fast in older children, start the test between 1600 and 2100 hours and take samples at 0900 and 1200 hours or 1600 hours the following day. In young children, or when hyperinsulinism is strongly suspected, do not begin the fast until 0900 hours.

The patient can be given water to drink during this time. It is advisable to check the plasma glucose level regularly and, if symptoms of hypoglycemia occur, either by laboratory assay or on the ward by means of a reliable bedside method, then terminate the test and treat with oral glucose or 2 mL/kg 10% dextrose over 3 min followed by an infusion of 0.1 mL/kg per min to keep the blood sugar between 5 and 8 mmol/L (90–144 mg/dL). If hypopituitarism is suspected, also give 100 mg hydrocortisone i.v.

SAMPLES REQUIRED

- Fluoride tube: glucose, lactate, alanine, free fatty acids, β-hydroxybutyrate and carnitine.
- Heparinized blood: cortisol, GH and insulin (plasma should be separated from cells promptly

and stored at –20°C). (In cases of possible factitious hypoglycemia due to insulin administration, measure C peptide along with insulin.) A chilled tube sent straight to the laboratory is required to measure ammonia levels in hyperinsulinism.

- Urine: sample as soon as possible after hypoglycemia for organic acids and acylcarnitines. (In cases of possible factitious hypoglycemia due to oral hypoglycemic agents, send urine for toxicology.)

INTERPRETATION
See Chapter 11.

PHOSPHATE EXCRETION INDICES

PRINCIPLE

There is a maximal rate (transport maximum, Tm) for the active reabsorption of some solutes by the renal tubule. Abnormalities in the Tm for phosphate (TmP) may have primary causes as in familial hypophosphatemic rickets or be secondary due to the effect of parathyroid hormone. Direct assay of PTH in combination with a calcium level may obviate the need for this procedure in many cases.

MATERIALS REQUIRED

Lithium–heparin containers for phosphate and creatinine estimation, and urine container.

APPROXIMATE LENGTH OF TEST
One to 2 h, excluding overnight fast.

PATIENT PREPARATION
Overnight fast.

SAMPLES REQUIRED

After an overnight fast, collect a urine sample over 1–2 h and a single blood sample. Assay phosphate and creatinine on each sample.

RESULTS
Calculate:
a) The phosphate : creatinine clearance ratio:

$$\frac{C_p}{C_{cr}} = \frac{(P_{cr} \times U_p)}{(P_p \times U_{cr})}$$

where P_{cr} is plasma creatinine, P_p is plasma phosphate, U_{cr} is urine creatinine and U_p is urine phosphate (all in mmol/L).

b) The tubular reabsorption of phosphate:

$$TRP = (1 - C_p/C_{cr}) \times 100$$

c) The phosphate excretion index:

$$PEI = (C_p/C_{cr}) - ([0.155 \times P_p] - 0.05)$$

INTERPRETATION

In familial hypophosphatemic rickets, the TRP and TmP/GFR (which can be estimated directly or is roughly equivalent to TRP $\times$ P_p) and the plasma phosphate concentration are low. The C_p/C_{cr} and PEI may be high.

Raised PTH concentration in hyperparathyroidism decreases TRP and TmP/GFR, and increases C_p/C_{cr} and PEI, causing phosphaturia.

In hypoparathyroidism TRP and TmP/GFR are increased, and C_p/C_{cr} and PEI are reduced.

hCG TESTS

PRINCIPLE

hCG is an LH-like compound that will stimulate testosterone production from the testes in the normal state. Testosterone is converted to DHT in the presence of normal 5α-reductase activity.

MATERIALS REQUIRED

Pharmaceutical

■ hCG (or recombinant LH if available).

Other

■ Lithium–heparin containers for blood estimations of testosterone and DHT.

APPROXIMATE LENGTH OF TEST

From 5 days to 3 weeks (see below).

SAMPLES REQUIRED

Blood for testosterone, DHT, androstenedione and DHEAS.

PROCEDURE

Give hCG 1500 units i.m. for an infant and 2000 units i.m. for an older child on days 0, 1 and 2. Take blood samples on days 0 and 3.

In situations of prolonged cryptorchidism, or where testicular damage is highly likely, give hCG 1000 units twice weekly for 3 weeks and take blood on day 0 and 48 h after the last injection.

INTERPRETATION

A rise in testosterone concentration from the baseline demonstrates intact testicular Leydig cell function. If a prolonged test produces a rise in testosterone, spontaneous puberty is possible (assuming normal gonadotropin function), although surveillance will still be required and long-term ability to virilize plus fertility may still be in doubt.

Failure of a rise in DHT level (testosterone: DHT ratio > 25 or absolute DHT level < 1 nmol/L) implies 5α-reductase deficiency. The differential rise of testosterone to DHEAS and androstenedione can be used to explore defects in testosterone biosynthesis (see Ch. 8).

GENETIC TESTS IN PEDIATRIC ENDOCRINOLOGY

Table A.2 gives only a few of the most important locations, or specific gene abnormalities, of relevance to pediatric endocrinology, and indicates where analysis may help in management.

NORMAL VALUES

The cautions given in Chapter 11 regarding interassay variation, inappropriate age-related values and heterophilic antibodies in immunoassays should be heeded. Ideally all values given in **Table A.3** should be interpreted against a validated local range. Drugs and diet can interfere with some assays. Acute ill health, stress during the sampling procedure and prematurity can also cause variation.

Levels of steroid precursors and urinary steroid profiles, IGF-1 and IGFBP-3 levels, are highly specific to the assay system used, the local population and age/pubertal status; thus normal values will not be quoted for these compounds.

Some peptide hormone levels are given as units per liter. Standardization of biologic equivalence of recombinant products to weight in milligrams is currently in progress, but older human and less pure preparations are still in use to validate assays, which makes exact conversion difficult.

Condition	Defect	Chromosome
Adrenal		
Adrenoleukodystrophy	*ADLP (VLCFA)*	Xq28 + other?
CAH (common form)	21-Hydroxylase	p21.3
Adrenal hypoplasia	*DAX1* (deletion)	Xp21
Cellular receptors/signaling		
Laron syndrome	GH receptor	5p
Testotoxicosis	LH receptor (activation)	2p21
Male pseudohermaphroditism	LH receptor (deletion)	
See Chs 4 & 10	Insulin receptor	19p13.3-2
McCune–Albright	G protein	20q13.2
Thyroid hormone resistance	Thyroid hormone receptor β	3p
Nephrogenic DI (dominant)	Aquaporin 2	12q
Nephrogenic DI (X-linked)	Vasopressin receptor	Xq28
Kallmann	*KAL1*	Xp
GH resistance	IGF-1	12q22-24.1
Intracellular receptors		
Androgen insensitivity	Androgen receptor	Xq12
Ovary/testis		
Male pseudo-hermaphroditism	*DAX1* (duplication)	Xp21
Hypogonadotropic hypogonadism	*DAX1* (deletion)	Xp21
Gonadal dysgenesis (some)	*SRY*	Yp11.3
Camptomelic dysplasia	*SOX9*	17q
AMH deficiency	*AMH*	19p13.3
Pancreas		
MODY1	HNF-4α	20q12-13.1
MODY2	Glucokinase	7p15-13
MODY3	HNF-1α	12q24.2
MODY4	Insulin promoter factor	13q12.1
MODY5	HNF-1β	17cen-q21.2
PHHI (some)	*SUR1*	11p15
PHHI + hyperammonemia	*GLUD1*	10q23.3
DIDMOAD	Wolframin	4p & 4q
Pituitary		
Septo-optic dysplasia (some)	HESX-1	3p21
TSH deficiency	TSHβ	1p13
LH deficiency	LH	19q
FSH deficiency	FSH	11p
Combined GH–TSH	*PIT1*	3q
Diabetes insipidus (some)	ADH	20p13

Table A.2 Some genetic test in pediatric endocrinology

Condition	Defect	Chromosome
Syndromes		
Prader–Labhart–Willi	Imprinting (SNRPN)	15q11
Noonan	PTPN gene	12q24
Beckwith–Wiedemann	Imprinting (IGF2 gene)	11p15.5
Marfan	Fibrillin	15q, 17q
Williams	Elastin	7q11.23
NF1	Neurofibromin	17
Leri–Weill	*SHOX*	Pseudoautosomal region of Xp
Thyroid/parathyroid		
MEN II	*ret* proto-oncogene	10q11.2 (1p)
MEN I	Menin (suppressor protein)	11q13

Table A.2 *Cont'd*

Hormone	SI units	Conversion factor (if relevant)
ACTH (early a.m.)	2–20 pmol/L	÷ 0.22 = pg/mL
ADH	1–5 pmol/L	÷ 0.992 = pg/mL
Epinephrine (adrenaline)		
Infant	<30 pmol/L	÷ 5.46 = ng/L
Child	<80 pmol/L	
Adult	<200 pmol/L	
Androstenedione		
Prepuberty	<3.5 nmol/L	÷ 0.0349 = ng/dL
Male	4.5–10.5 nmol/L	
Female	4–10 nmol/L	
C peptide	20–50 nmol/L	÷ 33.3 = mg/dL
Calcitonin	<30 pmol/L	÷ 0.29 = ng/L
Cortisol		
Early morning	120–660 nmol/L	÷ 28 = μg/dL
Midnight	Up to 280 nmol/L	
FSH		
Prepubertal	<3.5 U/L	
Pubertal, follicular	2–7 U/L	
Glucose	3.0–6.5 mmol/L	÷ 0.057 = mg/dL
GH		
Stimulated	>7 μg/L	(1 mg = 3 IU standard)
Suppressed	<0.3 μg/L	
HbA1c (assays vary)	<6%	
hCG	<5 IU/L	
17α-Hydroxyprogesterone		
Males	<12 nmol/L	÷ 3.0 = μg/L
Females	<10 nmol/L	
(increased in sick and premature neonates)		
Insulin	<10 mU/L	
(interpret w.r.t. glucose in hypoglycemia)		
Lactate	<2.5 mmol/L	÷ 0.1 = mg/dL
LH		
Prepubertal	<2 U/L	
Pubertal, follicular	<12 U/L	
Pubertal, mid-cycle	<70 U/L	
Norepinephrine (noradrenaline)		
Infant	<100 pmol/L	÷ 5.91 = ng/L
Older	<900 pmol/L	
Estrogen (E_2)		
Prepubertal	<60 pmol/L	÷ 3.67 = pg/mL
Adult male	<250 pmol/L	
Adult female, mid-cycle	Up to 1500 pmol/L	
Osmolality (plasma)	275–295 mmol/L	= mOsmol/L
Prolactin (unstressed)	<800 pmol/L	÷ 44.4 = μg/L

Table A.3 Normal values

Hormone	SI units	Conversion factor (if relevant)
Progesterone		
Prepubertal	<1.5 nmol/L	÷ 3.18 = µg/L
Pubertal, follicular	<5 nmol/L	
Pubertal, luteal	15–90 nmol/L	
PTH (intact)	2–8 pmol/L	÷ 10 = ng/mL
SHBG		
Male	20–45 nmol/L	÷ 2.0 = µg/L
Female	50–80 nmol/L	
Testosterone		
Prepubertal and female	<1.0 nmol/L	÷ 0.035 = ng/dL
Pubertal male, post hCG	10–25 nmol/L	
TBG	N/A	7–17 mg/L
TSH (high sensitivity)	0.3–5.0 mU/L	
Thyroxine		
Free	9–23 pmol/L	÷ 12.9 = ng/dL
T_3 (free)	4.5–8.0 pmol/L	÷ 0.015 = ng/dL
Urinary free cortisol	<250 nmol/day	÷ 2.8 = µg/day
VMA (24 h urine)	<40 µmol/day	÷ 5 = mg/day

Table A.3 *Cont'd*

Index

Numbers in bold print refer to illustrations and their captions

Malignancies 43, 66, 107, **2.4**
 screening survivors 229–230, 231
 see also individual conditions
Malnutrition 103, 106, 206–207, **4.1–4.7**
Marasmus 103, **4.1–4.2**
Marfan syndrome 87, 246
 arachnodactyly **3.7**
 high arched palate 17–18, **1.70**
 increased joint mobility **1.18–1.21**
 lens dislocation 30, **1.119**
 pectus excavatum **1.87**
 sex hormone treatment 101
 tall stature 100, **3.4–3.6, 3.35**
Marshall–Smith syndrome 87, 94, 100
Masculinization *see* Virilization
Mauriac syndrome 123, 200, **4.17–4.18**
Medroxyprogesterone 155
Menarche 26, 133
 premature 142
Menkes' kinky wool hair syndrome 108, **4.15**
Metabolic disorders 64, 108, **2.49–2.50**
Metacarpal index 100
Metformin 201
Methyloxidases 218
Microalbuminuria 198
Microcytosis 74
Micropenis 172–173, 162, **8.13, 8.44, 8.50**
Midline brain structures 41
 absent 75, **2.81, 2.83**
Midline cleft 16, 42, **1.66–1.67**
Mineralocorticoids
 excess 221
 replacement 170
 secretion 218
Moon face 57, 64, **2.45**
Morquio syndrome
 (mucopolysaccharidosis type-4) 53, **2.30**
Mosaicism, tissue 35, 157, **1.137**
Mouth examination 16–20, **1.65–1.79**
Mucolipidosis type-3 53, **1.23–1.24, 2.63–2.64**
Mucopolysaccharidosis
 type-2 (juvenile Hunter syndrome) 53, **2.28–2.29**
 type-4 (Morquio syndrome) 53, **2.30**
Müllerian ducts 157, 161, 174, **8.8, 8.46**
Müllerian inhibiting factor (MIF) 157, 169
 deficiency **8.1, 8.4**
Multiple endocrine adenomatosis
 (neoplasia) (MEN) syndromes 191
 Investigations 100, 226, 246
 neuromas 18, **1.72–1.73**
 thyroid carcinoma 191
 treatment 101, 191
 type-2b 97, 99, **1.72, 3.33**

N

Nails
 Sotos syndrome 12, **1.41, 3.13**

Ullrich–Turner syndrome 12, **1.42–1.43**
 Weaver syndrome **3.16**
Neck
 loose skin 14, **1.50**
 palpation 20–21
 short 14, **1.52–1.54**
 webbing 14, **1.51**
Necrobiosis lipoidica 38, 199, **10.12**
Nelson syndrome 35, 83, **1.138**
Neonates
 achondroplasia **2.23**
 breasts 23, 132, **1.97–1.98**
 IUGR 50, **2.22**
 lymphedema **1.43**
 measurements 2, **1.3–1.5**
 neck skin 14, **1.49–1.50**
 pelvis **6.9**
 withdrawal bleeding 132, **6.8**
Nephrocalcinosis 226
Nephropathy, diabetic 198
Nesidioblastosis 228, **11.33**
Neurofibromatosis
 café-au-lait spots 33–35, **1.130, 1.132, 1.135**
 exophthalmos 14, **1.63–1.6**
 neuromas 18, 33–34, **1.72, 1.131–1.134**
 optic glioma **6.46**
 precocious puberty 135, **6.22**
 scoliosis **1.89**
Neuromas
 multiple endocrine adenomatosis 100, **3.33**
 neurofibromatosis 18, 33–34, **1.72, 1.131–1.134**
Neuromuscular disease, congenital 7
Nevi, pigmented 34–35, 93, **1.136–1.137, 3.22, 3.24**
Nevus of Ota 30, **1.121**
Nifedipine 229
Nipples, accessory 23–24, **1.102**
Non-alcoholic steatohepatitis (NASH) 121, **5.13**
Noonan syndrome 246
 features 48,49–50, **1.153, 2.17**
 neck webbing **1.51**
 pectus carinatum **1.88**
 ptosis **1.61**

O

Obesity *see* Overweight 115
 Cushing syndrome 57, **2.41–2.43**
 GHD 44, 123, **1.124, 2.9**
 hypothalamic tumors 94, 97, **5.14–5.15**
 Laron syndrome **2.3**
 measurement 1, 4–5, 126
 nutritional 59, 94, 117, 121, 128–129, **2.48, 3.30**
 Prader–Labhart–Willi syndrome
 pseudo-Cushing syndrome 59, **2.48**
Occipitofrontal circumference (OFC) 4, **1.9**

Octreotide 101, 229
Optic atrophy 29, **1.111**
Optic chiasma/nerve compression 29, 86, **9.10, 1.111, 1.113**
Optic glioma 34, **1.134, 4.24, 6.20–6.22, 6.46**
Orbit 14, **1.60, 1.63–1.64**
Orchidometer **1.105**
Orchidopexy 171, 174
Organomegaly 22–23, **1.93, 3.19**
Orlistat 130
Osmoregulatory system 214–215
Osteogenesis imperfecta 30, 66, **1.21, 2.53, 2.61–2.62**
Osteoporosis 106, 225, **11.28**
Ovaries
 age-related changes 131–132, **6.1, 6.4, 6.6, 6.9–6.10**
 cyst 138, **6.25–6.26**
 enlarged **6.44–6.45**
 genetic disorders 245
 torsion 135, **6.44**
 tumor 176, 178, **1.109, 6.34–6.35, 8.62–8.65, 10.9**
Overweight 115–117, **5.1–5.8**
 causes 121, **5.9–5.13**
 CNS 123–124, **5.14–5.16**
 endocrine 32, 122–123, 126, **1.124, 2.9, 4.17–4.18, 9.5**
 genetic 124–125, **5.17–5.19**
 iatrogenic 125
 immobility 117, 125
 psychosocial 125
 epidemiology 117
 evaluation 125–128, **5.20–5.21**
 physiology 117, 121
 treatment 128–130, **5.22**
 see also Obesity
Ovotestis 161, **8.9–8.11**
Oxandrolone 154

P

Palate
 cleft 16, 106, **1.65–1.67, 1.69**
 high arched 17–18, **1.70**
Pallor 12, **1.45**
Palms
 single crease 7, **1.17**
 yellow 12, 86, **1.44**
 red 12, 37
Pancreas 227
 in diabetes 204–205, 207
 exocrine failure 114
 genetic disorders 245
 nesidioblastosis 228, **11.33**
Pancreatectomy 229
Panhypopituitarism **2.76, 7.11**
 cleft lip/palate **1.65**
 micropenis/cryptorchidism 228, **8.12**
 treatment **2.90**
Papilledema 29, **1.110**
Parathormone 221–223, 226